T0202084

Music, Evolution, and the Harmony of Souls

Music, Evolution, and the Harmony of Souls

Alan Harvey

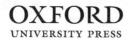

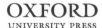

UNIVERSITY PRESS

Great Clarendon Street, Oxford, OX2 6DP,
United Kingdom

Oxford University Press is a department of the University of Oxford.
It furthers the University's objective of excellence in research, scholarship,
and education by publishing worldwide. Oxford is a registered trade mark of
Oxford University Press in the UK and in certain other countries

Published in the United States of America by Oxford University Press
198 Madison Avenue, New York, NY 10016, United States of America

British Library Cataloguing in Publication Data
Data available

Library of Congress Control Number: 2016958451

ISBN 978–0–19–878685–6

Printed and bound by CPI Group (UK) Ltd, Croydon, CR0 4YY

To Paulien, Christopher and Peter;

To all the brilliant, dedicated, and hard-working scholars
and researchers who have devoted their time and energies
to the precious study of music, and whose data form
the basis for this book;

To my wise mentors in human biology, Charles Oxnard
and the late Len Freedman, and to my early guide to the wonders
of neuroscience, the late Dr Geoff Henry;

To everyone who has shared with me the
joy of creating and making music;

And to some of those special few who have enriched
my life beyond measure, and whose music and souls
accompanied me as I wrestled with this ambition: Nick Drake,
The Beatles, Edward Elgar, Sergei Rachmaninov, Jean Sibelius,
Jackson Browne, Franz Schubert, Antonín Dvořák, Karla Bonoff,
Bonnie Raitt, and the incomparable Sandy Denny.

Foreword

Do you know that our soul is composed of harmony?
—Leonardo da Vinci[1]

This is a book about the importance of music in human evolution and its continued relevance to modern-day human society. How, from our very beginning as a species, musical communication has acted as a necessary counterweight to our other, newly evolved communication system—language,[2] and why music continues to be an essential part of the cognitive well-being of each of us and our society in the twenty-first century. It is about why music should form a core element of our children's education, and why music should gain traction as an important therapeutic tool in clinical practice and rehabilitation. I hope this book is of interest to all sorts of people, including clinicians, psychologists, allied health professionals, anthropologists, teachers, and musicians—anyone at all interested in who we are, where we came from, and how our species has grown from several thousand to seven billion members in perhaps less than 5,000 generations ... all of us still linked by the universality that is music.

The usual disclaimer—this book is inevitably incomplete! In attempting to accomplish such a broad and ambitious enterprise, I have had to explore a diverse but extraordinarily rich literature. I have found myself immersed in many disparate topics such as anthropology, brain imaging, sociobiology, linguistics, neurogenetics, neonatal communication, mechanisms of evolution, auditory processing of complex sounds, and so on. I have sometimes felt like the great Sir David Attenborough or the Australian naturalist Harry Butler, turning over rock after rock and discovering dauntingly complex layers of life under each one. Each time I mined the literature of a topic I uncovered what often seemed to be a never-ending constellation of new facts, new hypotheses, new controversies. I could have gone on forever, or at least until my body ceased to allow it. Perhaps that, and the fear of saying something daft, is why this book has taken so many years to write! But if you keep turning more and more rocks over, day after day, you never get to see the horizon. Perhaps it has ever been thus. To quote Sir Isaac Newton: "but to myself I seem to have been only like a boy playing on the sea-shore, and diverting myself in now and then finding a smoother pebble or a prettier shell than ordinary, whilst the great ocean of truth lay all undiscovered before me."[3]

Harvard Professor David Haig wrote in an essay devoted to discussing Richard Dawkins' concept of memes (units of ideas, of culture, passed from one person to another, within and across generations) that: "Many ideas have competed for inclusion during the course of writing. ... The final version contains the ideas that have grabbed my attention. It has sometimes seemed that they are using me for their ends. What fraction of these ideas are my own and what fraction borrowed from others? The web of intellectual influence is complex and it is unclear whether I ever have a truly original idea."[4] I know how he feels. I first started thinking about writing this book at the end of the last century, several years after fortuitously coming across two (for me at least) explosive books while browsing in the music section of a well-known bookshop on Tottenham Court Road in London. These books were Critchley and Henson's *Music and the Brain*[5] and Anthony Storr's *Music and the Mind*.[6] In 2008, I wrote what was essentially a précis of this book for *Music Forum*, a publication of the Music Council of Australia, and a chapter entitled "Evolution, music and neurotherapy" in a book about the modern-day relevance of evolutionary theory to our species.[7] After that, I even got as far as discussions with a couple of publishers, but I continued to prioritize lab work, grant writing, neurotrauma research, and doctoral teaching—the denouement has been far too long in coming!

During this protracted gestation period, an ever-increasing number of erudite, insightful, and informative books and reviews have been published that address many of the issues I have written about in *Music, Evolution, and the Harmony of Souls*. At times, a new book or substantial scientific review on any, or all, of the topics of music, evolution, and/or language have made me lose heart. But I have tried to make this new book different from any other, for example by not focusing quite so much on the rudiments of music and analysis of modern-day musical styles. "Distinctions between the surface complexity of different musical styles and techniques do not tell us anything useful about the expressive purposes and power of music, or about the intellectual organization involved with its creation. Music is too deeply concerned with human feelings and experiences in society."[8] Rather, the emphasis is more on the evolution of modern humans, how humans may have evolved their unique cognitive architecture, how music is processed in our brains, and why two complementary but distinct communication systems—language and music—remain a human universal. In this way, by laying out my ideas about the evolutionary importance of music as a driver of cooperative and interactive behavior throughout human existence, I wish to create the foundation for a primary aim of this book: what this evolutionary imperative means to twenty-first century humanity and beyond, from cultural, social, educational, and medical/neurological perspectives. I hope to convince the reader that music is not just serious and wondrous stuff, but that it needs to become more widely accepted in our community as a mainstream educational and therapeutic tool.

I am accustomed to generating my own data, and have sometimes been hesitant when writing and talking about data and ideas that have been generated by others...but as someone suggested to me, I should perhaps think of myself as an investigative reporter or maker of a tapestry, hopefully seeing new patterns and links that those inside their own work may not always see. I hope I have done justice to these dedicated researchers and scholars, and do not annoy them by my wandering into their chosen and well-tilled fields of interest. And I also obviously hope that readers of this book appreciate the approach that I have taken. In any case, and I trust the authors and editors of other recent books and articles will agree, the more frequently the message about the seminal importance of music in contemporary human life is broadcast, the better for us all. I want this book to be a "good news" story about how music, from our very beginning, has played such an important role in fostering prosocial, cooperative behaviors, and why music remains a core element of our makeup.

I am a neuroscientist by training, and having taught and researched the subject for many years I appreciate how difficult it is for others to wade through and remember the complex terminologies, and appreciate the brain's three-dimensional architecture and connectivity. Pictures and diagrams can help a great deal, and I am enormously grateful to my friend and talented artist Martin Thompson for generously giving of his time to interpret my rough sketches and create the figures that grace this book. I also thank The University of Western Australia for approving two periods of sabbatical during which much of the book was written.

In attempting the task of writing this book, I am especially grateful to those who gave of their precious time to exchange ideas and/or who read drafts of parts of the manuscript, suggesting corrections and pointing out errors and omissions. I should also acknowledge the book by Nat Shapiro, *An Encyclopedia of Quotations About Music*[1], a wonderful source of quotations and comments that drives home the unrivalled impact that music has always had on our species. The creative process was painfully slow—I took to measuring progress based on the size of the bulldog clip needed to hold the manuscript together, and friends and colleagues provided constant nagging and jocular quips about my seemingly always hypothetical deadlines. I am grateful to them all, and I acknowledge their helpful advice during the writing of this book—here they are in no particular order except alphabetical: Nicholas Bannan, Avinash Bharadwaj, Stuart Bunt, Jim Chisholm, Geoff Cooper, Jane Davidson, Len Freedman, Stuart Hodgetts, John Jory, Debra Judge, Colette Moses, Charles Oxnard, Rob Patuzzi, Don Robertson, Jennifer Rodger, Linc Schmitt, and Terry-ann White. I am especially grateful to Nicholas Bannan, Len Freedman, Silvana Gaudieri, Cyril Greuter, Stuart Hodgetts, Carmen Lawrence, Concetta Morrone, Charles Oxnard, and Don Robertson, who read and critiqued various draft chapters, and a grand bouquet to Danii Baron-Heeris for helping to organize and proof my bibliography. Of course any oversights or errors that remain are my sole, reprehensible responsibility.

Contents

List of Illustrations

Chapter 1

Introduction: What is Music? What is this Book About?

The senseless happiness of music engulfed me like a golden bath; it's a happiness that never depends on the objective, only the subjective, and perhaps it has a more profound link with the humanness of things because it's altogether senseless: the strenuous production of certain nonsensical sounds—that are no good for anything—for no explicable reasonable purpose.

—Josef Škvorecký, *The Bass Saxophone*, Picador

"he sensed as much as saw the men in the room begin to loosen, not moving, not swaying, certainly not dancing but some reassembling taking place as the melancholic music completed its work upon them and reduced them to essential men—the dirge played out was for each of them alone even as it sang of their brothers, of their others, of all mankind around them and all those come before and all following."

—Jeffrey Lent, *Lost Nation*, Grove Press

Musicologists and anthropologists tell us that all human cultures and social groups on the face of this earth participate in, and respond to, music and dance.[1,2] Music seems to be a "specific biological competence,"[3] and from the earliest age we humans are responsive to its charms. While it is true that in the twenty-first century there are now many different types of music and many different modes and scales, played on many different types of musical instruments, they all appear to be governed by the same physical laws of fundamentals, overtones, and harmonics when producing sound—the so-called harmonic series. Unlike the spoken word, "the use of fixed and discrete pitches seems to be fundamental and unique to music."[4] In his recent book about the prehistory of music, Iain Morley nicely summarizes what he believes is the common ground that links all musical forms: "musical behaviours amongst all humans involve the encoding of sounds into pitches (usually between three and seven) which are unequally separated across the scale, including the perfect fifth, favouring consonance and harmony over dissonance, and organizing sequences of sounds so that they have a deliberate temporal relationship to each other."[5] And we shall see that music's universality extends beyond the structural components of pitch and rhythm, extending to cross-cultural roles in "facilitating group coordination and cohesion."[6]

Most of us are aware of the complex and often strong emotional impact that music can have on us, and almost everybody enjoys or appreciates some form of music. There are, of course, notable exceptions to this; for example, the neurologist and author Oliver

Sacks tells us that the author Vladimir Nabokov thought music a sequence of arbitrary, irritating sounds.[7] I also enjoy the quote by US President Ulysses S. Grant, who apparently said: "I know only two tunes; one of them is "Yankee Doodle" and the other isn't."[8] As discussed in Chapter 2, such individuals may in fact have had a condition known as amusia, possessing underlying differences in brain circuitry, perhaps akin to those with color blindness. Nonetheless, despite these exceptions, music has been a source of wonder to the human species for many thousands of years, certainly for at least as long as musical instruments have been made—which at the last count was about 45,000 years. Music has the mysterious power to coalesce the past, present, and future into singular moments of transcendence—or as the influential ethnomusicologist and sociologist John Blacking put it, music has the power "to create another world of virtual time."[1] When I listen to a piece of classical music I love, for example, I can sometimes conjure up thoughts about the composer; his/her inspiration during the act of creation; the first musicians to play the work; the conductor and musicians who performed the recording; my own experience and emotional responses to this particular piece; and how the music will echo on into the future, affecting other listeners' hearts and minds.

A brief survey of Nat Shapiro's uniformly excellent and enlightening *Encyclopedia of Quotations about Music*[8] quickly reveals just how many of the famous and wise have commented on and proffered opinions about music, and have marveled at, and been inspired by, its beauty and power. Why does music allow us to glimpse beauty and the infinite, transcend time and space, and generate such moods and physical emotional responses? Confucius, in 500 BC, said that "music produces a kind of pleasure which human nature cannot do without"; Aristotle pondered: "Why do rhythms and melodies which are mere sounds resemble dispositions, while tastes do not, nor yet colours or smells?"; Martin Luther wrote that: "music is the art of the prophets, the only art that can calm the agitations of the soul; it is one of the most magnificent and delightful presents God has given us"; and according to Samuel Johnson, "it is the only sensual pleasure without vice."[8] Charles Darwin and the English philosopher and theorist Herbert Spencer fought a long battle over the evolutionary origins of music and language.[9] Darwin thought music was "of the least use to man in reference to his daily habits of life," that it was mysterious and preceded speech, and that "man possessed these faculties at a very remote period."[10] Herbert Spencer, however, thought that music was the language of passion derived from speech: "a physiological phenomenon, arising through an exaggeration of the emotional characteristics of human speech."[11] To Spencer we owe one of the better statements about the impact of music on our species: "Music must rank as the highest of the fine arts—as the one which, more than any other, ministers to human welfare."[12]

Dictionaries tend to define music in more prosaic ways. For example, the *Oxford English Dictionary* describes music as "that one of the fine arts which is concerned with the combination of sounds with a view to beauty of form and the expression of emotions." The *Chambers 20th Century Dictionary* on my office bookshelf defines it as "the art of expression in sound, in melody, and harmony, including both composition and execution; sometimes specially of instrumental performance to the exclusion of singing." These are useful definitions, but in some ways I confess I prefer Aldous Huxley's: "after silence, that which comes nearest to expressing the inexpressible is music,"[13] or Leonard Bernstein's poetic and limitless description: "Music … can name the unnameable and communicate the unknowable."[14] As the nineteenth-century classical composer Felix Mendelssohn wrote in a letter, in response to a question about the meanings of some of his *Songs Without Words*: "There is so much talk about music, and yet so little is said. For my part, I believe that words do not suffice for such a purpose, and if I found they did suffice I would finally have nothing more to do with music" (letter to Marc-André Souchay, 1842—quoted in Morgenstern[15]).

Music is a form of universal communication that, in our culture at least, clearly differs from language and articulate speech, yet as discussed more fully in Chapter 2 (under the heading "Harmony—musical syntax?"), music has a somewhat similar organizational nature to language, with structural principles and processes (a type of syntax) and the possibility of hierarchically embedding phrases within phrases (recursion). In humans, music affects arousal, it entrains neural activity, it has the extraordinary capacity to stimulate our emotions, and it can elicit substantial internal (autonomic) and overt physiological responses.[16] The autonomic nervous system monitors and controls the internal environment of our body, its visceral functions. Everyday examples of autonomic function include control of heart rate and blood pressure, digestion, respiration, and the apparatus of sexual arousal. Most autonomic functions are involuntary but they can often work in conjunction with the somatic nervous system—the part of the nervous system that gives us our sensations of the world around us—and with the brain regions that control voluntary movement. Music seems to have "gold pass" access to this autonomic network. Thus, many physiological changes linked to emotional responses are elicited when listening to favorite pieces of music, including changes in cardiovascular function (eg heart rate and blood pressure), goose bumps, chills, and tears.[17,18,19] Positive internal emotions can include joy, triumph, amazement, and feelings of vitalization, consolation, spirituality, and calmness.[20]

Of course we are all aware that music is intimately linked to movement and dance.[21,22,23] There is an intrinsic, almost unbreakable coupling between perceptual musical experience and the various motor actions that are elicited,[24] and the predictability of time and pitch, seemingly unique in our species, makes communal music-making possible.[25] *Homo sapiens* is the only living species in which individuals co-coordinate movement to a rhythmic pulse—humans have "the ability to follow precise rhythmic patterns so as to permit group singing, drumming and dancing."[26] Darwin suggested that music—including singing and dance, and therefore perhaps the positive selection of fitness attributes and the type of brain which creates and coordinates these activities—was the means by which humans could attract potential mates. Music and sex often seem to belong together; we remember that special song that was playing when we first met an important partner, perhaps our wife or husband, or when we first shared breakfast with a significant other. If most guys who are old enough to have seen the movie "*10*" are like me, then Ravel's "Bolero" is now inextricably linked with the sight of Bo Derek running in slow motion down the beach towards her improbable beau, Dudley Moore.

In addition, and of critical importance, music and dance create or at least facilitate more widespread social interactions that are associated with communal physiological arousal states, which can promote the collective expression and experience of emotion between individuals within a population. Participating individuals are yoked together in mood and activity—in harmony if you like; thus music can promote social cohesion and help to define, as well as separate, social groups.[26,27,28] When two or more people play what one person could play, they are deliberately sharing a social experience where "individuality is community."[1] Some thoughts about how and why music does this will be discussed in detail in Chapter 5, but the capacity for music to bind us together may be its most important evolutionary rationale.

Music (and sometimes dance) also forms a core component of ceremony and ritual. Most cultures and ancient civilizations had (or have) gods dedicated to music, for example Bes and Ihy in ancient Egypt, Apollo in Greek (and Roman) mythology, and the Hindu goddess Saraswati. Some scholars have suggested that early in human history unified, transcendental states induced by chanting and synchronous music-making may have been especially needed to bond groups together during times of conflict with other groups.[29,30] Many of us participate in group musical events, whether this involves singing the national anthem at a football match, singing the club anthem, singing hymns in church, or responding to music at a wedding or a funeral. Whether we ourselves are involved in choirs, karaoke, or rock 'n' roll jam sessions ... it doesn't matter; music is embedded in our lives. My colleague Nicholas Bannan has listed some reasons when and why we sing:[31] for personal amusement; for teaching purposes and the social development of children; as a means of recalling information; as an efficient carrier of sound across distances or in noisy environments; for display or entertainment purposes; as a means of communication with animals; to soothe infants; to introduce states of mind appropriate for specific activities; to heighten speech in a ritual or to an audience; as an accompaniment to work; and finally, as a cohesive force in social and political organizations. Singing together in choirs rapidly creates mutually satisfying bonds between strangers, "bypassing the need for personal knowledge of group members gained through prolonged interaction."[32]

Leaders—whether of nations, political parties, armies, or religious denominations—have long understood the power of music to influence the so-called masses, for good or for ill. In the fourteenth century, the organ was called "the devil's bagpipe" and by the fifteenth century most organs had been destroyed in England. Nat Shapiro includes this remarkable excerpt from a 1642 English Act of Parliament: "If any person or persons ... commonly called Fiddlers or Minstrels shall be taken playing, fiddling, or making music, in any Inn, Alehouse or Tavern ... or shall be taken entreating any person ... to hear them play ... that every such person shall be adjudged rogues, vagabonds, and sturdy beggars ... and be punished as such."[8] Hmm, I remember in the 1970s buskers being turfed out of the London Underground for entertaining the passersby ....

Dictators such as Hitler and Stalin knew the potentially subversive (to their way of thinking) impact of music on a population, hence their control over the types of music that they allowed to be played and the types of music that people were permitted to hear. Hitler banned jazz and would not allow music by Jewish composers such as Mendelssohn to be played, and most Soviet composers in Stalin's era lived anxious, precarious lives. They were expected to write populist, optimistic music deemed suitable by the party propaganda machine. In a speech in November 1935, Stalin said: "Life has improved, comrades. Life has become more joyous," and socialist realism meant that art, including music, had to serve the purposes of the communist state, had to be understood by, and in turn glorify, the achievements of the proletariat. Abstract, expressionist, and/or decadent music was frowned upon, and viewed as a perilous activity. Presumably, music that induced feelings of spirituality or transcendence, anger, disaffection, melancholy, or even lust was just too powerful to be let loose on the masses. Music can inflame passions and revolutionary zeal. Even today, music (and dance) is actively suppressed by certain religious groups and/or political organizations in various parts of the world. Such autocratic suppression is surely a sign of weakness, a symptom of an insecure ideology, depriving the populace of perhaps their most vital social binding agency, music.

Thankfully however, recent history can also provide powerful and heartening examples of the unifying and restorative power of music for humanity. For example, in 1914 the Germans and allies in their respective trenches sang Christmas carols to each other across no man's land, thus beginning the famous Christmas truce of that year. In more modern times, because "music-making is a safe place for people to 'be' together and rebuild trust,"[33] various music-based initiatives have been developed in regions of conflict and extreme social disharmony, such as in the Balkans and in Africa.[33] In the Middle East, the West-Eastern Divan Orchestra—an ensemble of Israelis, Palestinians, and Arabs—was created in 1999 by Daniel Barenboim. In an interview published in July 2012 in *Limelight*, an Australian Broadcasting Corporation magazine, Barenboim responded this way to a comment that the orchestra was created to promote a dialogue between Israel and other countries in the Middle East: "Yes, but our project is not a political one.... It's a project between Israelis and Palestinians and other Arabs, but still it's not political, because it doesn't have a political line. We believe it's exactly the opposite: that the Israeli and Palestinian conflict is not a political conflict. This isn't a conflict between two nations; it's a conflict between two peoples who are deeply convinced that they have the right to live on the same piece of land. This is a human problem. And therefore it cannot be solved militarily; it cannot be saved politically; it can only be solved with human understanding and with the acceptance of the rights of the other. That's what we in the orchestra strive to practise, and it provides us with an alternative way of thinking. But, you know, it's like many things—alternative medicine takes much longer than antibiotics." We shall come back to the therapeutic power of music and Barenboim's alternative medicine analogy in a couple of pages.

If the aforementioned diverse impacts of music were not already sufficient to impress upon the reader the importance of music to modern-day *Homo sapiens*, there is more.

In the educational field, researchers have shown that music structures time and provides mnemonic frameworks that help learning and memory. Many of us can remember the lyrics of songs for example, but may not remember much, if any, prose. Somehow attaching words to music makes the words easier to remember, something of critical importance and usefulness as we get older. And the benefits of music extend well beyond the musical domain. As discussed in detail in Chapter 7, music education increases verbal skills, enhances general cognitive and perceptual abilities, and facilitates a child's overall social development.

Yet, when peering into the dim shadows of our past and thinking about music in the context of human evolution, reasons for the transcendental power of music and its universality remain elusive and controversial. Yes, music makes our bodies move, and yes, it hooks into emotional circuitry within our brains, involving a complex group of interconnected cortical structures that are given the collective name of the "limbic system," a term first coined in the nineteenth century by the French physician Paul Broca (who also gave his name to the specific part of the brain long thought to be the motor speech area). But, as the eminent English psychiatrist Anthony Storr wrote in his excellent book *Music and the Mind*,[34] music is not usually propositional—it does not put forward any testable hypotheses; it promulgates no doctrines and preaches no gospels. Music does not convey information in the same way as language or speech. As described in the writings of Cambridge scholar and musician Ian Cross, music has no immediate or evident efficacy—it "neither ploughs, sows, weaves nor feeds."[35] According to the philosopher Schopenhauer (quoted in Storr[34]), music is "a copy of the will itself, music speaks of essence, the inner spirit." Such properties don't feed or clothe a family! So at its most basic and fundamental level, what exactly is music for? Why do humans make music and respond to it, and why does music remain such an important part of our lives—an integral component of our social architecture? Why is it, again quoting Anthony Storr, "a permanent part of our mental furniture?"

In his book *How the Mind Works*,[36] Steven Pinker suggests that music is merely auditory cheesecake, "a biologically pointless challenge," a "cocktail of recreational drugs" that aurally activates and stimulates our pleasure circuits. Is it secondary? An accidental by-product? What Stephen Jay Gould and Richard Lewontin called a "spandrel"? A spandrel is a space next to or between arches that may be filled in with beautiful ornamentation, but which has no structural relevance. Recent functional imaging studies of the human brain do indeed show that pleasure and reward centers in the brain are stimulated when we listen to pleasurable music. This is discussed in more detail in Chapter 5. But the essential point to make here is that drugs and addictions are usually, in the long run, debilitating to the individual. As David Huron suggests, what he terms non-adaptive pleasure-seeking behaviors, such as drug use, are not usually conducive to ongoing reproductive success: "poor health and neglect of offspring are infallible ways of reducing the probability that one's genes will be present in a future gene pool."[37] Drugs often lead to isolation and introspection, and if too many members of the population indulge there will almost certainly be a loss of social order and cohesion. Even when opening the gates of perception, drug-induced hallucinations cannot be shared, even with an identical twin. ... It seems to me that music, and with it dance, are the very antithesis of this. This is surely *not* what music was, or is, about.

Unravelling the evolutionary relevance of music to our species is the key; despite all of the writing and theorizing, and the centuries of scholastic endeavor, most in agreement that music has a weird and wonderful power over our species, there remains a lack of consensus as to exactly why humans, seemingly throughout their history, have responded so positively to music. Many questions remain. Is there a broader context of music? What, if any, adaptive advantages did music give to *Homo sapiens* from an evolutionary perspective as our founders migrated out of East Africa to rapidly colonize the world? What collection of circuitries and abilities was needed to generate and underpin what we define as human musical behavior? Our numbers increased perhaps by a thousand fold between 60,000–70,000 and 10,000 years ago, and increased yet a further thousand fold after the transition from hunter-gatherer to farmer. Why does music continue to remain important to all human cultures, thousands of generations after the founders of our species evolved?

Finally, there is the thorny question of the relationship between music and language. The modern human brain is clearly wired to deal with both forms of communication, in a sensory-perceptual as well as motor capacity, but how do these forms interact? From an evolutionary point of view, did music come before language, did language come before music—or was there some common progenitor that somehow separated into two distinct yet still overlapping strands when *Homo sapiens* evolved, with both types of communication retained? If this was the case, then why were both retained? Why were both communication systems needed? Was music an important ingredient in the phenotypic recipe that contributed to the survival of our newly evolved species? Why are we the all-speaking, all-singing, all-dancing creatures of our planet?

In this book, in suggesting possible answers to these questions, I will take you on a wide-ranging journey that encompasses anthropology and archaeology, genetics, neuroscience and behavior, brain imaging, neurology, and modern-day neurotherapies. Bringing these various strands together I hope to convince you that music (and with it, dance) was there at our beginning, in our founder population, and is a unique and special communication system that continues to promote the collective expression and experience of emotions. Music fosters cooperation and social cohesion. Our recognition of, and emotional responses to, consonance (tones that sound good together, for example octaves or fifths) and dissonance (tones that are slightly different and that interfere with each other, causing an unpleasant sound that we find difficult to resolve), to pleasant and unpleasant music, seems to be universal and expressed even in very young infants,[38,39,40,41] although exposure to music increases our appreciation of consonance and "harmonicity."[42] Music, or perhaps the elements in any type of vocalization that signal emotion or emphasis of some kind,[43,44] may be an important way of helping to bond with infants prior to the ontogeny of articulate speech, and "happy voice quality"—irrespective of whether speech or singing is involved—is the most important element in gaining an infant's attention.[45] Excitingly, responses to music appear to be independent of our cultural upbringing.[46] Modern neuroscience research confirms that the appreciation and processing of music has a real and consistent structural foundation in the human brain. As each decade passes, we learn more and more about how such music-related circuits differ from, or overlap with, other pathways involved in cognitive and emotional processing. Of particular importance is the realization that brain areas associated with positive responses to music are closely aligned to networks associated with reward behaviors and acts of social cooperation/altruism, consistent with earlier ethnomusicological descriptions of music as "a product of the behaviour of human groups."[1]

In close association with the evolution of the modern sentient mind, I will propose that music was an essential attribute of our early ancestors. It acted as a counterweight to the new and evolving sense of self, to the emerging sense of vulnerability in all of us as we began to appreciate our mortality—a realization that grew along with the evolution of the modern brain and newly acquired language capability. In arguing the case, and noting the inevitable danger of "spinning untestable 'just so' stories" that cannot be proved or disproved,[25] I hope to persuade you that music remains just as essential to *Homo sapiens* now in the twenty-first century as it was perhaps 80,000 years ago. Music can be a source of joy and excitement, a bringer of tranquility and enlightenment, and a vehicle for reconciliation and unification. It is important for both social and cognitive development in children. Music is cathartic. It helps sustain our health and overall sense of mental well-being, our sense of community, and our sense of belonging, and it has potentially great power as a therapeutic tool. To quote a great title of an earlier essay by Ian Cross: "Is music the most important thing we ever did?"[47]

Back in November 1997, I gave a talk on the basic principles described in this book at a local meeting known as the Western Australian Neuroscience Colloquium. The next day I listened to a talk by an eminent Australian neurologist about "the clinician's approach to neurodegenerative diseases" and was surprised to discover that music, and in particular a patient's cognitive and affective reactions to music, did not normally form part of the clinician's armamentarium, and was not used to help decipher mood and emotional responsiveness in patients. Today, in the minds of most people, music therapy remains a branch of "alternative" medicine. In recent times the phrase "nonpharmacological" rather than "alternative" therapy has gained currency in some quarters and is perhaps an improved descriptor, but it still implies something outside the mainstream.

Any brief online search will show how music therapy, especially in the treatment of chronic pain or anxiety, is so often grouped together with other so-called alternative medical treatments such as acupuncture, hypnotherapy, aromatherapy, balneotherapy (treatment of disease by bathing), thermotherapy, magnetic therapy, homeopathy, relaxation methods, massage, prayer/meditation/yoga, lifestyle or dietary changes, herbal treatment (eg green teas), vitamins, "ethnomedicine" (eg treatment with garlic, lime juice), reflexology, hydrotherapy, and pet therapy.[48,49,50,51,52,53] I am sure that champions of any of these "alternative" therapies wish that their favorite treatments were accorded more conventional clinical status. I am convinced that this is the status that should be afforded to music therapy, with its beneficial effects on the mental and physical health of the great majority of the human species.

By compiling this story and putting musical processing fairly and squarely into an overarching evolutionary, neuroscientific, and sociological context, I hope to convince you that music should be recognized as being less specifically "arty"—less "alternative"—and should be recognized as being central to human cultural and intellectual experience. My hope is that this book is of interest to a wide range of readers from different backgrounds, all interested in why music is a human universal, its possible role in our recent evolutionary history, and why music: (i) remains important for the welfare of human society in the twenty-first century, (ii) is an essential element in early education, and (iii) should be viewed as a proven and reliable therapeutic tool for use by neurologists, neuropsychologists, and rehabilitation specialists when treating neurologically and/or physically challenged patients. But before addressing these twenty-first century "big picture" issues, we must first consider how and where music is processed in our brains, and after that when and how *Homo sapiens* evolved, and why our species continues to possess two interrelated but distinguishable communication systems: music and language.

Chapter 2

How the Brain Processes Music

It is essential to understand our brains in some detail if we are to assess correctly our place in this vast and complicated universe we see all around us.
—Francis Crick, *What Mad Pursuit: A Personal View of Scientific Discovery*

It is worth restating that in modern humans, at least in our culture, language—usually but not necessarily communicated via the spoken word—is regarded as the major and universal form of communication between individuals. It is a unique attribute of *Homo sapiens*. But then so is musicality; why is music also a universal form of communication? Is music merely an accidental by-product of evolution, just a hang-over from our forebears, or is it, in partnership with language, an essential part of our cognitive and emotional makeup?

To address this core question, we need first to understand the extent to which music and language differ from each other. How do modern-day musicologists and linguists define and describe the various intrinsic properties of our two communication streams? Of course the phenomenon of music, like language, has a number of essential psychological and physiological elements—creation (mind/imagination), performance (motor), and perception (sensory). Broken down into its basic constituents, music contains pitch changes, tonal relationships, melodic contour and harmony, changes in volume, and changes in stress/emphasis. There is also what is termed "timbre," or the particular sound quality of tones. Music has beat, meter, and rhythm. It has a regular pulse that invariably elicits involuntary or voluntary movements in the listener. As most of us appreciate, music is inextricably and universally linked to physical movement and dance, especially in a social context. It is particularly revealing that some societies do not have a word that distinguishes between music-making, singing, and dancing, even ceremony—it is all one and the same.[1] This music–movement alliance is clearly an important evolutionary relationship, something that is discussed in more detail later in this chapter. Finally, music also has a hierarchical structure, with various rules and constraints, which requires the processing and prediction of phrases and extended musical sequences, and with that comes the need for efficient and reliable classification, recognition, and memory systems.

While music has the well-known capacity to affect human emotions, human language also has what are termed "prosodic elements." These include pitch range and variation, voice quality, loudness, and rhythm of delivery that convey information about the emotional state of the speaker or that color an utterance in some way (for example, whether what is spoken is a question or a command, praise or sarcasm, threat or plea). But language also supports literal and scientific content; it is a primary medium through which we store, catalog, and transmit data and knowledge.[2] Language has grammar (nouns, verbs, adjectives, etc) and a complex set of hierarchical principles (syntax, recursion) that underpin the construction and arrangement of words (the lexicon) into meaningful sentences, clauses, and phrases. These underlying rules seem to be instinctive in us,[3] and are learned by each individual in order to be able to produce meaningful sentences and recognize that a particular combination of words is grammatical and makes sense: "Comprehending a sentence involves identifying the structural relations among its words and phrases. By assigning grammatical functions and thematic roles to different arguments of the verb, syntactic structure of a sentence indicates who is doing what to whom."[4] Remarkably, language is not exclusively the domain of speech and audition. Thus the congenitally deaf, who have a morphologically normal volume of auditory-related cortical areas with typical asymmetry between left and right temporal lobes,[5] also possess the virtual cognitive architecture that enables them to babble with their hands as infants, eventually learn to use signing, lip-reading, and so on, in adulthood, and apparently communicate via "standard" language networks in the brain.

Language is propositional; it is referential in that meaningful interpretation requires additional knowledge or experience—sometimes termed "external referents." Language is expandable in content and facilitates the virtual creation and manipulation of symbols, the meaning and relevance of which vary depending on context. It permits intuitive reasoning and the expression of thoughts and ideas, and facilitates planning and choice-making. Language contains past, present, future, and conditional constructions (was, is, will, may, might, should, could) that allow descriptions, and a shared appreciation, of time and its possibilities. It is not necessarily representative of anything real and can be used to convey information about objects or occurrences that are not necessarily "here and now." As my late friend and esteemed colleague Dr Len Freedman once said to me: "language both defines and defies time." For many scholars, and this is a key point, the creation of language in *Homo sapiens* must have been intimately associated with the evolution of the modern mind.

The biologist and cognitive scientist Tecumseh Fitch has put forward some possible design features that characterize and distinguish music from language.[6] Based on the early work of Charles Hockett, who argued that there are 13 design features of language (and only the human language possesses all 13), Fitch suggests that music—specifically vocal music—is "speech minus meaning." The lack of referentiality and semantic meaning in music gives it special "affective and aesthetic power" that can have different connotations to different individuals.

There is considerable evidence in support of the proposal that the basic circuits needed to learn language are innately wired—are "a distinct piece of the biological makeup of our brains"[3]; however, these networks require social and cultural experience and training during critical periods of early life in order to develop them to their full potential, as evidenced by the rare occasions when human infants are raised by non-humans. The extraordinary tale of the two Indian girls discovered in the 1920s who were raised by wolves in the Bengal jungle is a classic case in point.[7] These so-called feral children did not, even when eventually reunited with humans, acquire many human characteristics, including articulate speech, although one surviving girl was eventually able to generate some words, but apparently not sentences or conversation. This disquieting human story is not unlike the maternal and social deprivation studies on baby rhesus monkeys carried out by the psychologist Harry Harlow and colleagues in the late 1950s/early 1960s. He found that early and sustained deprivation caused profound and long-term physiological and behavioral dysfunction in animal subjects.[8]

Perhaps the clearest example of how refinement of an innate neurological potential requires appropriate environmental input at the appropriate time comes from the primary visual cortex. In animals like us, with frontally placed eyes, each eye is in a different position in the head and thus views the world from a slightly different perspective. The visual cortex can combine these images from the two eyes, and by comparing the two inputs, generates a binocular three-dimensional reconstruction of the outside world—giving us the perception of depth, or stereopsis. But this remarkable facility cannot be harnessed if early visual experiences are abnormal. If, during the first four to five years of life, a child's eyes are misaligned relative to each other (squint), then the signals to the visual cortex are desynchronized and binocular processing is not established. If the eyes are subsequently aligned correctly, but after this critical developmental period, it is then too late and stereoscopic depth perception is permanently lost. The potential circuitry was there, but the input triggers were not. So, too, does effective and appropriate maturation of language circuits also require early experience, and the same appears to be true for many aspects of music-making. Importantly, as discussed in Chapter 7 on music and education, early musical training has diverse developmental and cognitive benefits that extend well beyond the purely musical domain.

Given that the sensory aspects of both music and speech require a sophisticated hearing apparatus and involve extraordinarily complex auditory processing within the brain, it is important to present a brief introduction to human auditory pathways, from the ear to the cerebral cortex. I will describe the essential elements of this sensory pathway and what is currently understood about the processing of complex sounds. I will then go on to describe what is known about where and how music is processed in the brain of *Homo sapiens*, and briefly compare this neural architecture with what is known about the processing of speech and language. Differences will be emphasized at this point, but we shall see in Chapter 4 that the circuits involved in the processing of music and language are not entirely separate, providing intriguing clues about the possible evolutionary antecedent of these two human communication streams.

The brain—an overview

At the most basic level, the human brain above the level of the spinal cord is divided into a number of major regions, from back to front—hindbrain, midbrain, and forebrain.

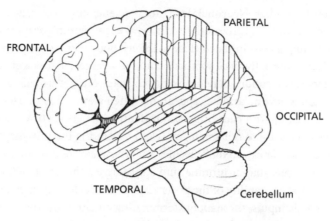

FRONTAL

PARIETAL

OCCIPITAL

TEMPORAL

Cerebellum

Figure 2.1 The major lobes (frontal, parietal, temporal, and occipital) of the human cerebral cortex and their approximate boundaries. The cingulate lobe/cortex can only be seen on the medial aspect of each cerebral hemisphere (see Figures 4.2 and 5.1).
© Martin Thompson, 2016.

Many important aspects of auditory (sound) processing are carried out in specific parts of the hind- and midbrain, as well as in part of a major sensory relay station, the thalamus, which is located deep in the forebrain below the cerebral cortex. The nerve cells (neurons) in this part of the thalamus then send information on to a number of auditory processing areas in a lobe of the overlying cerebral cortex, called the temporal lobe (Figure 2.1). These small sensory areas of the superior temporal cortex are involved in the initial processing of sound, and transmit information on to so-called higher level cortical regions involved in music and language processing, as well as to regions concerned with affective/emotional responses and motor control. Beyond auditory cortex there are also interactions with complex multimodal cortical regions that are the presumed repository of higher cognitive and social functions, including the long-term storage and recollection of autobiographical memories, assorted facts, and other types of stored knowledge.

The nervous systems of our body contain different types of cells, essentially divided into two major classes: neurons and glia (the latter from the Greek word meaning "glue"). All these cells have typical—what is termed "eukaryotic"—features, which include a nucleus containing the genetic code within chromosomes, cytoplasm, and intracellular organelles such as mitochondria, Golgi apparatus, and endoplasmic reticulum, all necessary for maintaining the long-term health of each cell. The central nervous system (CNS, brain, and spinal cord) comprises a huge range of neuronal types, defined morphologically by the size and shape of their cell bodies and the three-dimensional shape of their cellular processes (dendrites or axons—see below). Neurons also differ in the chemicals they contain and in the complement of receptors and various ion channels located on their membrane surface. This in turn influences how they receive and respond to information exchanged with other nerve cells. Neurons are the obviously electrically excitable cells in the brain; they process and then transmit signals either locally or over long distances, from one brain region to another. Neuronal dendrites are generally the receivers of information (the antennae if you like) from other cells, whereas a neuron's output signal (action potential or nerve impulse) is initiated close to the cell body and is then propagated along the axon to influence the activity of another neuron or a target such as a gland or muscle. Anatomically, large aggregations of neurons into clusters or layers are called "gray matter" because these regions have a dark(ish) appearance when viewed postmortem.

Neurons communicate with each other and with other targets via tiny structures called synapses. At these sites, there is a small gap (cleft) separating the presynaptic side from the postsynaptic side. Neuroactive molecules (neurotransmitters or neuromodulators) are released from the presynaptic terminal and diffuse across the cleft to either increase or decrease the electrical excitability of the postsynaptic cell. Each neuron can receive many thousands of synaptic inputs, these inputs terminating on either the dendrites or the cell body itself. At any given time the physiological state of the neuron will be affected by different combinations of excitatory or inhibitory inputs, and by how these active inputs are spatially distributed around the cell. Whether or not a given neuron then generates its own action potential depends on whether the overall integrated drive to that neuron is sufficient to excite the cell. If inhibition prevails, the neuron is silent for that period of time.

Glial cell types are also diverse. The main cell type is the astrocyte, originally named because it has a star-like appearance. Classically, its role is both structural and functional, especially in the maintenance of a barrier between the bloodstream and the brain, and in providing substrates needed by neurons, and subsequently, in eliminating any breakdown products (metabolites). Astrocytes are now understood to be a heterogeneous population, and we shall in Chapter 3 (under the heading "Chemistry and plasticity") that this traditional "housekeeping" role undoubtedly does not do justice to the physiological importance of astrocytes in the modern human brain. It is also possible that subtle changes in astrocyte function occurred in our ancestors that contributed to the eventual evolution of a thinking, talking, musical *Homo sapiens*. To speed up the transmission of signals in the brain, many axons are insulated with a fatty sheath called myelin, which is produced by another glial cell called the oligodendrocyte. Regions that contain bundles or tracts of large numbers of myelinated axons look white in cut sections of the brain; hence these tracts are called "white matter." Immune responses and reaction to injury and disease involve a third glial type: the microglial cell. Remarkably, these cells originate from the bone marrow and can continue to colonize our central nervous system throughout life, helping to maintain brain health.

In all mammals, the cerebral cortex is the gray matter on the outside of the cerebrum. It is where the cortical neurons are located and is divided into two huge masses in the left and right cerebral hemispheres of the brain. These two halves differ significantly in their functionality and capability. Many parts of the left and right cerebral cortices are interconnected by a massive white matter tract called the corpus callosum, estimated in humans to contain about 100 million axons.[9] The cortex receives axons from, and sends axons to, subcortical structures, and vast and complex association white matter tracts interconnect cerebral cortical regions on the same side of the brain. There have been many estimates of neuronal number in the gray matter of human cerebral cortex, ranging from 16 billion to 23 billion.[10,11] Perhaps surprisingly, the smaller cerebellum (Latin for "little brain"), which is situated at the back of the brain (Figure 2.1) and is involved in motor learning and the coordination and synchronization of movement, contains far more neurons (69 billion) than the cerebral cortex.[10] This is because cerebellar neurons are much more closely packed together and there are far fewer glial cells.

Within each hemisphere, regions of the cerebral cortex can be defined anatomically and functionally. For example, certain areas are involved specifically in sensory processing, such as the primary and secondary auditory cortical areas, primary and secondary visual areas, and areas relating to touch sensation and proprioception (awareness of the position of our limbs) (Figure 2.2). In addition, other areas are involved in the control of movement, and yet another area is specialized for the control of eye movements. Multimodal association cortical areas integrate all this information via complex interconnecting circuitries; other cortical regions are involved in learning and memory, the planning and processing of ideas, as well as in many other higher-level cognitive functions. This functional localization has been acknowledged for some time, but until recently information was obtained primarily through analysis of the effects of injuries such as stroke or trauma. Modern techniques that measure neural activity, such as electroencephalography (EEG; electrodes on the scalp measure voltage changes due to electrical activity in the brain) or magnetoencephalography (MEG; measures magnetic fields produced by electrical currents in the brain) and diverse ways of functionally imaging the living brain, have vastly expanded our knowledge about how the brain works.

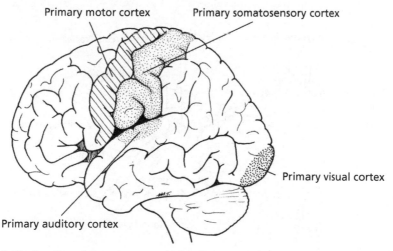

Figure 2.2 The location of the primary cortical regions processing movement, somatosensation (touch, pain, etc), sound, and vision.

© Martin Thompson, 2016.

Anatomy and physiology of the human auditory system

Auditory pathways differ from some other sensory pathways in that they involve many synaptic relays as they ascend through various regions of the brainstem on their way, via the thalamus, to cerebral cortex. Ascending pain pathways may also make connections in the brainstem en route to higher centers, whereas the projection from the retina in the eye to visual cortex is more direct and involves only one major relay in the thalamus. Auditory pathways therefore potentially have access to the reticular formation and autonomic brainstem areas, regions that influence the way our bodies physically respond to arousal and emotions. In fact, there is good evidence that autonomic responses can be synchronized with music.[12] It is tempting to speculate that such potential interactions with brainstem circuitries are not accidental and may reflect a long evolutionary history of the potent impact of sound on emotions and affective social behaviors.[13]

The human ear comprises three parts, classically divided into an outer, middle, and inner part (Figure 2.3). The outer or external part is called the pinna or auricle and is mostly made of cartilage. This structure is highly specialized in mammals, and is movable in most species, including many primates, but not in the so-called *Hominidae* (the great apes—chimpanzees, bonobos, gorillas, orangutans, and us!). In each human, the shape of the pinna is subtly different, and our brains seem to adapt to these shape variations in order to best process incoming auditory information. The pinna helps to facilitate sound localization and to resolve so-called front-back ambiguities (the ability to determine whether the sound source is in front or behind).[14] Of course, localization of sound

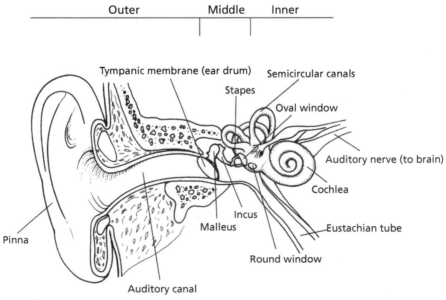

Figure 2.3 The human ear and auditory apparatus.
© Martin Thompson, 2016.

is facilitated by turning the head towards that sound, and in the horizontal plane is perceptually achieved by reference to the timing of inputs to the left and right ears, and interaural intensity differences due to head shadowing effects. The pinna is thought to be especially important in localizing sound in the vertical plane and may also be important in aiding the processing of speech.

The auditory canal or external auditory meatus is about 2.5 cm long and leads to the tympanic membrane or ear drum. The canal can amplify certain frequencies of sound. The ear drum, which lies at an angle to the canal and is circular in shape, separates the outer from the middle ear (Figure 2.3). It has elastic properties, and air pressure changes (sound waves) entering the ear cause the drum to vibrate. There is air in the middle ear, and the pressure on either side of the ear drum is usually kept fairly constant because the middle ear is connected to the nose and throat via a tube called the Eustachian tube. When that tube becomes blocked, owing to a heavy cold for example, this equalization of pressure cannot occur, and thus any external pressure changes such as we experience during takeoff or landing in an aircraft can be very uncomfortable!

The middle ear bones, or ossicles, form a hinged chain ("ossicular chain") that transmits vibration or mechanical energy from the eardrum to the inner ear, where the energy is transduced into electrical signals for transmission to the brain. The malleus (hammer) is firmly attached to the ear drum; the incus (anvil) is next, and the stapes (stirrup) is the last in the chain. This small bone then contacts a structure known as the oval window, an opening in the bone that separates the middle ear from the chambers of the inner ear, which in turn are filled with fluid. The area of the stapes footplate on the oval window is about 17 times smaller than the area of the ear drum, and the ossicular chain plays an important role in magnifying the mechanical energy per unit area as the sound energy moves from "floppy" air to the stiffer fluid medium in the inner ear. It has been suggested that these middle ear ossicles may also have eventually become useful in reducing the interference from internally generated sounds such as chewing and crunching.[15]

The inner ear

The inner ear is contained within a labyrinth of bone in a part of the skull called the petrous bone. It consists of a number of specialized structures that encode information about sound (the cochlea) or head position and head movement (the vestibular apparatus) (Figure 2.3). The cochlea is a highly specialized sensory apparatus that transduces mechanical energy into electrical signals. In humans, the cochlea is about 35 mm long and resembles a snail shell (hence its name—of Greek origin) with two and one half-spirals, from base to apex. Along its length, the cochlea is divided into three fluid-filled chambers: the scala vestibuli, cochlea duct (scala media), and scala tympani (Figure 2.4). The first two named ducts are separated by a thin membrane, and the cochlea duct and scala tympani are separated by a complex structure that includes the so-called basilar membrane. On this membrane is the organ of Corti, where the receptors are located and the transduction process begins. The two scala chambers are continuous at the apex of the cochlea (the opening is called the helicotrema), and both contain a clear fluid called

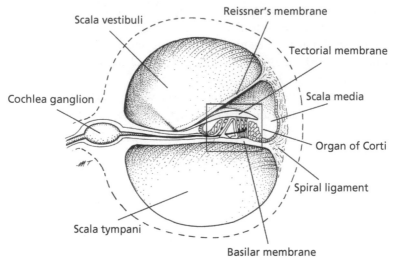

Figure 2.4 A high-power view of a section through the cochlear spiral showing the various fluid-filled chambers, the basilar membrane, and the organ of Corti, containing the receptors needed to transduce vibrational energy into electrical impulses that are subsequently perceived as sounds.

© Martin Thompson, 2016.

perilymph. By contrast, the cochlea duct contains a fluid called endolymph that contains a comparatively different concentration of sodium and potassium ions—essential for the ongoing activity of the inner ear receptors. Endolymph is made by specialized cells in a structure known as the stria vascularis.

Vibrations that enter via the oval window travel all around the cochlea until the energy is eventually dissipated back into the middle ear at another membranous window known as the round window. These vibrations cause the basilar membrane to oscillate in a travelling wave towards the helicotrema. The width of this membrane is about ten times wider at the apex than at the base. Anyone who has played a stringed instrument will know that the shorter the string, the higher the note. Similarly, high frequencies preferentially cause the basilar membrane to vibrate at the base, whereas the membrane at the apex is sensitive to low frequencies. This, together with progressive changes in the mass and stiffness of the membrane, results in a place code on the basilar membrane, from high to low. Receptors located at different positions along the length of this membrane, and that are activated by vibrational energy, therefore respond optimally to different characteristic sound frequencies (the number of times a waveform repeats itself per second) (Figure 2.5). This place code is used to assist in the neural coding of frequency and in the formation of frequency maps that are found throughout the various stages of auditory processing all the way up to auditory cortex. This ordered representation of sound frequency is called "tonotopicity." The range of frequencies heard by humans is about 20–20,000 Hz, and not all frequencies are heard with the same degree of sensitivity; there is inter-individual variation, and the

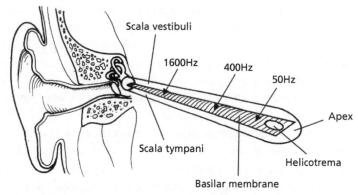

Figure 2.5 The basilar membrane extended out as a sheet, showing its increase in width from base to apex of the cochlear spiral, and its concomitant sensitivity to different sound frequencies (high to low).
© Martin Thompson, 2016.

frequency range diminishes with age, especially at the high frequency end of the sound spectrum.

The organ of Corti, located on the basilar membrane, is a very complex structure containing not just rows of receptors (hair cells) but an array of supporting cells (Figure 2.4). There are both inner, and a greater number of outer, hair cell arrays, the former seeming to be the primary receptors signaling activity to the brain. The tips of the hair cells (stereocilia) are embedded in a gelatinous mass called the tectorial membrane, which is hinged at one end. There is relative movement and oscillation between the underlying basilar membrane and the overlying tectorial membrane, which sets up shearing forces that mechanically deform and deflect the receptors. This conformational change induces ionic currents and a graded electrical signal or receptor potential in the hair cells, a signal that is eventually transmitted up to central processing regions. Interestingly, at least in animals, the sensitivity of the cochlear hair cells to sound can be altered by central commands originating in the brain, but the exact role that this "efferent" control of the peripheral sensory apparatus plays in human auditory perception is still not fully understood.[16]

Central pathways

Sensory fibers that synapse on the receptor hair cells in the cochlea derive from neurons located in a structure called the spiral or cochlear ganglion. If the potential change (called a "depolarization") in the receptors is sufficient, calcium flows into the cell, resulting in the release of neurotransmitters that excite the nerve terminals, generating an action potential—the neuronal code. Each sensory auditory neuron is sharply tuned to a particular frequency and has a central axonal process that projects through the auditory branch of the eighth cranial nerve to the brainstem. Once in the brain, the 30,000 or so axons in each human auditory nerve first terminate in the cochlear nuclei in the brainstem, where they form synapses with a diverse population of neurons. Axons from these neurons then project rostrally via a number of pathways towards the midbrain and forebrain (Figure 2.6). These pathways are very complex, and involve projections that can either stay on the same side of the brain or cross over and ascend in bundles on the opposite side. A number of relays take place, and at each level there appears to be feedback to earlier stages including, as mentioned earlier, central projections all the way out to the receptors in the cochlea itself. At various stages along the auditory pathway there is convergence and integration of information from the two ears, necessary for the localization of a sound source. Remarkably, there is evidence that the structures in the inner ear that process balance (the saccule and utricle, parts of the vestibular apparatus mentioned earlier) can also process loud sound and vibration.[17] This sensitivity, also associated with connections to brainstem regions, may well contribute to our external and internal physical responses to music.[18]

Axons in all ascending auditory pathways originating from the cochlear nuclei eventually converge on, and form synapses on neurons within, a midbrain structure called the inferior colliculus. These neurons then project their own axons forward to the auditory part of the thalamus, a structure called the medial geniculate nucleus, or MGN

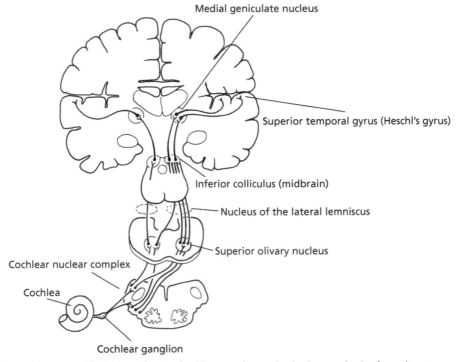

Figure 2.6 A simplified view of central auditory pathways in the human brain, from the cochlea—via relays in the brainstem, midbrain, and thalamus—to primary auditory cortex in the superior gyrus of the temporal lobe (Heschl's gyrus).
© Martin Thompson, 2016.

(Figure 2.6). It should be noted that in this context the term "nucleus" refers to a group of neurons, sometimes containing millions of cells that are usually anatomically distinct and that together subserve a particular function. Neurons in the MGN then relay auditory information to cells in the primary auditory cortex in the superior part of the temporal lobe. As seems always to be the case when studying human cerebral cortex, there is considerable inter-individual variability in the exact gyral and sulcal patterns that make up the superior temporal lobe; however, in the great majority of people the primary auditory cortex is located in the anterior transverse gyri, or Heschl's gyrus (named after the Austrian anatomist Richard Heschl, who first described these transverse protuberances in the superior temporal gyrus) (Figure 2.7).[19,20,21] Again, there are also very important feedback loops, with axons originating in neurons in auditory cortex projecting back to cells in the MGN and inferior colliculus. In the context of the way music can affect human emotions and alter our physiological responses (eg heart rate), it is worth noting here that ascending auditory projections also have various connections with a complex gray matter structure known as the amygdala, important in processing valence, or emotionally relevant information (see Chapter 4).

The human auditory cortex contains numerous auditory fields in and around Heschl's gyri in the superior temporal lobe (Figure 2.7).[19,20,21,22,23,24] As alluded to earlier, primary auditory cortex and some other auditory areas on the medial aspect of the auditory cortical region have a tonotopic organization and thus contain organized maps of frequencies ranging from low to high. There are two (some suggest three) tonotopic maps in primary auditory cortex in which the responses to different frequencies are narrowly tuned. Primary auditory cortex is usually divided into two zones (termed A1 and R), each with a tonotopic map that is essentially a mirror image of the other, the reversal occurring at the A1/R border, where low frequencies are processed. Primary auditory cortex is flanked by numerous so-called belt and parabelt regions that possess broader and weaker frequency tuning characteristics, all sub-regions containing some

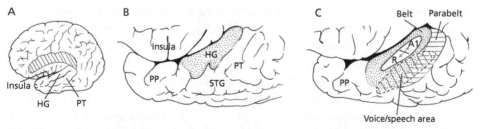

Figure 2.7 A, A cut-away image showing the location of the superior temporal gyrus. B, Higher power view of the superior temporal gyrus (STG) showing the location of Heschl's gyrus (HG), the planum polare (PP), and the planum temporale (PT). C, Primary auditory cortex (divided into A1 and R) and surrounding belt and parabelt auditory regions (modified from Moerel et al, 2014). The region that processes voice/speech is also shown. The arrows show the reversal of the tonotopic map at the A1/R border, with the arrowheads pointing towards increasingly higher frequencies.
© Martin Thompson, 2016.

form of tonotopic organization.[21,22,25,26,27,28,29,30] While these multiple tonotopic maps derive, to a large extent, from the frequency place maps that are established peripherally along the basilar membrane in the cochlea within the inner ear (place coding), groups or arrays of auditory nerve fibers can cooperate to provide phase-locked information about a particular stimulus frequency (the "volley-coding principle"), which is especially important at low frequencies. The maximum rate of phase locking decreases as pathways ascend through the midbrain and thalamus, and it has been suggested that "the form of the neural code changes at least twice as the information progresses from cochlea to cortex."[31] Neurons in these regions may also respond preferentially to sounds of particular intensities and locations. The complex issue of pitch processing is considered further in the "Frequency/pitch" section below.

There is evidence that the left and right auditory cortices are organized somewhat differently in humans.[21] Morphologically, the left cortex has a different cellular and fiber architecture, and is functionally capable of finer and more dynamic temporal resolution, whereas the right auditory cortex displays better frequency and spectral resolution.[32,33,34,35] These differences are almost certainly pertinent to the known bias of music and language processing to the right and left hemispheres respectively, a critical issue considered further below (under the heading "An introductory word on the processing of language and speech") and again in Chapter 4.

In secondary belt and parabelt auditory association cortical areas (Figure 2.7), sound-responsive neurons analyze natural sounds and complex acoustic stimuli,[36,37] not just frequency and intensity, including spectral and timbral features, clicks, bursts of noise, and "kissing" sounds. Some neurons preferentially respond to the spatial location of the sound source.[15,38] The more lateral parts of the human auditory cortical complex in the superior temporal gyrus are less "influenced by acoustic features but rather respond to behaviorally relevant complex sounds such as speech and are strongly modulated by attention."[19] More recent research has confirmed preferential responses to the human voice and acoustic properties thought to be unique to language/speech in populations of neurons in non-primary auditory cortex, lateral and anterior to primary auditory cortex (Figure 2.7),[21,23,39,40,41] although (interestingly) not necessarily exclusively left-lateralized. Responses to particular aspects of language (phonemes, words, phrases) have also been reported.[42] Another study revealed that preferential responses to voice and speech occurred mainly in regions processing sound at the lower frequency end of the spectrum.[28] This low frequency information may be an important factor in how we perceive emotional content in speech.[43] Building on imaging studies that identified regions in anterior superior temporal cortex responsive to musical instrument sounds or components of speech,[36,39,44] a population of neurons that apparently selectively respond to natural speech sounds has been confirmed in non-primary auditory cortex, a population that appears to be distinct from one responding to music.[45]

The extent to which the processing of music and language involves separate versus overlapping areas of neural circuitry has important evolutionary implications, and is an issue discussed at length in Chapter 4. At this point, however, it is useful to summarize how auditory processing influences neural activity well beyond the confines of the superior temporal gyrus. These outputs have particular distributions to parts of frontal and parietal cortex (Figure 2.8) and are associated with even higher level processing, including interactions with other sensory modalities and links to motor systems controlling vocalization. A ventral stream originating in anterior auditory areas projects to parts of inferior frontal and prefrontal cortex and "plays a general role in auditory object recognition, including perception of vocalizations and speech"[44]—a "what" pathway—while the dorsal stream originates from more caudal auditory belt regions, connecting with inferior parietal cortex, premotor cortex, and dorsolateral prefrontal cortex, and "plays a general role in sensorimotor integration and control"[44]—a "do" pathway. These auditory networks are important not only in language and speech processing but are also thought to be important in the perception and performance of music-related activities,[35] presumably with some left versus right bias for speech and music respectively (see also Chapter 4).

I introduced some of the core physical elements of music at the beginning of this chapter. Over the next couple of pages I will describe these basic constituents in a little more detail, along with our current knowledge about their processing and analysis in auditory pathways of the brain. For those interested, a book by John Powell (*How Music Works*)[46] provides a useful and intelligible introductory guide to the science of music. Sound waves are complex and energetic, with a particular frequency (measured in Hertz) and amplitude (intensity of sound, in decibels). These sound waves are rarely

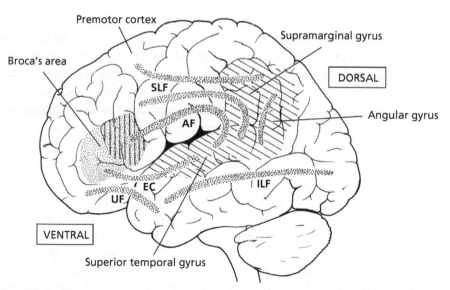

Figure 2.8 The complex white matter tracts in humans (shown as dotted bands) that interlink different parts of the temporal lobe with specific regions in parietal, frontal, and occipital cortex. AF, arcuate fasciculus; SLF, superior longitudinal fasciculus; UF, uncinate fasciculus; EC, extreme capsule; ILF, inferior longitudinal fasciculus; SMG, supramarginal gyrus; AG, angular gyrus.
© Martin Thompson, 2016.

purely harmonic in shape, and the complexity of waveforms is the physical basis for the perception of timbre, or how the note *sounds*. Each one of these elements can be modulated independent of the others, and although music is a universal, different cultures use these elements in different ways and with different emphasis, resulting in subtle inter-cultural variation in musical sound and structure.[47] Of course, sensory responses to music involve widespread interactions with pathways associated with the control and initiation of movement—movement to the beat, or "dance." In fact, the interactions between regions of the brain that perceive sound and those that plan, control and synchronize movements seem to be especially developed in our species.[48] This is a most important aspect of music, and involves not just dancing but singing, humming, and playing an instrument. The emotional and more psychosocial aspects of responding to, and participating in, music are also of the most fundamental importance, and form much of the basis of the content of Chapters 4–6.

Frequency/pitch

Pitch is not the same as frequency; each successive octave-increase in pitch (eight white keys on a piano) corresponds to a doubling of frequency. Pitch is not represented in the peripheral apparatus (cochlea) but is the perceptual or subjective correlate of frequency—a note that is constructed from a harmonic series of frequencies (spectral content) that are related to what is termed the "fundamental frequency," the lowest harmonic component in the periodic waveform. Pitch, together with amplitude and timbre (the color or tonal quality of the sound) interact, influencing the way that we perceive the pitch of a particular note.[49] Complex sounds can produce a sensation of pitch when there is no acoustic energy present at the perceived pitch frequency, thus sometimes you can "hear" the fundamental frequency in a note even if it is not actually present in the waveform. Remarkably, in human auditory cortex separate populations of neurons exist that respond to multiple frequency bands that are harmonically related and exactly one octave apart, suggesting an intrinsic network that explains why notes an octave apart sound pleasant and somewhat similar in pitch, despite the halving or doubling of frequency.[50,51] Nonetheless, this may not be a feature unique to our species.[52]

Temporal organization

Hearing in time is an essential aspect of musical perception and appreciation.[53] Rhythm is the regular pattern of accents (stresses) and temporal intervals between sounds that creates a perception of stronger and weaker beats/pulses. Beat is the underlying temporal regularity, giving us the perception of metric organization—strong beats usually elicit motor responses such as finger or foot tapping. Meter is the perception and anticipation over time of a repeated series of beats, accents, or pulses derived from a recurring rhythmic pattern. Tempo is the speed of beat and meter. The responses of populations of neurons can be entrained both to beat and to meter, the cells perhaps resonating at the beat frequency in a complex dynamic of synchronized activity combined with perceptual expectation.[54]

Loudness or intensity

The firing rates of groups of neurons with different thresholds and dynamic range code for sound intensity or loudness. Loudness is a subjective measure that is related to, but by no means identical to, sound intensity. The latter is the amount of energy emanating from a source, whereas the perception of loudness also depends on several other parameters. At the low frequency end, bass can often be perceived as "loudness," perhaps owing to additional vibrational energy that is detected by other sense organs such as receptors in the vestibular system.[17]

Timbre or tonal color

Timbre is a complex attribute that is related to the spectral envelope (energy/power at each constituent frequency) and temporal components of a sound.[15] The perceptual basis for timbre perception has recently been modeled.[55] To distinguish one voice from another, or one musical instrument from another, requires four basic components: analyses of the sound frequency (requires tonotopicity), the spectral envelope and temporal modulation (including how a sound begins and decays), and finally, the time needed to acquire sufficient information to process and then recognize these various attributes.

Harmony—musical syntax?

As briefly mentioned in Chapter 1, music has a hierarchical organization—with particular rules and constraints—that requires the processing and prediction of phrases and extended musical sequences over time. It is generally believed that this constitutes a musical lexicon, with a type of syntax that underlies our context-dependent understanding of musical structures and sequences, and so forth, and also allows the recognition of errors. The concept of a musical syntax is significant because it points to potentially shared resources with language, and this in turn has important evolutionary implications. It is important to note, however, that there are those who question this relationship, proposing that musical syntax is more like an "an emergent property of auditory memory" and that "musical rules organize the perceptual effects of sound while conceptual information dominates language processing."[56] It is suggested that some of what people have called musical "syntax" may be more to do with the storage of, and access to, acoustic information in auditory short-term memory (memory that has a limited storage capacity and is available for active recall for only a limited period of time), whereas true language syntax deals with much more abstract representations and cognitive processing at a higher level. While neonates also seem to react to "errors" in expectancy of what comes next in a musical sequence, and at least our basic responses to dissonance versus consonance seem to be a universal, I wonder if the more conceptual aspects of musical syntax as we understand them are a relatively recent processing phenomenon, since music has become more intellectually and rationally organized over thousands of generations? I will return to the thorny but important issue of musical and linguistic syntax in Chapter 4.

Of course, in the real world there are other sounds being processed when listening to music, yet our brains can organize and perceive the musical sound stream in a coherent fashion. In general, how do we abstract meaningful information from background noise, and listen and attend to a particular voice in the midst of many others—the so-called cocktail party phenomenon? Is this an ability that we are especially good at? And did it require any additional changes in human cortex? Recently, studies using natural sounds as stimuli have enabled the development of models and theories that might help to explain how we detect relevant complex sounds in a shifting auditory landscape.[50] But are there any special features needed for acquiring speech recognition capacity or for recognizing a voice or instrument in a musical presentation? It is generally presumed that our peripheral machinery was already sufficiently sophisticated to encode the building blocks, prior to the evolution of articulate speech and language as we know it. This capacity is remarkable because we need to be able to recognize vowels, syllables, and so on, irrespective of factors such as frequency/pitch, amplitude, and timbre. We understand words and phrases whether voiced by a child or an adult, male or female, or whether spoken out loud or whispered. It is a skill of adaptation and scaling that appears to be built into our auditory system,[31] requiring "a dynamic speech-processing network" that involves a number of areas in the superior part of the temporal lobe, on each side of the brain.[57] Each voice is unique, a characteristic part of the person—how I dislike foreign language overdubs of Michael Caine or Sean Connery! And I suspect we all have the ability to recognize and appreciate a good impersonator/impressionist, and switch off a bad one?

The processing of music

Neurologists and neuroscientists have long sought to understand where music's essential building blocks (pitch, timbre, rhythm, etc) are processed in our brains, and which regions and neural circuits are associated with musical perception and communication. The post-mortem examination of ostensibly normal brains, a seemingly common pastime for neurologists in the nineteenth and first half of the twentieth centuries,[58] has revealed some interesting facts. For example, citing the work of Geschwind and Levitsky,[59] the Nobel Prize winner Sir John Eccles suggested that asymmetries in the temporal lobe were related to intrinsic abilities in either speech or music: "we would suggest that the enlargement of the right planum temporale is a measure of the musical ability built into the brain by genetic coding."[60] The planum temporale is the region of cortex just caudal to Heschl's transverse gyri (Figure 2.7). In the left cerebral hemisphere of almost all right–handers, it forms part of the region known as Wernicke's area (named after the German physician who first identified this region's role in language), which is important for sensory aspects of language processing.

Until recently, before the development of modern imaging techniques that allow us to visualize the living brain as it performs various activities, most of our understanding about where music and language are processed was mainly derived from the correlation of functional loss and behavioral dysfunction after injury or stroke with subsequent post-mortem neuropathological examination. This is by no means a perfect and exact science. From a musical perspective, there is clearly a distinction between the physical characteristics of the sound stimuli themselves and the "objects of perception, those things that carry the perceptual properties we attribute to sounds such as pitch, timbre, spatial location, and so on and so forth."[61] Thus tones, tonal relationships, melodic contour, harmony, pitch, duration, timbre, intensity, and rhythm are descriptors that reduce music to its essential physical components when studying the psychophysics of music, yet for most of us they do not figure in our own, very personal, appreciation of music. When we listen to a piece of music, most of us at least do not consciously deconstruct the sounds into all their core elements; the total experience ("gestalt") is everything. What we hear depends on context—the relationships between sound components—and music perception requires a rapid abstraction and analysis of multidimensional stimuli: "...music includes not only sound, but also organization, both in sound, space and time."[61]

Not surprisingly then, musical perception and performance entails "processing demands that are realized by a cerebral network distributed over four cortical lobes and the cerebellum."[62] Into this network we should also add structures such as the basal ganglia—a complex of nuclei located below the cerebral cortex in the forebrain—and the so-called limbic system involved in our emotional responses to music. But in an integrated multi-directional network, one in which it is not entirely clear what does what and to whom, damage to one region may throw the entire system out of balance, with broad functional changes that only partially reflect the role of the region that was initially damaged. If a completely ignorant alien orders a legless animal to walk, and the animal does not move, does that mean the animal needs legs to locomote, or does the animal not respond because its legs are its hearing organs? Or is the auditory system intact but it needs to communicate via the legs as an intermediary in order to drive the locomotor apparatus, wherever and whatever that is?

This is a silly example I know, but I hope it makes the point. Interpretation of the function of a specific region based on damage to only one part of the network may be misleading. We shall see that there are similar, if not identical, risks when interpreting neural activity in living brains using sophisticated neuroimaging techniques. Nonetheless, and despite potential interpretative difficulties, the study of acquired amusias (the loss of functionality—ability, expression, and/or appreciation—in the musical domain) and aphasias (the collective term for speech/language deficits) has proved highly informative, and more recent imaging work tends to support many of the conclusions drawn from these studies of neuropathology and neurological dysfunction. Oliver Sacks wrote a popular and widely read book documenting a number of interesting cases of musical disorders, including amusias as well as cases of musicogenic epilepsy and auditory hallucinations.[63] Musicogenic epilepsy is rare. It occurs perhaps in about 1 in every 10,000 people with epilepsy and always involves the temporal lobe, more often in musically talented people.[64] During the seizure, the person may hear specific types of music, sometimes even a particular piece!

Acquired amusias associated with random traumatic injury, stroke, or neurodegenerative disease, or as a by-product of a necessary neurosurgical procedure, must be distinguished from so-called congenital amusias, or true tone deafness, in which people are seemingly born with deficits in the perception and processing of pitch, resulting in a lifelong inability to really appreciate and produce music. In some instances, congenital amusia may be inherited within a family.[65] Such individuals of course have great difficulty in hearing and recognizing tunes. The eminent music researcher Isabelle Peretz has developed a test (the Montreal Battery of Evaluation of Amusia) that can distinguish between these two types of amusia. I will first discuss acquired amusias in more detail, and will return to the intriguing phenomenon of congenital amusia later, after describing how the musical brain is analyzed using various neuroimaging techniques.

Acquired amusias

During the nineteenth century, neurologists became increasingly interested in the presence or absence of musical abilities in aphasic patients, but it was the German physician and anatomist August Knoblauch in about 1888 who first used the term "amusia" to describe the syndromes associated with impaired capacity for human musical activity.[66] He even proposed a cognitive model of music processing and suggested that there existed a large number of disorders of music production and perception. These days, acquired amusias are categorized into six major types: oral expressive (eg singing, humming), instrumental amusia (performing music on an instrument), musical agraphia (writing music), sensory/discriminative, amnesic amusia (cannot identify familiar tunes), and musical alexia (reading a score).

Aphasias are—at least in right-handed people—generally a result of damage to the left hemisphere. Music was, for some time, also thought to be primarily associated with the left hemisphere, but Brenda Milner's careful psychological studies in the 1960s on patients who had undergone surgical temporal lobectomies as a treatment for epilepsy pointed to an important right hemisphere role for processing non-verbal auditory signals that was related more to music perception.[67] For example, such patients exhibited decreased discrimination of tonal patterns and impaired judgment of timbre. Similar work carried out in the 1990s examined the perception of pitch, melody, and rhythm in right-handed individuals in which either the right or left temporal lobe had been surgically removed.[68] A more recent study of acquired amusia described a right temporal lobe lesion in an individual that resulted in the selective inability to perceive the quality or color of sounds, but only those produced by keyboard or percussion instruments.[69] Overall, acquired amusias are usually right hemisphere biased, although lateralization for music can be less absolute than that for speech.[70,71,72] Expressive amusias generally involve anterior lesions in the frontal lobe, whereas receptive/recognition amusias are generally associated with temporal lobe pathology. There is also a strong link between damage to the right temporal lobe and altered emotional reactions to music, an association that is presumably mediated through the limbic system, as we shall see in Chapter 4.

A thorough and informative overview of the disorders of musical listening was published by Lauren Stewart and colleagues in the prestigious journal *Brain* in 2006.[73] It is worth bearing in mind that the perception and processing of music requires complex neural analysis and the rapid integration of many features, including initial acoustic processing and the subsequent analysis of tone, pitch, timbre, and rhythm. As summarized in the Stewart review, acquired injury studies suggest that loss of most aspects of musical processing involves the right cerebral hemisphere, especially in and around Heschl's gyrus and the planum temporale in the superior temporal lobe and the area around the border between the temporal and parietal lobes (the temporo-parietal junction). There is also left hemisphere involvement when amusias are associated with loss of rhythm sense or the inability to discriminate certain global aspects of pitch/melody, or to recall familiar tunes.

It has been estimated that about 30% of patients who suffer from an acquired amusic condition do not display any form of aphasia.[74] Similarly, there may be language deficits following a neurological injury, but musical capacities remain essentially normal. In his article in the excellent *Music and the Brain*,[74] Arthur Benton gives some interesting examples, such as individuals who can still play an instrument but who are aphasic. The deficits can be subtle, such as the patient who was word-deaf but could still recognize melodies and apprehend the prosodic elements of speech. There are examples, too, of patients who can speak, read music, play scales, and recognize melodies, but are unable to whistle or hum a tune. Alternatively, a person may no longer be able to read music but can still read and comprehend words in text.

There are some famous examples of dissociations of this type. The Russian composer Vissarion Shebalin suffered a stroke in the left temporo-parietal cortex and remained severely aphasic for the rest of his life, yet he continued to write and compose music of some quality.[75] Maurice Ravel suffered a stroke that left him with a Wernicke (sensory) type of aphasia with typical deficits in language comprehension and also some motor dysfunction. He stopped composing but apparently "his internal invention, affectivity and aesthetic sensibility were undisturbed. It was difficulty in playing the piano and in using musical signs which hindered his production."[58] It has also been suggested that Ravel may have had a presenile, progressive neurological illness that caused aphasia, motor problems, and—later on perhaps—dementia-like symptoms.[76] A recent study reported the case of the excellent preservation of musical memory in a professional cellist with severe impairment of other types of memory as a result of encephalitis.[77] Because amusias are sometimes found not to be associated with concurrent deficits in language, this dissociation between loss of musical versus language abilities has historically been used as an argument that music and speech must be processed in different parts of the brain, involving different circuits. We shall see that this is in part true, but the more recent neuroimaging data discussed in Chapter 4 will show that this separation is by no means absolute.

Altered affective responses to music occur after damage to the amygdala and insula, the latter a region of cerebral cortex buried deep within the lateral fissure that separates the temporal lobe from frontal and parietal cortex (Figures 2.1 and 2.7). The amygdala is a large gray-matter structure buried towards the base of the forebrain, and has long been associated with a person's mental state and emotive responsiveness to external events. The amygdala is active when stimuli have high affective valence (psychologists use the term "valence" to describe the subjective aversiveness or attractiveness of an event, object, or situation). Electrical stimulation of this structure in humans produces emotions such as fear, sadness, anxiety, or happiness, the nature of the emotional responses varying depending on whether the left or right amygdala is stimulated.[78] The amygdala is active when aversive or fearful stimuli are presented, although subjective valence with pleasant or positive attributes also influences amygdala function.[79] It forms part of the limbic system and—as discussed again in Chapter 4—is integrated into circuitries that are activated when responding to emotional content (prosody) in both music and speech.

Other methods used to study the neural substrates of music

In the 1940s and 1950s, a series of groundbreaking human studies was carried out in Montreal, Quebec, by the American-born neurosurgeon Wilder Penfield.[80] Using local anesthetics at all wound sites, Penfield studied the responses of conscious patients undergoing neurosurgery for epilepsy. He passed small currents through electrodes (electrical probes) to stimulate discrete regions of the patients' cerebral cortex. These small "shocks," depending on where they were delivered, could cause a muscle to twitch, evoke a sensation of some kind that was verbalized by the conscious patient, affect speech itself, or even evoke autobiographical memories. In this way Penfield and his colleagues were able to generate maps of the sensory and motor cortices of the human brain. Similar methods are still used to map the cortical regions involved in different aspects of language processing.[81] Hallucinations were sometimes elicited in patients who had "experiential responses" after stimulation of the superior or lateral aspect of the temporal lobe—occurring more often when the right lobe, rather than the left, was stimulated.[82] It was also possible to induce recollection of music by stimulating parts of the temporal lobe. Electrical stimulation of the primary auditory cortex produced buzzing or whistling. Others neuroscientists injected a drug such as sodium amytal into one of the carotid arteries in volunteer test subjects. Henson stated that injection into the right carotid caused defects in singing, while injection into the left one affected speech the most.[71] However, a later study found that injection of local anesthetic into either hemisphere disrupted singing.[72]

Neuroimaging

Over the past three decades, the development of modern imaging techniques such as positron emission tomography (PET), magnetic resonance imaging (MRI), and functional MRI (fMRI) has revolutionized the study of the human brain. Using very complex engineering and powerful computational methods, these technologies now enable neurologists and neuroscientists to accurately map the human brain—permitting, for example, measurement of the inter-individual variation in cortical organization.

PET involves the injection of biologically active molecules that contain short-lived radioactive isotopes into the bloodstream. As the isotope decays, gamma rays are produced and are detected using specialized coincidence detection systems. If, for example, a positron-emitting analogue of glucose is used in PET, then it is possible to measure uptake of glucose in different parts of the brain and thus determine regional metabolic activity. A disadvantage is the need to have a cyclotron close by to produce the short-lived radioactive compounds. This technique can be combined with the structural information gained from other forms of imaging, such as MRI.

For MRI, a powerful external magnetic field aligns protons of (usually) hydrogen nuclei. Radio waves are then pulsed to alter the alignment of the nuclei, and as these nuclei relax to their previous state, energy is released that is detected by 3D scanning coils. Using MRI, it becomes possible in living subjects to quantify the volume and density of gray and white matter in different parts of the brain, and then compare inter-individual morphological differences using an assortment of behavioral, psychological, or pathological data.[83] In the human brain each white matter tract may contain millions of axons, and represents the interconnections between one part of the brain and another. Because these tracts contain huge numbers of aligned nerve fibers, the diffusion of water and other molecules is constrained more in some directions than in others (anisotropy), enabling researchers— using procedures known as diffusion tensor imaging (DTI) and tractography—to identify and model the structure and organization of white matter. This is a powerful technique now widely used, although this method in itself does not necessarily provide information about the direction of a given pathway; are tracts or fascicles running to or from a particular region, or are nerve fibers coursing in both directions?

Consistent with numerous earlier post-mortem brain studies, individual differences in the architecture and relative size of particular brain regions have now been documented using MRI. In fact, detailed and complex MRI mapping of the human cerebral cortex carried out by David Van Essen and his group at Washington University in St Louis has revealed surprisingly large variation in the areal dimensions of numerous cortical regions between individuals of our species.[84] Variation in size can sometimes be linked to functional differences. For example, for some basic percepts, such as those involving visual illusions, the ability to experience such illusions is correlated with the connectivity and dimensions of specific cortical regions, in this case the size and organization of the primary visual cortex, termed V1.[85,86] I previously mentioned that there are left-right differences in the cellular and fiber architecture of human temporal cortex, and MRI has confirmed gross structural asymmetries in both the lateral temporal and parietal cortex. There is an increase in the size of the left angular and supramarginal gyri (Figure 2.8) and a much larger left planum temporale,[84] although in this particular study neither handedness, nor musical ability and training, were taken into consideration.

Modern-day imaging and computational technology is remarkably powerful, but it should be noted that the analysis and processing of MRI images require many assumptions. Observed effects may be small, and studies often use relatively low numbers of subjects, meaning that the studies are underpowered.[87] The ability to detect tracts can critically depend on the calculations and assumptions used to interpret the imaging data.[88] Furthermore, the reasons behind altered tissue volume or increased gray or white matter density have not been entirely resolved. Increased gray matter density may indicate higher cell numbers, more neuronal processes, or different types or sizes of neurons (or even glia), while altered structure of white matter may reflect the number or diameter of axons, and/or the amount of insulation (myelin) around them, and the presumed efficiency (and strength) of signal transfer between one region and another. And to further muddy the waters (please keep these caveats in mind as we move on through the neuroimaging descriptions that come later), increased gray matter density may *not* necessarily mean improved or better function. Sometimes the inverse is true, perhaps because during maturation of the brain the wrong, or least appropriate, connections were inadequately pruned.[83]

Functional MRI

In addition to the analysis of gray and white matter anatomy in the living human brain, neural activity can be functionally imaged by measuring blood flow and oxygen utilization to different regions. PET can be used for this, as can functional MRI (fMRI), which allows the comparison of magnetic signals that originate from oxygenated versus deoxygenated hemoglobin. Because the function of nerve cells is critically dependent on oxygen and energy supplies, metabolic activity and blood flow automatically and locally increase in regions with increased levels of neural activity, and it is therefore possible to identify areas of the brain that are more "active" when subjects perform, or just think about undertaking, a specific task. In blood oxygen level-dependent (BOLD) fMRI, increased blood flow or oxygenation is presumed to indicate greater activity in that area. The temporal definition provided by these techniques is imperfect and nowhere near the millisecond timescale required to reflect temporal patterns of neural activity; nonetheless, these imaging techniques not only provide an unprecedented window into the workings of the normal human brain, but also enable clinicians and scientists to study brain organization in individuals with different types of neurological dysfunction, such as amusia or aphasia. I will first discuss a number of human neuroimaging studies that provide useful and intriguing information about how music is processed in our brains, and then briefly relate this information to language, and in Chapters 4 and 5 to other forms of human behavior.

Using fMRI it is possible to gain some insight into how different brain regions are interconnected and interrelated by analyzing spontaneous correlative activity between these regions ("resting state MRI"). This is a technique that is applied when a subject is not being specifically tested in one way or another—that is, when he/she (and his/her brain) is "at rest."[89,90] However, most BOLD fMRI analysis of brain activity requires individuals to actively repeat a specific task or trial many times. During these repetitions, enormous computational power is required to average and then abstract relevant signals from control conditions and/or background noise. But scanners can be claustrophobic and they are noisy.[91] Changing the rate of background scanner noise can alter activity in cortical regions associated with auditory and language processing, especially in males.[92] The interpretation of fMRI data thus requires great skill, and even today exactly what some of the computed changes in BOLD fMRI signals mean in terms of neural activity in the brain is not completely understood, and results may sometimes be over-interpreted.[93,94,95,96,97,98,99,100,101]

Discrete regions of the brain can be activated or deactivated during tasks or during repetition of tasks, but the extent to which these changes reflect local or long-distance connectivity, or reflect excitatory versus inhibitory activity, or even neuronal versus glial cell activity, remains controversial.[102,103,104,105] A study in animals directly comparing BOLD signals with electrophysiological recording of activity in the same neural tissue concluded that most of the BOLD response was not related to input or output activity per se, but due to the "input-dependent interplay of principal and inhibitory interneurons,"—in other words, both excitatory and inhibitory synaptic activity in local circuits.[106] A study comparing BOLD fMRI to MEG signals in human subjects (in this case, reading various forms of text) revealed significant differences in the spatial localization of activity in the brain when using the two techniques.[103] Remember that MEG measures magnetic fields from *naturally* occurring, synchronous electrical activity in the brain whereas BOLD fMRI uses external magnetic pulses to reveal relative levels of oxygenated versus deoxygenated blood—it is a hemodynamic measure. As the authors discuss, one difference may be that BOLD fMRI is influenced by non-synchronous neural activity, or perhaps owing to its longer timescale the MRI signal may be summing a broader set of activations. In this context a colleague well-versed in MRI methodology told me that much of this measured activity may in fact be due mostly to changes in glial cell activity—especially in the networks of astrocytes in our brains. Finally, in yet another cautionary note, recent complex statistical analyses of a great many fMRI trials suggest that there is a bias in the reporting of data from these studies, with potential for the reporting of false-positives, especially when using a cohort of subjects that is too small to allow meaningful statistical comparisons.[100,107,108,109]

In addition to such technical and interpretative uncertainties, as I mentioned earlier the musical experience is a complete, multidimensional percept, yet until recently neuroimaging studies have usually attempted to map activity driven by isolated acoustic features chosen by the experimenters—features such as discrimination of pitch, timbre, intervals, or melodic contours, or the processing of beat, meter, or rhythm. Such an approach using music's specific building blocks may not yield a percept we would necessarily call "musical," but it does provide a controlled stimulus environment with which to study specific patterns of neural activation and monitor inter-individual variation. Peretz and Coltheart proposed a "modular functional architecture for music processing" that consists of a number of interrelated and interactive modules, some of which they suggested may overlap with aspects of speech perception and production.[110] In proposing another cognitive model of music perception, Stefan Koelsch[111,112] acknowledges that such modules—or "stages" as he now calls them—may "also serve in part the processing of language," and his model sets out to further integrate "different domains (such as music, language, action, and emotion) within a common framework, implying numerous shared processes and similarities."[112] Presumably however, this overlap must be incomplete. How else to explain the neurology of amusias and aphasias?

Professor Koelsch's model, involving as it does increasingly integrated domains of auditory processing, memory, "vitalization" (physiological and emotional responses), initiation of movement, and so on, has implications for the evolutionary origins of music, to be considered in more detail in Chapter 4. In the present context, the presence of such frameworks makes it difficult to isolate experimentally the various perceptual and expressive elements, and know exactly what is being tested when the brain is being scanned for processing/listening to music. Furthermore, music is associated with short-term as well as more long-term memory processing, triggering the recall of autobiographical memories.[113,114] Moreover, a subject's often complex and highly subjective emotional responses also have to be taken into account. The psychologist John Sloboda argued that to explain adequately the power of music, scientific studies "must investigate music as it is actually experienced" using "complete, authentic musical objects, such as whole songs, rather than impoverished or machine-constructed stimulus segments," and should take into account the preferences and past experiences of each experimental subject.[115] This was an important insight, and more recent imaging studies, as we shall see in Chapter 4, do indeed show that brain activity varies depending on whether the music being played is, or is not, to the listener's liking.

From a motor or performance perspective there may be real (or imagined) singing, playing of a musical instrument, and/or movement in time to the beat, ranging from foot tapping to full-on dancing. Potentially, these motor aspects of music can also add to interpretative difficulties when analyzing sensory processing of music. In particular (because in an MRI machine you are supposed to stay as still as possible), the listening subjects may engage in mental imagery of singing, humming, or involuntary or instinctive rhythmic body movements or tapping of hands or feet, all capable of generating a sort of internal activity that is not truly related to the sensory side of the musical perception. "Even when lying perfectly still, listeners in fMRI studies show activation in those regions of the brain that would normally orchestrate motor movement to music, including the cerebellum, basal ganglia, and cortical motor areas—it is as though movement is impossible to suppress."[116] Finally, the neural networks involved in processing harmony and melody vary depending on the amount of musical training a subject has experienced and the sophistication of the trials,[117] and as I have previously mentioned there is evidence of practice-dependent effects on the actual morphology and neural architecture of a musician's or singer's brain.[118,119,120,121,122,123]

Despite this seemingly endless list of caveats and deficiencies it is nonetheless possible, based on a plethora of brain imaging studies, to discern a consensus as to which parts of the brain are activated when listening to music. Other brain regions are implicated in musical imagination/creation, and in our emotional and motor responses to music, but for now the emphasis will be on sensory processing.[35,116,124,125,126,127,128] The perception and processing of music involves, as might be expected, a complex network of many interrelated cortical areas, including the temporal, parietal, and frontal lobes. Subcortical regions are also activated, for example in the thalamus and basal ganglia, as well as certain areas of the cerebellum and parts of the brainstem. We shall see that, consistent with acquired amusia data,[73] melodic and temporal content appears to be processed in different regions of the brain, and likely involves different types of network.[129]

Because music generally has fixed intervals and scales, and contains melody and harmony, there is a need to accurately encode pitch information. However, as discussed earlier, the perception of pitch is a complex phenomenon that requires responses to the frequency of incoming tones but then also involves the coding and analysis of other acoustic and harmonic parameters. I have already discussed the observation that we possess clusters of acoustically responsive neurons that respond to harmonically related frequency bands separated by octaves.[50,51] Of course, pitch is important not only in music but also in speech: "rising and falling pitch contours help define prosody and in tonal languages, such as Mandarin and Cantonese, pitch contours help define the meaning of words."[49] Prosody acts as an obvious link between music and language, and lesion studies suggest that both the left and right auditory cortex can detect changes in pitch.[130] Yet there are subtle differences in perceptual processing, thus patients with epilepsy-related surgical excision of Heschl's gyrus in the right hemisphere found it difficult (but not impossible) to judge the *direction* of pitch changes.[131]

Even today, exactly where and how our brains process pitch, and especially relative pitch and melodic contour, are not entirely settled.[29,49,61,97,132,133,134] Pantev et al[135] had earlier reported that tonotopic maps in humans may be maps of pitch, supported by other neuroimaging studies, suggesting that there is cortical representation of pitch in parts of primary and non-primary auditory cortex,[125,136,137] "partially overlapping the low-frequency field of primary auditory cortex."[134] However, others failed to find unequivocal response selectivity for pitch,[138] these differences seemingly due to differences in the exact nature of the harmonic stimuli that are used.[29,134] In agreement with many earlier studies,[21,35] Leaver and Rauschecker[24] reported that tonotopic organization in early auditory cortex is mostly associated with frequency analysis, but they obtained confirmatory evidence that more laterally placed auditory areas also encode pitch, consistent with observations from acquired amusia subjects.[73]

In comparative human and animal studies, different techniques are used to study the neural mechanisms of pitch perception.[132] In addition, the way pitch is processed may differ across the sound spectrum. For example, in a study on a New World monkey, the marmoset, cues in the periodicity of the temporal envelope are used to extract information about lower pitch sounds, while spectral patterns (variations in amplitude with frequency) are used to perceive higher pitch sounds. Thus it seems that pitch can be extracted using a combination of acoustic features,[139] and more recent work suggests that pitch perception mechanisms in marmosets are in fact similar to those in humans.[140]

Pitch discrimination is usually relative rather than absolute, and combinations of pitch constitute harmony (or disharmony!). The analysis of pitch intervals and relations between them is of critical importance in music as well as in speech, and requires memory retention and recall in sequential pitch comparison tasks. Predicting what is likely to come next is also very important. Without this cognitive capacity, appreciation of melody and the overall contour of a sequence of notes (the relative change in pitch over time and the direction of that change) would not be possible. Judgments about pitch relations and melody perception are associated with increased neural activity in a number of belt and parabelt areas in the superior temporal gyrus, posterior and anterior to Heschl's gyrus, and mostly biased to the right hemisphere. Individual pitch height and detection of the separation between pitches are predominantly processed in specialized systems in the right superior temporal cortex, particularly the right planum temporale,[35,127,141,142] with activity also reported in a region known as the intraparietal cortex.[143] Anterior regions of the superior temporal cortex show greater activity when processing pitch chroma—that is, "the cycle of notes within the octave" needed for recognition of acoustic patterns.[141] The perception of melody per se requires complex hierarchical processing, and has been reported to involve not only the planum temporale but also regions within the planum polare.[31] Recognition of familiar tunes also appears to reside in the right superior temporal sulcus.[144]

I noted earlier that, compared with the left hemisphere, evidence from imaging and lesion studies indicates that the right superior temporal cortex is capable of finer frequency and spectral resolution, likely important in the early stages of music processing. Nonetheless, in studies of patients lacking either the right or left temporal lobe, while confirming that the processing of contour, pitch patterns, and melody was affected in subjects with right superior temporal gyrus surgery, some aspects of interval discrimination were also affected following left temporal lobe surgery.[68] It is also intriguing to note that melody discrimination has been reported to result in increased cerebral blood flow in *visual* association cortex in the occipital lobe.[124] Finally, the perception and analysis of harmony and timbre—remember the latter containing frequency, and spectral and temporal information[55]—involve distributed systems predominantly in the right, but perhaps also in the left, hemisphere, again usually with involvement of regions in the superior temporal gyrus.[73,127,145]

Absolute (or perfect) pitch is a rare but intriguing phenomenon. Individuals with absolute pitch can analyze and identify the pitch of a note without reference to any other tone or sound. They just intrinsically know it. Absolute pitch ability is slightly more common in people who speak tonal languages such as Mandarin or Cantonese. This ability seems to differ from the "pseudo-absolute pitch" learned by someone who, through considerable practice and experience, is able to identify notes in particular contexts. Having absolute pitch is not necessarily a blessing—at school I shared a study with an incredibly gifted young musician with this ability, but listening to belt-drive turntables that played records at not exactly the correct speed drove him, as he used to say, "completely (expletive deleted) nuts."

Outstanding musical ability is associated with increased leftward asymmetry in the planum temporale of superior aspect of the temporal lobe, especially in musicians with absolute pitch capability,[119] perhaps owing to an increase in that hemisphere or perhaps a reduction in volume in right hemisphere auditory structures.[146,147] A later imaging study using DTI and tractography revealed increased white matter connectivity within sub-regions of the temporal lobe, especially on the left side.[148] As well as differences in gray matter thickness in primary and secondary auditory cortical areas in musicians with absolute pitch, changes in dorsolateral prefrontal cortex outside auditory areas have also been reported,[121] perhaps suggesting that absolute pitch capability involves differences in encoding pitch/notes as well as an altered working memory capacity. By the latter I am referring to the theoretical neural framework that allows us, for short periods of time, to mentally monitor, organize, select, and manipulate information needed for various cognitive tasks. There seem to be a number of different components to working memory, including an attentional control system, separate verbal (phonological) and visuospatial buffers, and an executive, integrative center.[149] Interestingly, absolute pitch is more commonly encountered in congenitally blind people, who seem to use different neural networks.[150] In functional imaging studies, compared with sighted musicians with the same musical ability, blind musicians with absolute pitch showed greater activity in bilateral visual association areas in occipital cortex, as well as in frontal and parietal cortices. In sighted musicians, however, there was relatively greater activity in the right primary auditory cortex and cerebellum. This is an intriguing example of how other sensory cortical systems can be engaged when a specific modality is absent or lost.

Analysis of how the auditory parts of our brain perceive and process rhythm (temporal grouping), beat (temporal regularity), tempo, and meter is just as complex, and depends to some extent on the task and nature of the sound stimulus. As alluded to earlier, interpretation of imaging data in particular is further muddied by the strong and pervasive, subliminal or overt, motor responses that are associated with the perception of rhythm and beat. As with pitch perception, rhythm is an important component of speech as well as music, although with the notable exception of reciting poetry, it is in music that the perception and prediction of beat and rhythmic patterns become so essential, so fundamental to musical performance and our capacity to synchronize movements with others.[48] These universal attributes are influenced by cultural background and an individual's familiarity with a particular musical style,[151] suggesting that our behavioral response to musical rhythm helps consolidate group identity and promote social cohesion.

The initial encoding of acoustic rhythm and timing occurs very early in the auditory pathway, in parts of the brainstem.[152,153,154] Fast rhythms can elicit feelings of excitement; slow rhythms induce calm.[155] In the cerebral cortex there is evidence from acquired amusia studies that perceptual aspects of timing, meter, and beat are mostly encoded in non-primary auditory cortical areas caudal to Heschl's gyrus in the right cerebral hemisphere, while perception of rhythm and underlying temporal grouping appears to be more bilateral and involve more distributed systems and networks.[73,127] More recent neuroimaging (PET scans) of the brain in right-handed musicians or "non-musicians" who were asked to discriminate changes in either meter, pattern, or tempo have revealed further details about the cortical processing of rhythm.[156] All three parameters resulted in increased neural activity in right, but sometimes also bilateral, areas of temporal, cingulate, parietal, frontal, and prefrontal cortices; however, there were subtle differences—especially in the right hemisphere—in the location of activity in temporal, inferior parietal, prefrontal, and frontal cortex associated with each temporal component. These differences were attributed to differences in the auditory, sensorimotor, cognitive, and executive processes that were required to achieve each discriminative task. Interestingly, compared with "non-musicians," musicians used "more higher level representations" in cerebral cortex, with a shift to activation in the left hemisphere,[156] and there is evidence for greater interactions between auditory and supplementary motor areas in musicians.[157]

Clearly, the neural activity associated with the perceptual processing of timing, beat, meter, and rhythm is widespread, yet it becomes even more distributed when motor-related representations are added to the mix. This integrative network is far more extensive than that seen for tasks that focus on melody discrimination, "consistent with the suggestion that neural representation of temporal features of music are more intrinsically multi-sensory than those of melody and harmony (perhaps tied to melody as implicit vocal singing, whereas rhythm involves more of the body)."[156] Others have reported that the encoding, memorizing, and retrieval of rhythmic temporal sequences is generally more bilateral when compared with the processing of melody, and involves auditory cortex as well as sensorimotor cortex and cerebellum.[129,158] The inherent coupling of musical perception and action/performance in humans is so strong that, even if a movement is only imagined,[116] listening to musical rhythm is associated with altered activity in motor and premotor areas in cortex, the cerebellum, and basal ganglia.[159,160,161,162,163] The latter two complex structures have long been known to be essential for the planning, initiation, control, and coordination of voluntary movements. The ability to tap to a musical beat in particular involves not only several regions in the cerebral cortex but also circuits in the basal ganglia, especially a subdivision known as the putamen.[157,164]

In the visual system the various submodalities such as color, shape, motion, and depth are processed in different regions of the visual cortex, and need to be synchronized or integrated somewhere (real or virtual place?) to produce a unified percept, a unified reconstruction of the visual world. Presumably, when listening to a symphony orchestra, jazz band, or even just a piano virtuoso, the different brain regions that are primarily responsible for the processing of information about pitch, melody, timbre, rhythm, etc., must also interact to again yield a unified percept of the musical experience. As pointed out by Israel: "classical and rock music are not that different from each other. Most low-level descriptors of the two would not be too far from each other—overall spectral range…, typical rates of spectral and temporal modulations."[61] Where and how these complex perceptual discriminations take place remain a mystery, although a music-specific region in the anterior part of the superior temporal gyrus (the planum polare, Figure 2.7) has recently been characterized, perhaps acting as "a second-order relay, possibly integrating acoustic characteristics intrinsic to music."[165] As noted earlier, others have also described selective music processing neurons in this part of the non-primary auditory cortex.[45]

I have already introduced the idea that the brains of experienced musicians differ from those of musically naïve individuals, reflecting perhaps the degree of musical training undertaken by an individual, and suggesting a degree of plasticity and adaptability in the cortical architecture of humans when they are young. Most studies have found that musical training and experience alter the pattern of activation, there being a shift towards increased processing in the left hemisphere. This increased emphasis on left hemisphere processing is especially obvious in two cortical regions, Heschl's gyrus and the supra-marginal gyrus, and the shift is greater with more frequent musical practice.[156,166] Some have reported that this increased activation of regions such as auditory association cortex in the left hemisphere correlates with the age at which training begins.[120] It is as if the right hemisphere processes general or holistic musical execution and faculty in the first instance, but with training and increased sophistication the left hemisphere starts to become more dominant; perhaps more cognitive, analytical processing elements start to take over during constant rehearsal and scrutiny of content?

Inter-individual variability in the size of Heschl's gyrus may relate to musical aptitude,[167,168,169] but at least some of this variation seems to be unrelated to experience because, for example, left-right asymmetries in the planum temporale and Heschl's gyrus are already present in one- to four-month-old "preverbal" infants.[170,171] Interestingly, individuals with a larger cortical volume of Heschl's gyrus are better at learning how to incorporate foreign pitch patterns into English words,[168] and more recent work has found a correlation between the size of this region and "frequency discrimination, reading, and spelling skills" in children.[172] Such comparisons are interesting, although it remains uncertain the extent to which such differences reflect developmental experiences or are the result of pre-existing genetic influences, or are a mixture of both. The nature versus nurture question continually arises when attempting to correlate inter-individual differences in the overall size, or gray or white matter density, of particular cortical regions with a particular function or skill—something that should be borne in mind throughout: "both nature and nurture contribute to individual differences in brain structure. However, a consensus regarding the extent to which morphology is genetically or environmentally determined ... has not yet been reached."[173] Longitudinal studies in which subjects are tracked over time from early life into adulthood are needed to satisfactorily address the perennial gene versus experience issue—which will almost certainly reveal complex and variable interactions between the two!

Studies on retention of music knowledge in two "expert" adult musicians with different forms of dementia suggest that there is a "relatively independent associative knowledge system for music," which is distinct from other kinds of non-verbal information but which "shares certain cognitive organizational features with other brain knowledge systems."[174] I imagine that such an experience-dependent reorganization and hemispheric shift make life difficult when experimenters are picking subjects to enroll in these types of studies—how easy is it to determine how musically adept a person is? More than half of the English and American population have had music lessons of some kind, and "the ordinary adult listener is a musical expert, although s/he may be unaware of this."[175] Thus the definition of what characterizes a non-musician versus musician may be critically important and may well depend on the individual's cultural and ethnic background (see discussion on

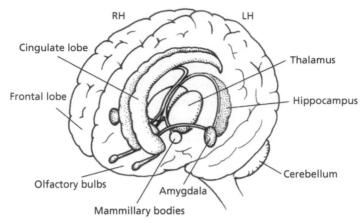

Figure 2.9 Major components of the limbic system. RH and LH, right and left cerebral hemispheres respectively.
© Martin Thompson, 2016.

"WEIRD" subjects in Chapter 3). Interpretation of any data may also depend on the complexity and sophistication of a particular musical trial.

Finally, neuroimaging studies have also revealed that the limbic system (which includes parts of the cortex, the amygdala, the hippocampus, and mammillary bodies—part of the hypothalamus, Figure 2.9), as well as areas of the brain associated with reward, can be activated when listening to music (see Koelsch 2014 for an excellent recent review).[18] These areas are generally associated with emotion, with reward systems associated with food, sex, and so on, and with linkages to our autonomic nervous system, all of this perhaps adding to the early evolutionary importance of music in social attachment and prosodic-like communication in our ancestors and cousins. These considerations are, I believe, important in understanding why music is a human universal, and will be considered further in Chapters 5 and 6.

Congenital amusias

To now return to the phenomenon of congenital amusia (tone deafness), neuroimaging studies reveal that such amusias are associated with remarkably discrete changes in brain structure. Hyde et al examined PET scans (horizontal sections) through the human brain in subjects with congenital amusia.[176] The work consisted of two studies that were conducted independently—one in Montréal, Quebec, and the other in Newcastle, UK. There was a remarkable concordance between these two separate studies, which revealed that there was a small and consistent white-matter deficit in people with congenital tone deafness. In this case the deficit was found in the right inferior frontal gyrus, a region that normally has extensive connections with the right auditory cortex. A subsequent paper showed that cortical thickness was actually greater in these amusic brains in the right inferior frontal gyrus and right auditory cortex,[177] findings confirmed more recently by Albouy et al in France.[178] Others have reported changes in the left frontal and temporal cortices in tone-deaf subjects, and suggest this may also reflect perceptual problems during singing owing to "an impairment in the auditory-motor feedback loop."[179]

One further study in "tone-deaf" individuals identified substantially reduced connectivity in the right cerebral hemisphere of a major white matter tract that interconnects the posterior part of auditory cortex with inferior frontal cortex, the arcuate fasciculus (Figure 2.8).[180] This is an important observation, even though recent work has suggested that interpretation of such white matter changes depends very much on how the MRI images are analyzed.[88] Nonetheless, such apparent deficits in circuitries that are believed to be essential components of an "action-perception network"[180] are consistent with findings that the brains of tone-deaf individuals can process "fine-grained" pitch differences pretty well, but they seem unaware of this neural capability and cannot use it to detect and then consciously perceive melodies and so on.[134,181,182,183,184] There is a mis-match between perception and production. In addition, short-term memory and retrieval is deficient when listening to melodic contours,[178] perhaps related to the previously mentioned deficits in white matter connectivity between auditory and inferior frontal cortex. Interestingly, congenital amusics are able to imitate and thus produce vocalized pitch changes in speech,[185] but they are less able to detect emotional content (prosody) in speech.[186] Any evidence of cross-talk in auditory perceptual and vocal capabilities between music and language domains is important when thinking about the evolutionary origins of these two communication streams in *Homo sapiens*; did they spring from a common source, or did they develop independently?

Overall, the data I have just discussed are consistent with a more general idea that changes in human cognitive capacity and processing are associated with changes in fiber connections in the white matter between cortical regions, and may also be affected by changes within the neuronal architecture of the cerebral cortex gray matter itself. The term "connectopathies" has been coined to describe developmental defects in the pattern, number, and proportion of interconnections between regions that may contribute to neurological disorders such as schizophrenia and autism.[187,188] Perhaps this is a term that can also be used when discussing the pathobiology of congenital amusia?

An introductory word on the processing of language and speech

Neurologists and neuroscientists have long sought to understand the relationship between music and language by examining the brain and working out which regions and neural circuits are associated with the two communication systems. Are they separate or do they share common networks? This is a critical question with profound evolutionary implications that will be discussed in some detail in Chapter 4. Here, however, it is worth providing an introduction to what is known about the neural circuitry associated with language. Similar to amusia case histories, in the early days information about language-related areas was obtained by examination of the brains of patients who exhibited some form of speech or language deficit (aphasia). More recently, researchers and clinicians have used electrophysiological methods or imaging techniques such as fMRI or PET to map areas in the brains of normal subjects that are activated when performing language-specific tasks such as speaking words or sentences, listening to and comprehending speech, processing syntax, or reading words.

Here, I will summarize processing in the cerebral cortex, but similar to structures involved in movement/vocalization in a musical context, in language—and especially in speech production—a number of other subcortical regions are also critically important in coordinating motor control, including the cerebellum, basal ganglia, and thalamus.[189] These structures are integrated into the distributed networks that mediate language processing and articulate speech production. In fact, the importance of the cerebellum in cognitive- and language-related tasks is increasingly being recognized.[190,191,192]

In 1861, Paul Broca published what is regarded as the first description of a correlation between deficits in motor aspects of speech, and degeneration of a specific part of the cerebral cortex. Twenty years before this, the famous French novelist Stendhal carefully documented his own very specific, temporary aphasias resulting from transient ischemic attacks.[193] Broca's patient, named Leborgne, had a motor or expressive aphasia, and examination of his brain at autopsy revealed a syphilitic lesion in the left inferior frontal lobe. This region is now named after Broca. Other aspects of language (eg language comprehension) were found to be processed in the posterior part of the superior temporal cortex (Wernicke's area, named after the German neurologist/psychiatrist Carl Wernicke, in 1874). Many subsequent studies built on this pioneering work; examinations were performed on the brains of aphasic patients after stroke or on traumatic brain injury patients. At McGill University, Penfield and his colleagues also identified cortical locations involved in language processing while electrically stimulating the brains of locally anesthetized but conscious patients undergoing neurosurgery; for example, stimulation of Broca's area resulted in the arrest of ongoing speech.[80]

Based on analysis of functional losses after cortical damage, in an estimated 95% of right-handed individuals the motor and ideational aspects of speech and language comprehension are processed primarily in the cerebral hemisphere on the left-hand side of the brain, the so-called dominant hemisphere. Extensive human electrophysiological studies by George Ojemann and colleagues showed that a large region of the left hemisphere is involved in speech/language, but surprisingly there can be considerable inter-individual variability in the size and location of these regions, and many neurons in the right cerebral cortex can also "fire" when subjects are undertaking language and speech-related tasks.[81,194] Similar to music processing, different aspects of speech/language are processed in different brain regions, and it is possible to distinguish circuits that are involved in the sensory, motor, or ideational aspects of speech and language, although with more and more research the simple motor-sensory distinction has become somewhat blurred.[4,66,195]

Historically, and largely based on acquired aphasia data, Broca's area in the left inferior frontal cortex (Figure 2.8) has been regarded as being primarily involved in speech production; as noted earlier, lesions here often (although not always) result in an inability to produce articulate speech. However, lesions in left inferior frontal gyrus may also lead to problems in understanding and processing certain syntactic elements of speech comprehension, and neuroimaging studies also suggest that Broca's area subserves additional functions (see especially Chapter 4). Following damage to Wernicke's area, speech remains fluent but has disrupted content and there are deficits in language comprehension (sometimes termed receptive or sensory aphasia). The left temporal cortex in particular appears to be part of the repository for word-processing circuits.[196] Broca's and Wernicke's cortical areas are among those that are functionally interconnected via the large white matter bundle of nerve fibers mentioned earlier, the arcuate fasciculus (Figure 2.8), which develops relatively late in childhood but is especially prominent in the human brain.[197,198,199] This tract can itself sometimes be damaged.

Hemispheric lateralization of language is less clear-cut in left-handers, who make up about 10% of the general population. About 75% of left-handers have left hemisphere dominance for language, while the remainder process language function on the right side or bilaterally.[200] Genetic linkage studies did not find "a major gene for left-handedness, atypical lateralization, or degree of language lateralization," but these complex traits did exhibit moderate heritability, influenced by independent sets of genes.[200] Interestingly, right hemisphere lesions can affect language in normally left hemisphere-dominant individuals because the prosodic, emotional quality of speech is often reduced and perhaps even absent; this is an interesting point that will be especially pertinent when I discuss the possible properties of the precursor of modern language and speech in Chapter 4. There have also been studies that seem to show that some aspects of language processing in females are less confined to one hemisphere, although interpretation of these data is controversial.[201]

It seems that early exposure to different languages can alter cortical architecture. People who learn a second language in early childhood (bilinguals) have larger gray matter volumes in the transverse gyri (Heschl's gyri) of left superior temporal cortex—part of the primary auditory cortex.[202] Plasticity in language-related white matter tracts seems to be greatest before the age of four years.[203] In addition, in bilinguals the overall cortical network involved in processing a second language can differ to some extent from the first language architecture.[175,204] According to Peretz,[175] because second language can be acquired at different ages and with different levels of experience, the areas activated may vary considerably between individuals, with cortical processing of first and second languages showing more overlap if both languages are acquired early in life, and if there is a high degree of proficiency in the second language.[205] Similar arguments may explain why inconsistencies in the cortical representation of music from individual to individual can be expected, between trained and musically untrained subjects. As discussed in Chapter 8, the increased "cognitive reserve" that seems to accrue as a consequence of musical training or bilingual capability lends some useful protection against cognitive decline as we get older.

Overall, the neuroimaging work on musicality confirms the substance of earlier neurological and neuropathological reports, providing evidence for distributed music processing networks in the brain of *Homo sapiens* that include multiple regions in the cerebral cortex, basal ganglia, brainstem, and cerebellum. Historically, the extensive neurological literature tends to emphasize and highlight differences in the cortical regions that are affected in amusic or aphasic patients, and modern neuroimaging data also point to some divergence in the networks that subserve music versus language. This idea of parallel, distributed neural circuits gains some support from the remarkable work of Robert Shannon, who amongst other interests has carried out research that relates to auditory/cochlear implants and how to make them even more effective in hearing-impaired people. Research in his laboratory suggests that music and speech require different types of peripheral processing and have different requirements for temporal and spectral resolution.[206,207] Speech is more of a "top-down" pattern recognition process by the brain. The rapid, short-duration components of speech are probably encoded not as individual elements but by the overall sound pattern: "Speech perception does not depend on the extraction of simple invariant acoustic patterns directly available from the speech waveform … instead, the speech sound's acoustic pattern varies in a complex manner according to the preceding and following sounds."[15] Speech can be understood even when there is substantial distortion or degradation of spectral cues, as long as dynamic temporal cues are still available, but music recognition and appreciation are affected even by only minor degradation.

Imaging studies support the idea of complementary cortical systems specialized for differential temporal integration and resolution of the spectral elements of sound. The left auditory cortex is capable of more dynamic analysis of temporal structure, whereas the right temporal cortex has better frequency resolution. These distinctions are perhaps related to an emphasis on rapid speech analysis in the former, and discrimination of pitch and spectral analysis of sound in the latter.[32,33,34,208,209] Acoustic energy peaks in the spectral envelope of speech are called formants and are usually related to vowels. Vowels can have a similar spectral structure to music, but consonants such as fricatives and sibilants often contain high frequencies and we understand whispered speech even when vocal cords are disengaged and vowel sounds are considerably diminished. Music often has significant low-frequency content, and perception via cochlear implants is poor,[210] although children who have some (normal) low-frequency hearing prior to implantation of the prosthetic device are better able to perceive certain aspects of music.[211]

Conclusion

In this chapter I have focused on how music is perceived and analyzed in the human brain, and in so doing I have emphasized differences in a number of the neural substrates that mediate the sensory and perceptual processing of music versus language and speech. However, as will be detailed in Chapter 4, at the network level this separation is not clear-cut; there is increasing evidence for at least some shared resources that encode features of both music AND language, although at the time of writing the extent and nature of this intersection and interaction still require clarification.[212] Research has revealed—perhaps not surprisingly—overlap in areas of the brain that control many of the fundamental motor aspects of singing and speech,[213] and there are similarities in the regions that process the prosodic and emotive content of these two communication streams, including the fundamental building blocks of pitch, loudness, rhythm, and so forth. There may also be some overlap in the regions of cortex involved in higher levels of melody and sentence generation. From an evolutionary perspective, if modern language evolved or piggy-backed on circuitries previously associated with a more "primitive" type of communicative activity, and if both music and language evolved from a common progenitor or precursor, then clearly some overlap in their neural processing networks is to be expected. This is a critically important issue that is considered in later chapters. First, however, we must take a detour into the fascinating but difficult, and always controversial, domain of human evolution—what we are, how we are different, who and where we came from, and when? It should become clear that our brains are unique, with newly evolved cognitive, linguistic, and memory capacities. But with that uniqueness comes danger and insecurity, and an ever-increasing need for social adhesion.

Chapter 3

Brains and the Evolution of *Homo sapiens*

The profundity of music shows us how unique the human brain is.
—Michael A. Arbib, *Language, Music, and the Brain*

Man is human because he can say so.
—Philip Lieberman and Edmund Credlin

Two fundamental questions posed in Chapter 1 that get to the heart of the universality of music are: what is the relationship between music and modern language, and why have we evolved and retained both forms of communication—communication systems that are interrelated yet distinct? Following on from this, is it possible to surmise the forms of communication used by our immediate ancestors? From an evolutionary perspective, did music come before language, did language come before music—or was there some common progenitor that somehow separated into two strands when *Homo sapiens* evolved, with both strands of communication retained?

Human language has many unique properties, properties that differentiate it from communication systems used by other animals, including other primates. In *"The Language Instinct,"* Steven Pinker describes non-human communication as being based on three designs—either a finite repertory of calls, a signal that registers the magnitude of some state, or a series of random variations on a theme.[1] Moreover: "The discrete combinatorial system called 'grammar' makes human language infinite (there is no limit to the number of complex words or sentences), digital (this infinity is achieved by rearranging discrete elements in particular orders and combinations, not by varying some signal along a continuum like the mercury in a thermometer), and compositional (each of the infinite combinations has a different meaning predictable from the meanings of its parts and the rules and principles arranging them)." And there is widespread agreement, considered more fully in the evolutionary synthesis section later in this chapter, that the evolution of language was a—perhaps *the*—critical event associated with the evolution of the modern human mind.

Given this seminal importance of language, how do we explain the remarkable universality of musical behavior in our species? It is my view that to provide a convincing rationale that accounts for the continued persistence of music as another type of human communication, we first need to consider how the language revolution came about. What new physical features, genetic or cellular mechanisms, or altered neural architectures and connectivity underpinned this stunning evolutionary transition and the remarkable advances in cognitive power? We can then ask whether any other evolutionary changes were needed to create the loquacious yet musical animal we are today. How do we do this? We do not have brain material from our ancestors or close cousins, but we can make useful comparisons with fossilized remains, including ancient genetic material from fossil bones. Comparative information can also be obtained by analyzing the brains, behavior, and genes in our closest living relatives in the great ape family, including of course chimpanzees. We can also trace lineage relationships in *Homo sapiens* to determine how genes, and the regulation of those genes, have changed over the millennia.

Brain size, laterality, and behavior

In the forebrain the two cerebral hemispheres (right and left) contain various types of cortical gray matter. The so-called archicortex is organized into three distinct layers and is regarded phylogenetically as the oldest. In mammals, this type of cortex is found in the hippocampus, a part of the brain essential for converting new experiences into long-term memories. The six-layered neocortex, comprising six stratified bands of cells from outside to inside, each with its own input and output characteristics, is an evolutionarily more recent addition to the mammalian forebrain. Neocortex makes up the bulk of the expansion of the cerebral gray matter in primates, with increased numbers of cortical, relative to subcortical, neurons (corticalization) in visual, auditory, and motor-related structures.[2,3,4] Our species possesses a particularly large volume of cerebral cortex, although as a proportion of total brain mass there is little difference between us and most other mammals.[5] In non-human primates, cognitive ability correlates well with absolute brain size, but not in terms of the so-called "encephalization quotient"—that is, the relative size of the brain when compared with the size of the host body.[6] Whole brain size is as good a predictor of cognitive ability as neocortical volume, although others have suggested an alternate correlation between the size of the neocortex, sociality, and the level of social complexity exhibited by a given species.[7]

In the *Homo* line, a relative increase in brain volume versus body mass began to emerge about 600,000 years ago.[8] This is clearly an important evolutionary trend; however, in *Homo sapiens*, as many males of our species have long opined, size is not everything. This is because the relationship between brain size and neuronal number is complex, with evidence that the scaling rules governing density and size of neurons in primates (including those of the family *Hominidae*) differ from those found in other mammalian orders.[5] In *Homo sapiens* there is little correlation between intelligence, creativity, and gross brain size/volume: "a difference in almost 50% of brain mass, with its billions of neurons and synapses, may have no functional significance in terms of intelligence."[9] In fact, the number of neurons in normal human cerebral cortex can vary considerably, ranging from 14.7 billion to 32 billion cells—a 118% range.[10] The cortical neuronal number constitutes about 25% of the whole brain number, a proportion that remains remarkably constant across species.[5] Analyzing the size of individual components (eg the cerebellum, the basal ganglia, the brainstem, or the different lobes of the cerebral cortex) can provide more useful, but not necessarily definitive, information about brain function and behavior. Brain sizes of our ancestors can be estimated from fossil skulls by measuring the volume of the cranial cavity using endocranial casts—essentially using the skull as a mold to reveal the external shape of the brain that is encased. Such casts reveal gross differences between Neanderthals and modern humans, including a larger cerebellum in humans and changes in the external forms of most lobes of the cerebral cortex, especially the parietal and temporal lobes, and parts of the frontal cortex.[8] Using rules that scale cell number to brain size in different primate species, including our own, it may be possible to estimate neuronal number in the brains of our extinct cousins.[5,11] As can be seen in Figure 3.1, modern *Homo sapiens* have large brains, but the brains of the now extinct Neanderthals were at least as large as ours[12] with possibly similar numbers of neurons,[13] although some have inferred—using other measures—that their brains were organized differently, with perhaps more emphasis on sensory processing.[14]

As briefly discussed in Chapter 2, in right-handed individuals the region defined as Broca's area is almost always located in the left inferior frontal gyrus, consisting primarily of two anatomical sub-parts: the pars opercularis and the pars triangularis. Endocranial casts made from fossil hominin skulls have been used in attempts to identify an equivalent overall region in our recent ancestors. Some anthropologists believe it is possible, by looking at the shape and size of the lobes as revealed by these fossil casts, to identify a region similar to Broca's area in the inferior frontal lobe. As a result, all sorts of suggestions have been made about when speech and language might have evolved, although of course this does not necessarily reveal anything about a principal concern of this book— the evolution of music as a communication system.

Interhemispheric asymmetries and lateralization or bias of a particular function to one or other cerebral hemisphere are not unique to our species,[15,16] and are by no means critical indicators as to when *Homo sapiens* first changed from a modern human to a modern, sentient, articulate human.[17] The prefrontal lobes of all great apes show morphological lateralization, with one study suggesting that humans are merely

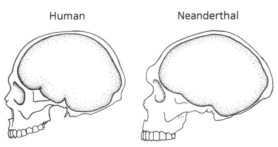

Figure 3.1 Representation of the brains of modern humans (A) and Neanderthals (B).
© Martin Thompson, 2016.

the extreme of that trend.[16] Nonetheless, if our immediate ancestors also had a right-handed bias, as evidence about tool making in Neanderthals may imply,[18] some have reasoned that the presence of some sort of specialization in the inferior frontal lobe of the left hemisphere could indicate a capacity for speech in a particular *Homo* line, many hundreds of thousands of years ago.[19] However it is now clear that Broca's area subserves numerous multimodal processing functions in *Homo sapiens*—not just the motor aspects of speech, and there is increasing evidence that language and speech may be biased to the left side, but by no means exclusively so.[20,21] In any case, I have looked at countless human brains during dissection labs for medical and science students, and while modern-day imaging reveals differences in gray matter architecture between male and female brains,[22] I cannot, by gross examination, necessarily tell the sex of that brain, let alone be certain whether the brain originated from a right- or left-hander. There is even lack of consistency in defining Broca's area in humans.[23] How much more difficult, then, to determine from such *external* features—especially vague in a brain cast—whether a particular fold in the brain is suggestive of speech processing in that long dead, ancestral individual?

Recently, careful quantitative MRI analysis revealed that there are indeed asymmetries in the human cerebral cortex that extend "over a large swath of lateral temporal and parietal cortex, centred on the angular and supramarginal gyri" (see Figure 2.8),[24] but such asymmetries do not *necessarily* correlate with handedness.[22,25] Another imaging study found no interhemispheric, macroscopic asymmetry in Broca's region in humans.[26] However, when brains are sectioned into thin slices, then stained and examined microscopically, some regions (such as superior temporal cortex, Broca's area, Wernicke's area, and primary motor/visual cortices) do show left-right differences. For example, histologically defined left Broca's area has slightly larger gray matter volume, contains more neurons with more complex nerve processes, and exhibits an overall increase in neuropil. Left-right asymmetries may also be the result of altered white matter volume, perhaps as a result of increased myelination of axons, important when rapid signal processing is required.[16,27,28]

Observed discrepancies between internal and external morphology led to the suggestion that: "... gross morphology of the frontal operculum is not a reliable indicator of Broca's area per se."[26] In fact, modern imaging technologies and intensive analysis of the human cerebrum reveal important gray and white matter features "that are not evident from visual inspection of individual subjects."[24] For example, the left primary auditory cortex has a slightly different fiber architecture from the right,[29] and there are human-specific white matter connections between Broca's area and middle and inferior parts of the left temporal gyrus that are buried within the brain.[30] In other words, it is really not possible to establish with certainty on which side a language-related area is located in a human brain merely by gross examination of the external anatomy, so to try to do so in ancestral fossil casts is speculative to say the least, if not impossible.

Simply increasing brain size as one means of increasing hard disk space and processing power is associated with a trolley-full of biological baggage. Bigger brains likely mean a larger head size, with associated biomechanical problems for the neck and shoulders. Furthermore, to make, nourish, and maintain a brain is a very energy-intensive exercise— there is a "trade-off" between the number of neurons in a brain, the energy required to nourish these cells, and body size.[31] Thus, possession of a large brain requires year-round access to appropriate food resources and lots of energy-rich foods, as well as the development of cognitive behaviors that encourage cooperative social strategies that result in reduced daily energy expenditure.[7,32] These behaviors include tool-assisted food processing,[33] hunting in groups, and then the storage, cooking, and sharing of food. The ability to function with proportionately less sleep might also have been important![34] The necessary dietary nutrients and the ability to process and use them efficiently are both necessary to sustain mature individuals, but of course these capacities are especially important when nourishing embryos in the womb and during prolonged human infancy and childhood when building the brain.[35,36]

Maximal brain growth in human children occurs in the last half of gestation and in the first two to three postnatal years. Most of this postnatal growth is related to the maturation of neurons as well as the ongoing production of glial cells.[10] Maternal stress and lack of adequate maternal nutrition will compromise fetal development and likely has long-term consequences for the health and cognitive abilities of offspring, well into adulthood.[37] Lack of vitamin D, for example, is linked to an increased rate of language impairment.[38] Presumably because "the high costs of human brain development require compensatory slowing of body growth rate,"[36] cooperative breeding strategies may have been needed to provide "energy subsidies for reproducing females and dependent offspring (that) can support increased brain size."[32]

As adults, it is estimated that we use 20–25% of our energy intake to maintain proper brain function. Bigger brains take more time to build during development, and if there is an accompanying increase in cranial capacity then this would likely necessitate the birth of even more immature offspring, before the head becomes physically too large. The alternative time-consuming exercise would be to redesign the human female pelvis, thereby potentially affecting locomotion and mobility, or otherwise accept that females might only rarely survive a first delivery! In fact, human females actually have a narrower pelvis than Neanderthals and may have required "both biological changes in the process of delivery and social changes in the level of support needed for modern human mothers giving birth."[39] This is all colorfully summarized by Robin Dunbar in his book *The Human Story*: "The cost of rearing an offspring with a brain of this size is enormous, and accounts for much of what differentiates our biology from that of other animals. Not only has the human brain played havoc with our anatomy in order to make gestation and birth possible, but it imposes monstrous demands on its progenitors after its arrival. It requires a long period of lactation and, beyond that, many years of nurturing and socialisation to turn what begins as little more than a wet lump into a half-decent human being."

If it is true that Neanderthal brains contained a similar number of neurons to the brains of modern humans,[5,13] and if the sheer bulk of the brain and its neuronal complement did not change significantly, whatever occurred in the nervous system during the comparatively recent speciation of *Homo sapiens* must have involved something more subtle. Fossil dental evidence suggests that Neanderthals matured more quickly and rarely lived to an old age,[8,39] presumably giving less time for early, as well as more mature, learning experiences. In modern humans, changes may not only have occurred in the number and perhaps type of connections between different parts of the brain, but also perhaps in the way neural circuits could be changed by experience, thereby creating a new and uniquely powerful learning machine. This would have led to an increasingly refined structure with new flexibility, a new capacity for selectively attending to particular events and stimuli, and a new cognitive power capable of virtual thought and able to accumulate and retrieve the vast stores of information necessary to acquire and retain a large vocabulary. Increased longevity due to enhanced social and cultural "buffering"[39] would also have increased the opportunity for transfer of information across multiple generations.

We do not know anything about the hardware or software in the brains of our immediate ancestors, whoever they were, or our recent "cousins" the Neanderthals. Brain endocasts suggest that they possessed smaller parietal and temporal lobes and larger occipital lobes,[14] but we have no actual brain material with which to work—soft tissue does not leave a trace in the fossil record. Unless artifacts survive across the millennia we also have no trace of behavior. Even then, as stated by the anthropologist Chet Sherwood: "Behavioral abilities … can only be glimpsed opaquely through material remains."[40] We can of course make some guesses about brain structure and function by studying our closest living hominid relatives, the great apes, including gorillas, chimpanzees, bonobos, and orangutans. Anatomical comparisons (whether post-mortem or using neuroimaging methods) are of course possible, and as we shall see a little later, such differences have been extensively documented; however, acute physiological studies on these wonderful primates are incredibly difficult and perhaps prohibitive, both ethically and practically.

Behavioral studies on great apes are of course possible, and there have been a number of intensive efforts to show that members of this family (eg chimpanzees such as "Washoe" and bonobos such as the famous "Kanzi") can learn to sign and can recognize and use hundreds of symbols, and that they have acquired at least some important elements needed for a rudimentary communication system some equate to language capability. However, with regard to grammar, even among the experts there has been controversy as to how to interpret Washoe's or Kanzi's remarkable skills, and to my knowledge there is no clear evidence for the consistent use of open, human-like hierarchical and recursive syntax in these non-human primates, and no convincing evidence that these trained animals can refer abstractly to past or future events. "Even putting aside vocabulary, phonology, morphology, and syntax, what impresses one the most about chimpanzee signing is that fundamentally, deep down, chimps just don't 'get it.'"[1] The new and undoubtedly interesting cognitive behaviors exhibited by these non-human primates take years of intensive training, and there is evidence of transfer of skills to offspring. Yet learning in such primates is perhaps two orders of magnitude slower than learning in children, who can learn at least ten words each day, with a resultant vocabulary that may contain on average about 20,000 word families, sometimes as many as 100,000.[41] Human creativity is special: "Having language is having the ability to use a limited set of symbols to generate a virtually unlimited number of combinations to form utterances, each of which has meaning."[42] Henry Plotkin estimated we have the potential to generate 10^{30} different sentences in a lifetime! And language is not alone in its potential profligacy—with 13 notes in an octave, and melodies of different length and rhythm, there are approaching 10^{20} possible tunes to write!!

But in any case analysis of these animals, while of great importance in gaining a greater understanding, and respect for, our living hominid relatives and their rightful place alongside us on this planet, may be misleading if an outcome of these long-term training programs is to divine the linguistic capabilities of our immediate ancestors. It has been estimated that separation of the genus *Pan* (chimpanzees and bonobos) line from the *Homo* line occurred as much as seven or eight million years ago.[43,44] Hominids have evolved and changed in important ways during that period—so too, I imagine, has the *Pan* lineage. We cannot assume that their brains and behaviors, as examined in the twenty-first century, necessarily reflect where our common ancestors were "at" all those millions of years ago. We have to make guesses—to quote Chip Walter from his intelligent and very readable book *Last Ape Standing*, "the illumination of our past is a little like trying to find a set of car keys in the Sahara with a flashlight."[45]

Nonetheless, despite all the unknowns and the dangers of a neophyte like me entering the contentious battlefield of evolutionary biology, I believe it is an essential part of my story to theorize about what may have happened to our brains during this critical period in human evolution. Although necessarily speculative, we need to ask what made *Homo sapiens* different from their closely related predecessors and thus, we must presume in classic evolutionary terms, more viable and capable of propagating and expanding the species? Many aficionados of evolutionary biology, building on the pioneering work of Nikolaas Tinbergen, emphasize the importance of distinguishing between so-called "proximate" versus "ultimate" causes when discussing the evolution of complex behaviors, especially in humans.[46] Ultimate explanations relate to the fitness of a particular behavior and the evolutionary pressures that influence its selection, while proximate explanations deal with the physiological mechanisms and environmental interactions that produce such a behavior. I do appreciate this distinction, and while perhaps annoying to some, I hope that the general reader will not mind me occasionally intermixing these explanations in the pages that follow.

According to the eminent philosopher Daniel Dennett: "most of the huge difference between our minds and the minds of chimpanzees is not due directly to the genetically controlled differences in neuroanatomy but to the vast differences in *virtual* architecture made possible by those minor differences in the underlying neural hardware. By becoming adapted to the transmission and rehearsal (internal replication) of a cornucopia of pre-designed cultural thinking tools, our brains became open-minded in a way that is apparently unavailable to chimpanzee brains no matter how intensively their cultural environment is enriched."[47] The genetic library of our immediate ancestors was very similar to that of modern-day humans, but as described later in the section on "Genes and their regulators", there is increasing evidence suggestive of important but subtle differences in how these genes are controlled, especially in the brain. I propose that there must have been some change, some co-evolution or co-adaptation of several small mutations, that perhaps subtly altered the wiring and functional adaptability of circuits, which proved to be the crucial cognitive tipping point. As we shall see, this change may have happened at an opportune time, a change that led to increased competitive advantage when it was needed, and resulted in a new type of rapid, positively selected, self-reinforcing evolutionary radiation.

Of cells and neural pathways

The classical Darwinian theory of evolutionary change involves the appearance of variant forms of an organism that are caused by mutations in the genome (the DNA in the genes), which is transmitted from parent to offspring. As famously elucidated by Watson and Crick, DNA (deoxyribonucleic acid) in the cell nucleus is made up of a double helical strand of sequences of simple organic molecules called nucleotides. DNA contains four different nucleotides in DNA, each with a different "nucleobase"—adenine (A), cytosine (C), guanine (G), and thymine (T). The two strands of DNA run in opposite directions, with C always pairing with G, and A always pairing with T. These nucleotides form a code (A, C, G, T) in the DNA, and a gene is: "a stretch of DNA whose linear sequence of nucleotides encodes the linear sequence of amino acids in a specific protein."[48] Thus the code can be read by copying the appropriate lengths of DNA into messenger RNAs (mRNA) by a process called transcription, and these mRNAs in turn are exported into the cytoplasm to make proteins of many kinds and widely diverse functions. The DNA is organized into chromosomes, which also consist of proteins that are needed for organizing and compacting the DNA helices. We will return to these vitally important proteins in the "Genes and their regulators" section of this chapter when discussing what is termed the "epigenome" and the "epigenetic" modification of "classical" genes.

Gene mutations are probably comparatively rare events; in humans there are estimated to be about 3.0×10^{-8} mutations/nucleotide/generation,[49] with perhaps 150–200 mutations in each of us in the entire genome. These mutations can be unfavorable or neutral in character, but positive natural selection occurs when a genetic change results in a phenotypic trait or characteristic that, in a particular environment, confers an adaptive advantage to the variant. This differentially affects genes and, of necessity, their carriers (Richard Dawkins calls these "replicators" and "vehicles") by enhancing survivability and reproductive success. Over successive generations, the frequency of this modified, relatively advantageous genotype and its adaptive phenotype increases in the population, a change that is likely to be significantly accelerated if the environment or habitat is also changing in a way that intensifies selection pressures. Eventually, over time and geographical separation, new species are established that cannot interbreed successfully with other species.

In re-examining the theory of evolution, Stephen Jay Gould and others have suggested that species go through periods of stasis, with little or no change, and that mutation and speciation occur intermittently but then very rapidly (so-called punctuated equilibrium).[50] There is always ongoing but slow evolutionary change involving natural selection, but there are also periods of more rapid evolutionary change. There is another important evolutionary concept, that of genetic drift, which describes a process in which the makeup of the genome of an isolated population, usually involving subtle variants of the genes (the different versions of a gene are termed alleles), slowly varies by chance over time. Evolutionary biologists tell us that the effects of genetic drift are greater when the populations in which it is occurring are small. These small, random changes in allelic frequency are often neutral and initially may have no substantive impact on the reproductive success of an organism. It is evolution without adaptation; it is not driven by environmental pressures and may, when examined retrospectively, look like a period of evolutionary stasis, where nothing of significance is happening. However, in classical Darwinian manner, a subgroup within a population subject to genetic drift may then be rapidly selected for because of some advantageous phenotype and increased reproductive success, presumably as a consequence of a sudden environmental/contextual change. Thus: "if an individual does not inherit its parents' environment along with their genes and other transmittable factors, it may not be well adapted to the conditions in which it now finds itself. But the altered environmental conditions may throw up variation that was previously hidden and from that may spring new lines of evolution. Active choice and active control by the organism together with its own adaptability may be all important additional drivers of evolutionary change."[51] Quantitative analysis of DNA variation in *Homo sapiens* does suggest that drift played a major role in determining genetic diversity in our species.[52]

With these basic evolutionary concepts in mind, let us now briefly but specifically consider *Homo sapiens* and the "origins of the modern mind."[53] What subtle variations in sequences of DNA in our genes (polymorphisms) were important during our recent evolution? Does knowledge about these changes help in any way as we try to understand the origins and antecedents of music, why music is a universal, and wonder at its continued presence alongside modern language and articulate speech in *Homo sapiens*? Is it too much to expect that there might be new types of language-related genes, gene mutations resulting in improved learning and memory, but in addition perhaps also gene polymorphisms associated with artistic performance such as dance and music?

As discussed earlier, our overall brain volume is probably not greater than the brain volume of our immediate ancestors, and on average our brains are slightly smaller than those of our extinct Neanderthal relatives. Thus if there were any mutations that influenced brain size they must have influenced the relative size, cell architecture, or interconnectivity of particular components within the brain.[9,54,55,56] Although the same scaling rules that relate cell number to brain size apply across primate species,[11] many differences between our brains and those of monkeys—including other members of our hominid family—have been documented although, as mentioned before, because our lines separated so many millions of years ago, such comparisons do not necessarily tell us anything about our immediate ancestors and should be interpreted with caution. For example, the human brain is about ten times bigger than the brain of a macaque monkey, and we have 150–200 distinct cortical areas per hemisphere compared with 130–140 areas in this species of monkey.[24,57] This is an interesting comparison, although it should be noted that it is neither straightforward to determine which areas perform similar functions between species, nor easy to determine whether there are novel processing regions unique to the neocortex of *Homo sapiens*.

Compared with our nearer relations the chimpanzees, *Homo sapiens'* brains also have relatively larger cerebral cortices as well as large cerebellar hemispheres, and sub-components of the basal ganglia and thalamus are also greater in volume. We have a far greater extent of multimodal association cortex—that is, an integrative cortex not directly involved in the immediate processing of sensory stimuli or motor control; this comprises regions with dense but distributed interconnections and a connectional flexibility that spans the cortex.[12] In adult humans, the lateral temporal cortex and parietal lobe are expanded, and our prefrontal cortex and inferior frontal cortex are enlarged and highly developed. The postnatal expansion in cortical regions such as prefrontal cortex is not related to the continued birth of neurons, which are born prenatally, but to the continued production of supporting glial cells, and the maturation and growth of neurons, their processes, and their multitude of interconnections.

The human prefrontal cortex is especially enlarged[58] and differs not only in the morphology of many of its constituent neurons, but also in the way in which cell populations are spatially organized, perhaps indicative of a greater amount of inter-cell connectivity within the gray matter.[59,60,61,62] In addition, our prefrontal cortex has a higher glial— neuronal ratio than other cortical regions.[56] Interestingly, these frontal regions—so important in human cognitive function—are associated with a high degree of variability in cortical folding (and surface area) and are relatively immature at birth, subsequently growing at faster rates than other cortical regions.[12,63] Remarkably, the maturation of neurons continues even after adolescence.[64] Some regions of human association cortex, including frontal cortex, are lightly myelinated (the insulation around axons that increases the speed of impulse conduction).[65] This relative lack of myelin in the gray matter is associated with higher metabolic activity and perhaps greater synaptic plasticity and adaptability.[66]

Prefrontal cortex (Figure 3.2) is an area critically involved in processing executive functions such as sociability, decision making, and the planning and selection of future strategies. Damage to this cortex may affect all of these higher level cognitive functions. Hill and colleagues suggest that the pattern of postnatal cortical expansion is similar to the pattern of human evolutionary cortical expansion, and hypothesize that "it is beneficial for regions of recent evolutionary expansion to remain less mature at birth, perhaps to increase the influence of postnatal experience on the development of these regions or to focus prenatal resources on regions most important for early survival."[63] Remarkably, in humans there appears to be an inverse relationship between the gray matter volume of anterior prefrontal cortex and the volume of primary visual cortex and primary auditory cortex.[67] The authors of that study suggest this reflects a trade-off between high-level cognition and basic sensation, but just why this should be the case is unclear—is high-level cognition associated more with imaginative thought than with real-world sensory information?

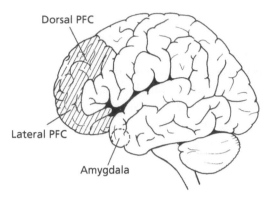

Figure 3.2 View of the lateral aspect of the human cerebral cortex highlighting dorsal and lateral prefrontal cortex (PFC) and the approximate location of the amygdala within the temporal lobe. © Martin Thompson, 2016.

With specific reference to communication and language, the inferior frontal cortex region (part of it comprising Broca's area in humans) is present in monkeys, but in *Homo sapiens* this area is much larger, and seemingly much more complex, with at least ten subdivisions that may be functionally distinct.[68] In fact, Broca's area shows one of the greatest relative volumetric increases of any neocortical region.[69] Species-specific calls in the macaque monkey have been reported to activate areas that may be homologous to language-related areas in humans.[70] In addition, and interestingly from an evolutionary point of view, stimulation of the proposed homologue of Broca's area in monkeys also results in hand and mouth movements—perhaps a precursor of the hierarchical organization necessary for gesture and vocal communication links used in *Homo sapiens*?[71,72,73] A ventral white matter pathway in non-human primates links these regions with more caudal auditory areas that are involved in processing (and recognizing) spectrally complex sounds such as vocalizations.[74,75] A similar ventrally located system is also present in *Homo sapiens*[76] and is already established at birth.[77] In humans there appear to be two ventrally located pathways involved in language processing (see Figure 2.8), including the processing of conceptual information, mapping speech sounds to the meaning of words, and perhaps certain aspects of syntax.[78,79,80,81] However, language function and speech production in humans are also critically supported by additional, more dorsally located fiber networks such as the arcuate fasciculus, which links parts of frontal, parietal, and temporal cortex (see Figure 2.8).

Initially discovered in ventral premotor cortex in macaque monkeys, some neurons discharge when performing a particular movement, or when watching another animal perform a particular movement. These are so-called mirror neurons, and it has been suggested that this region and the adjacent inferior frontal cortex contain a "vocabulary" of motor actions related to movements of the mouth and face, as well as use of the hands.[82,83] Mirror neurons are found in bird species as well as in primates, and as their name suggests, these nerve cells modulate their activity when an action is performed by self, or when the same action is performed by another, potentially providing a "mechanism that unifies action production and action observation, allowing the understanding of the actions of others from the inside."[84] In monkeys, attention to, and perception of, another's action are strongly influenced by an individual monkey's own personal experience,[85] and the activity of mirror neurons varies depending on social cues and the subjective value that the monkey associates with an object that is grasped by another,[86] as well as on the direction of the other's gaze.[87]

Mirror neurons have also now been found in other regions such as the parietal cortex, and can have a range of properties, including responses to various modalities such as sensation (touch), hearing, and sight.[88] The existence of the fronto-parietal mirror system may explain why some primates such as chimpanzees and bonobos apparently possess a perception of self in that they are capable of recognizing themselves in a reflection from a mirror (although of course this would be an inverted image ...). However, while most, if not all, monkeys possess mirror neurons, not all primate species have this self-recognition capability.[89,90]

Recognition of, and interpretation of, the mental state of other members of your species constitute a core element in empathy, in what is termed "Theory of Mind." Theory of Mind is our ability to imagine and understand others' intentions, desires, and so on, with the presumption that others have a mind similar to one's own. There is evidence that primates share with humans some of the basic neural networks that process social cognition and influence how individuals interact with each other,[91,92] although the extent and type of prosocial behavior can differ between primate species.[93] Nonetheless, understanding the primate mirror neuron network in the frontal and parietal cortex, and how it links to limbic pathways and centers involved in vocalization, may provide important clues to the evolution of complex communication systems, the capacity for empathy and imitation, and multimodal mimetic social interactions that involve sensation and movement—for example hand gestures, facial expression, and posture.[94,95,96,97,98,99]

Others have suggested that the multimodal mirror neuron system and the need to connect with other individuals formed an emotional and interactive network allowing "affective engagement" with others, important in the emergence of music as a social enterprise.[100] These are intriguing ideas although, in relation to the evolution of speech and language, fMRI studies show that visual and motor components of the human mirror system—while located in cortical regions similar to those in primates—are bilateral, not lateralized or biased to the left hemisphere.[101,102] There are also problems with working out how mirror neurons could have led to the development of symbols and syntax.[103] Nonetheless, it seems highly likely that our speech and language circuits were superimposed on, and augmented, existing communication and hierarchical visuospatial processing systems involving vocalization, gesture, and facial expression, of which the mirror neuron network was almost certainly a part.[74,104]

While it is true that different components of the "mirror" system are active when viewing mouth movements or speech-associated gestures,[105] and that this system is active when human subjects recognize happy faces[106] or mimic happy, angry, or sad facial expressions,[107] others propose that human communication is much more sophisticated and requires much more than just the mutual recognition of sensorimotor signals using the mirror neuron system. This is because a sender must "select a communicative action appropriate to convey a specific intention to the receiver" that must predict and take into account the receiver's knowledge and beliefs.[108] Based on functional imaging of subjects carrying out what is known as the "Tacit Communication Game," these authors propose that a region in the right posterior superior temporal sulcus is modulated by the inherent ambiguity—not sensory input or motor output—of a communication, and that this region thus encodes both the "selection and recognition of a communicative behaviour in senders and receivers respectively."[108] Amazingly, this same, lateralized cortical region has been reported to have a higher gray matter density in people who have a greater number of friends/contacts on the web-based social network *Facebook*![109] We shall come back to concepts of "Theory of Mind," social cooperation, and how we reciprocally model/predict/infer each other's beliefs and intentions in Chapter 5.

An intriguing addendum to the role of mirror neurons and the evolution of human speech and Theory of Mind considerations comes from a study showing that a mirror-like system also develops in the congenitally blind.[110] The authors of this study used fMRI to scan the brains of congenitally blind subjects as they were presented with, and asked to recognize, auditory sound samples of actions, and to pantomime movements/manipulations associated with those sounds (eg hammer, scissors). In both situations, in blind individuals there was enhanced activity in a network involving the premotor temporo-parietal cortex that overlapped the mirror system and motor regions activated in sighted controls. In other words, the human mirror system can develop in the absence of sight, and visual imagery seems not to be a "necessary precondition to form a representation of other's actions."[110] Interestingly, it is known that various Theory of Mind concepts are delayed (but not prevented) in congenitally deaf children,[111] as in blind children, although in the latter case at least, the neural networks develop normally.[112] There is a redundancy in the systems we use to learn how to interact with, and interpret the actions of, others. I wonder if this is another unique feature of the social human brain, perhaps linked to our enhanced communication and (perhaps) empathic capabilities (see Chapter 5)? Basic imitation can only go so far; it cannot lead to the sharing of "propositions, beliefs, institutions and goals."[42]

In addition to the previously described, language-related ventral fiber pathways that interconnect part of the inferior frontal gyrus to the temporal lobe, there are additional, dorsally located fiber tracts that interlink posterior superior temporal cortex with regions in the frontal cortex and inferior parietal cortex (see Figure 2.8).[30,76,78,80,81,113,114,115,116] The way in which these various dorsal fiber tracts and their pattern of connections differ between non-human primates and humans has been the subject of considerable recent research.[78,80,115] Not all of these pathways are language specific; nonetheless, taken as a whole, the dorsal pathway in the left hemisphere (for right-handers), which also includes the arcuate fasciculus, has clearly been modified during evolution—with a broader distribution from the temporal lobe—and "is likely to be the pathway most essential for higher-order aspects of language such as syntax and lexical-semantics."[114]

Developmentally, the ventral language-related pathways are established at birth, but there appear to be two distinguishable sub-components of the dorsal language network.[76,77,113,117] One of these is also established at birth and connects the temporal cortex to premotor cortex, forming an initial sensorimotor network needed for early auditory-motor integration, and the acquisition and memory of complex motor patterns required for articulate speech. Most importantly, the second pathway—part of the arcuate fasciculus—matures later in childhood (it is present in 7 year olds) and is the "classical" pathway associated with the acquisition of more complex linguistic processing (syntax, hierarchy, etc). It is unique to humans and connects superior temporal cortex to part of Broca's area, a pathway that is especially prominent on the left-hand side. Interestingly, this pathway and working memory performance have been reported to share common, heritable genetic factors.[118]

The homunculus

At a finer organizational level, within the already described primary motor and sensory cortical regions (see Figure 2.2), are ordered topographic maps that are representations of the particular functionality that is being processed. So, for example, motor cortex and somatosensory cortex contain coherent functional maps of the musculature and body surface respectively (somatotopicity), visual cortex contains a map of the retina and visual field (visuotopicity), and auditory cortex is organized into a frequency map (tonotopicity). But these are not faithful one-to-one representations—the maps are grossly distorted such that the parts of the cortex that process a particular aspect of the modality domain are greatly expanded compared with others. Moreover, these distortions are species-specific. In *Homo sapiens*, over half the gray matter of primary visual cortex processes information from the foveal region, the part of the retina that we use when fixating and focusing on objects. In human motor cortex and somatosensory cortex, the regions that process information to and from the hands, face, lips, and tongue are massively expanded compared with the regions that process information to and from other parts of the body—an arrangement represented by the cortical homunculus ("the little man inside the brain").

While there is now known to be a surprising degree of inter-individual variability in these "maps," in general the consequence of these expanded representations is a huge increase in the neural machinery devoted to processing information to and from the head and hands—a sizable increase in hard drive capability and computational power. To me, these virtual distortions of the real world within the cerebral cortex provide the clearest indication as to what is most important to that particular species, what is evolutionarily most critical. Hence, in humans the emphasis is on visual depth perception, fine-tuned sensorimotor control of the hands (thumbs and fingers), and expanded representations of the face and the oral cavity (facial expression and vocalization). As Sherwood et al point out, the relative increase in size of particular sub-regions of the human neocortex would likely have allowed greater voluntary control over certain critical behaviors.[40]

Chemistry and plasticity

Differences in the spatial organization of neurons in the cerebral cortex of humans, compared with those of chimpanzees, have already been discussed. These differences are especially evident in prefrontal cortex, and reflect altered connectivity as well as an increase in the complexity of dendrites of human pyramidal neurons.[61] What about the chemistry of the nervous system—how does that vary between us and our primate relatives? Neurons can either excite another nerve cell or inhibit its activity, and they communicate with each other over long or short distances via mostly chemically mediated synaptic connections. In different parts of the nervous system, in addition to neuronal number, the relative number, location, and type of excitatory versus inhibitory neurons are now understood to be important parameters in shaping activity and influencing the computational power of the brain.[9] A series of studies have compared the cerebral cortical distributions of neurochemical systems that modulate cognitive function in global ways.[119,120] Compared with classical neurotransmitters, these systems act over a longer timescale, are more diffuse, and utilize molecules such as acetylcholine, dopamine, and serotonin. The authors of these studies found many similarities between humans and anthropoid apes such as chimpanzees, but there were also subtle changes in the organization of the dopamine system, which may have functional implications.

However, a comparison of the local circuit, inhibitory population of neurons (interneurons) in prefrontal cortex failed to reveal morphological or neurochemical differences between primates and humans,[121] leading the authors of this study to speculate that "other significant modifications to the connectivity and molecular biology of the prefrontal cortex were overlaid on this conserved interneuron architecture in the course of human evolution." These modifications seem to be more in the excitatory domain, because Chet Sherwood's group has found significant evolutionary changes in primate genes that code for various components of the glutamate signaling pathway, the main excitatory transmitter in our brains, leading them to suggest that: "an overall upregulation in neural activity through excitatory mechanisms may have coevolved with greater cognitive capacities across primates."[122]

We shall see later, when discussing the role of genes in influencing cognitive power and neural plasticity in *Homo sapiens*, that there are indeed links between genes and subtle changes in the architecture/density of both gray and white matter regions in the brain, changes that are consistently associated with intelligence. In addition, over the past hundred years or so many physiological and functional studies in the brain have been directed at understanding how neurons are wired up and how they "talk" to each other in specific patterns of interconnectivity. Neurons are often very, very noisy; you can hear them chattering away when a recording electrode is inserted into neural tissue. They are—if you like—the dominant cell type, the show-offs. But glial cells may well be just as important. You cannot hear them easily with recording electrodes because they generally do not fire off action potentials. But there are more glia than neurons in a human cerebral cortex, and they could well turn out to be just as important players in normal and abnormal brain function as the chatty neuron.[123,124]

Probably every synapse between the processes of connected neurons has at least one associated astrocytic process. Astrocytes are linked together by special junctions, forming networks that can signal over quite large distances.[125,126] Amongst other things, astrocytes control the amount of space between neurons, they buffer the concentration of ions such as potassium and hydrogen (and therefore control pH), they can take up and release neurochemicals that modify how neurons fire, and they are needed to control the flow of blood to different brain regions depending on the level of activity in those regions.[123] Astrocytes can also supply energy resources (glycogen) to highly active regions of the brain for a brief period if glucose and oxygen are temporarily in short supply. They can modulate neuronal excitability and influence the strength of signal transmission between neurons, and they play an important long-term role in how individual synapses change their signaling strength as a consequence of ongoing neural activity.[126,127,128,129] Astrocytes therefore play a crucial role in plasticity associated with learning and memory, and perhaps also influence aspects of human cognition.[125] For some time, I have viewed astrocytes as the "yin" to the neuronal "yang," physiological partners in our dynamic central nervous system.

It may therefore be of evolutionary significance that human astrocytes have unique morphological and functional features that set them apart from astrocytes found in all other species.[130] Human astrocytes are generally larger, more diverse, and morphologically more complex, and can conduct waves of calcium at high speed, and compared with cells in other species a human astrocyte can support and modulate a greater number of individual synapses (perhaps twenty times as many as in rodent brains). This affects the size of the functional unit encompassed by each astrocyte, leading Oberheim et al to suggest: "By integrating the activity of a larger contiguous set of synapses, the astrocytic domain might extend the processing power of human brain beyond that of other species."[131] Pereira and Furlan use the term "Master Hub"[125] to define the concept of an astrocytic network that modulates neuronal systems and acts "as vehicle for whole-brain integration of information and support for the formation of conscious episodes." I believe it is also very meaningful that, while the numbers of neurons and glia in the human brain as a whole are about equal (about 170 billion cells in total), in the gray matter of cerebral cortex, neurons have a lower packing density with far more processes, and the glial-neuron ratio is about 1.5:1,[10,132] and even higher in our all-important frontal cortex.[56] Recent research has also revealed that microglia, the resident macrophages in CNS tissue, can help to both create and prune synaptic connections, and perhaps even modulate their strength.[124]

Any alteration in the way synapses function, and especially how they change structurally and chemically with experience, will have significant consequences on our learning abilities and presumably enlarge both our short- and long-term memory storage capacities. By long-term memory I refer to those memories that can be stored for long periods of time, memories that can last a lifetime. Psychologists usually partition long-term memory into what are termed procedural (implicit) and declarative (explicit) memory systems. Procedural memory is associated with the acquisition of perceptual and automatic motor skills. Declarative memories can be consciously recalled; they comprise stores of general factual information (semantic memory) and autobiographical memories of personal experiences (episodic memory).

The excitability of neurons and their interconnections can be strengthened or weakened over time depending on the location of the synaptic input and the timing of action potential firing and associated excitatory (or inhibitory) synaptic activity.[133,134] Analysis of how the timing of neural activity alters synaptic transmission in a part of the brain called the hippocampus, which is widely thought to be necessary for turning short-term memory into long-term memory, has revealed that there is a wider inter-spike tolerance for strengthening synapses in human tissue compared with rodents: "A wider temporal window for strengthening of synapses in the human brain may allow for the association of larger variety of events with less emphasis on the temporal order."[135] Our circuits thus appear to be more flexible and adaptable, and astrocytes may contribute an important role. Amazingly, when precursors of human glial cells were transplanted into the brains of neonatal mice that lacked a normal immune system response, the grafted cells survived, many turned into astrocytes, and there was improved "long-term potentiation" of synaptic performance as well as enhanced learning and memory. The term long-term potentiation is used to describe the increased strength of a synapse as a result of previous neural activity, with enhancement of the signal sometimes lasting for minutes or even days. Long-term depression also occurs, and reflects a persistent decrease in synaptic strength. Unlike human glial precursors, grafted glial precursors derived from mice did not enhance host performance, so: "human glia differentially enhance both activity-dependent plasticity and learning in mice."[136] Overall then, it seems clear that evolutionary changes in both neurons and glia opened up new possibilities for greater integrative complexity and more nuanced plasticity in the developing and mature human brain.

Genes and their regulators

There seems little doubt that subtle genetic variants could have resulted in altered developmental patterning as well as changes in the relative volume of regions of gray matter or altered neural circuitry between different parts of the brain of *Homo sapiens*. There are indeed links between genes and the dynamics of cell birth and cell death in the developing mammalian brain, including the cerebral cortex, which in different species may alter how fast different parts of the brain are built and their eventual size, thus influencing the final neural architecture.[137,138] In humans, a recent example of this is the variation in a gene encoding an immune-related protein called interleukin-3, which has been reported to correlate with brain volume[139] and may have been the subject of "weak or modest positive selection in the evolutionary history of humans."[140] However, we have already noted that brain size is not everything, and while there is, in humans, increasing evidence for some correlation between aspects of gray and white matter architecture and general intelligence[141,142,143,144,145] it must always be remembered that, based on fossil endocasts, the Neanderthals had brains at least as large as those of *Homo sapiens*.

A recent report noted that the number of DNA sequence changes "that distinguish modern humans from our nearest extinct relatives is comparatively small"—translated into only 87 proteins with fixed amino-acid changes.[146] Some of the changes that were seen in the archaic human material related to genes also expressed in the developing forebrain, and may impact on cell proliferation and differentiation during development. In addition, there were also likely to have been critical, positively selected mutations in DNA that altered the function of genes involved in the molecular and cell biology of individual cells, and in particular how brain cells exchange information with each other.

Small changes or variants (termed polymorphisms), sometimes involving the substitution of a single nucleotide (single-nucleotide polymorphism or SNP, pronounced *snip*) in the sequences of certain genes and their associated proteins, are increasingly being identified in the modern human population. In the nervous system, researchers have linked these mutations to, among other phenotypic characteristics, altered brain volume (see above), the relative size of certain brain regions, altered connectivity between cortical areas, altered learning and memory performance, and changes in speech capability. Overall, the genetic code of *Homo sapiens* possesses about 98% similarity with the code of our nearest living relative, the chimpanzee.[147,148] Importantly however, while many genes in the brain are conserved between human and chimpanzee, a critical subset of expressed sequences—mostly relating to brain function and especially development—differ in the human cortex compared with chimpanzees and appear to have evolved relatively rapidly.[149,150,151] As discussed earlier, we should be cautious in over-interpreting these data because, although chimpanzees are our closest relatives, evolution has still had seven to eight million years to continue to work on the genomes of the respective lineage. The hominin line as a whole does share some genotypic features, suggesting that hominins have positively (and quite rapidly) selected for various genes that enable greater metabolic capacity in brain tissue and enable increasingly large numbers of neurons and glia to generate aerobic energy more effectively/efficiently, thus allowing for potentially higher rates of sustained neural activity.[148,152,153,154] Humans have rapidly evolved high metabolic efficiency in the brain, seemingly at the cost of our skeletal muscles,[155] thus during childhood, at the peak of neural plasticity and learning, metabolic needs are so high that general body growth is slowed in compensation.[36]

Comparisons between human and non-human primates using expression profiling of genes further suggest that there has also been a more rapid, accelerated evolution of so-called transcription factors in *Homo sapiens* than in other primates.[138,154,156,157,158] Transcription factors are proteins made by regulatory DNA that bind to other specific DNA sequences (promoter or enhancer regions) upstream of a gene, and either recruit or block the cellular machinery that is responsible for mRNA transcription. The genetic flow of information from DNA to mRNA largely determines which proteins are produced and utilized by a given cell, at any given time, at any given place. Transcription factors, working alone or in combination with other proteins, are thus able to dynamically control whether a given gene is switched on (activated) or switched off (repressed). Gene expression regulation by transcription factors is critically important during brain development but is also relevant to the plasticity and adaptability of the brain during adult life.

In a study comparing human and chimpanzee genomes,[159] the authors ranked genes that showed significant evolutionary acceleration ("human accelerated regions"—HARs). A dramatic example was HAR1, part of a transcriptional regulation gene expressed in a specific type of nerve cell during an important period in the development and construction of the cerebral cortex. The authors estimated that there were 18 substitutions in the HAR1 region in human lineage since the human-chimpanzee common ancestor—a rate of change sixty to seventy times higher than expected. In another study, Uddin et al also found high expression of a cluster of what they term "human ancestry-specific" (HAS) genes, which are adaptively evolving and appear to be specifically associated with the prenatal environment, and may be involved in the formation of nerve connections.[154] HARs have also been analyzed in archaic humans (a Neanderthal bone), revealing many of these genes in our ancestor, but with numerous new, fast-evolving polymorphisms in HARs that may have been positively selected in *Homo sapiens*.[160] It is therefore of evolutionary significance that mutations in HARs are closely associated with altered human-specific social and cognitive behaviors, including links to autism spectrum disorders.[161] A very recent report found even more (524!) accelerated sites within human DNA likely to be involved in regulating DNA transcription, especially in the brain.[158]

When comparing gene expression during the postnatal development of human, chimpanzee, and rhesus macaque monkey brains, some striking differences were found in the human cortex, particularly during maturation of the prefrontal cortex and to a lesser extent the cerebellum.[162] Genes showing human-specific expression were those involved with synaptic function; the timescale of maximal expression of these genes was extended from less than a year in chimpanzees and macaques to about five years in humans, allowing a vastly increased opportunity for plasticity in early childhood. The authors also suggested that this change was very recent, and "may have taken place after the split of the human race and the Neanderthal lineages." Intriguingly, human-specific changes in metabolite concentrations and their corresponding enzymes, which influence levels of neural activity and plasticity, have also evolved most rapidly in human prefrontal cortex, the region involved in reasoning, executive planning, social interactions, and so on.[163] Such changes presumably contribute to the formation of even more complex and adaptable circuits in this critical part of the cognitive human brain.[164] Overall then, it is clear that modern humans have a much more active or dynamic brain environment, both during development and in adult life, and we possess a more complex and more regulatable transcription profile.[165]

But before we move on, some additional and very important provisos are needed here that are especially pertinent to our interpretation and understanding of evolutionary changes in brain function and plasticity. There is an almost unimaginable complexity in the way genes and their products operate and are expressed, and how they can interact with each other, within and outside the nucleus of a cell. It is increasingly difficult to see how genes can work in "splendid" isolation from each other, especially in the brain.

Yet until very recently the great majority of genetic comparisons between humans, and between humans and the closely related great apes, have been based on the "classical" genome—on genes and the DNA sequences within them that are the template for mRNA and the proteins that are produced. But of the almost 93% of human genome that is transcribed into RNA, much less than 2% actually codes protein sequences.[166] A recent study suggests that the human genome contains only 19,000 functional protein-coding genes, and that these are highly conserved across evolution.[167] What is the remaining RNA doing? What is it for? It turns out that the DNA-binding transcription factors described above are just one example of how genes control and influence each other. The effects of a given gene, and when and where they are expressed, are now understood to be influenced by many other, perhaps even more subtle, controlling factors that further enable cells to differ from each other phenotypically, even when they are genetically identical.

There are various types of so-called non-coding RNAs, of different lengths, and they are more prevalent in the brain and have evolved most rapidly in humans.[168] Similar to identified transcription factor sequences, this "non-coding transcriptome" may undergo important changes during evolution as the complexity of an organism, and its need for phenotypic flexibility, increases. There is evidence that some non-coding RNAs are regulated during development; they regulate other genes by cleaving mRNA or repressing translation, which in turn controls the expression of classical protein-encoding genes. The specific pattern of developmental gene expression in humans has evolved three to five times faster than in chimpanzees. The changes are most obvious in prefrontal cortex and are thought to be driven by altered expression of a small number of key regulators of neuronal gene expression, including several non-protein-coding RNAs called microRNAs.[169] These microRNAs usually suppress translation from mRNA to protein, and there is increasing evidence of their involvement in fine tuning aspects of neural development and connectivity.[170] In the more mature brain, suppression of one of these microRNAs is necessary for the structural plasticity associated with long-term memory.[171]

Non-coding RNAs, as a colleague of mine suggested to me, are like the genetic equivalent of dark matter—not easy to see, but tremendously powerful, and just maybe the key to everything! It is worthwhile quoting a passage from the abstract of John Mattick's insightful and informative review in full—it is challenging and far reaching in its implications: "It appears that the genetic programming of humans and other complex organisms has been misunderstood for the past 50 years, due to the assumption that most genetic information is transacted by proteins. However, the human genome contains only about 20,000 protein-coding genes, similar in number and with largely orthologous functions as those in nematodes that have only 1,000 somatic cells. By contrast, the extent of non-protein-coding DNA increases with increasing complexity, reaching 98.8% in humans. The majority of these sequences are dynamically transcribed, mainly into non-protein-coding RNAs, with tens if not hundreds of thousands that show specific expression patterns and subcellular locations, as well as many classes of small regulatory RNAs. The emerging evidence indicates that these RNAs control the epigenetic states that underpin development. Moreover it appears that animals, particularly primates, have evolved plasticity in these RNA regulatory systems, especially in the brain. Thus, it appears that what was dismissed as "junk" because it was not understood holds the key to understanding human evolution, development, and cognition."[168]

And there is still more! Increasing numbers of studies are focusing on so-called epigenetic regulation of gene expression, biochemical modifications that alter gene expression in a cell nucleus without changing the DNA nucleotide (A, C, G, T) sequences themselves. DNA does not sit naked within the nucleus; it is tightly packaged in association with special proteins—these proteins and DNA given the overall term "chromatin." Anything that modifies chromatin structure can alter the accessibility of the associated DNA to molecules needed for gene transcription. True epigenetic modifications are heritable, meaning that modifications to the chromatin structure can be preserved over cell divisions. However, rapid and dramatic epigenetic remodeling also occurs, especially during development and cell differentiation. Modification of DNA by a process called methylation reversibly alters certain sites or islands in promoter regions, which can physically block the transcriptional machinery and transcription factors from accessing the DNA, or attract DNA-binding proteins that impede transcription, leading to gene silencing or repression. The amount of methylation increases during development and maturation of the brain.[172] There are specific DNA enzymes associated with this transcriptional repression, and mutations in these enzymes are associated with impaired synaptic plasticity, impaired learning, and certain neurological disorders in humans.[173,174] Interestingly then, DNA methylation maps in prefrontal cortex differ between humans and chimpanzees, with likely functional and phenotypic consequences.[175]

Methylation and another process called acetylation are also common ways of reversibly modifying histone proteins in chromatin, proteins essential for organizing and packaging the DNA within the nucleus. Histone acetylation tends to loosen chromatin, facilitating gene transcription (activation), while histone methylation can have either an activating or repressing effect on gene expression, depending on the type of histone that is modified and the site of modification. Both processes can result in ongoing changes in the phenotype and behavior of an organism, including the facilitation of learning and memory.[172,176,177,178] Importantly, the pattern of histone methylation in neuronal chromatin from the prefrontal cortex also differs between humans and both chimpanzees and macaque monkeys, changes that may have occurred as a result of positive selection.[179]

Finally, once made, mRNA can be targeted and degraded by so-called microRNAs and can be sequestered within nuclear compartments, and the message can be degraded at different rates. mRNA can also be spliced into different forms, where exons from a gene can be either included or excluded in the processed mRNA, meaning a single gene can encode multiple mRNA splice variants and hence (potentially) multiple proteins. RNA editing to modify the transcriptome (the set of all RNA molecules being made in a cell or tissue) is more common in humans than in other primates, and most importantly, this editing differs between tissues and occurs most frequently in the brain.[169,180] And as if that wasn't enough, proteins are also subject to extensive modifications; after production from mRNAs in cellular structures called ribosomes, proteins can be cut into various lengths and chemically modified in a variety of ways (eg by phosphorylation) to alter their activity and efficacy. Knowing our complement of genes, and comparing it with living relatives and with dead ancestors, is obviously important and instructive, but I hope by now you are convinced that such knowledge reveals only a fraction of the story, and cannot tell us about the limits of phenotypic plasticity in our brains.

New neurons, learning, and memory

One other factor may also set us apart. It is well established that neurons continue to be created (neurogenesis) in the hippocampus of adult mice and rats, and that this neurogenesis is important in some aspects of learning and memory behavior in these species.[181,182] Exercise and environmental enrichment increase plasticity and the number of new neurons that are born in adult rodents,[183] as do social interactions and behaviours,[184] while social deprivation and stress have negative effects,[185,186] and there may be a link between altered neurogenesis and depression in humans.[187] Excitingly, it is now clear that new neurons are indeed produced in the human hippocampus. An ex-graduate student of mine, Kirsty Spalding, in association with numerous colleagues, proved this by developing a complex technique that measures the amount of carbon isotope 14 (C^{14}) in the DNA of cells obtained postmortem from humans.[188] C^{14} levels in the atmosphere peaked during the period of above-ground atomic bomb tests in the 1950s/early '60s, and have declined ever since. When cells divide they incorporate carbon into the newly formed DNA, so measurement of how much C^{14} is in the DNA gives an indication of when the cells were born. Neurogenesis in the adult human hippocampus (see Figure 2.9) occurs at surprisingly high levels and, unlike rodents, continues into old age. The cells are born in a sub-region of the hippocampus called the dentate gyrus, which is critically involved in the formation and consolidation of new memories. This sub-population of adult-born neurons lives for a shorter time than other cells in the hippocampus, but there is continued cell renewal. Spalding and colleagues estimate that we make about 1,400 new neurons per day, and in the renewing fraction there is an annual turnover of about 1.75% of cells. This proportion of "exchangeable" neurons is much higher in humans than in rodents, and levels are similar in males and females.

New neurons in the dentate gyrus form new connections that are highly plastic, and may allow us to "cope with change and novelty" and might even "prominently contribute to the individualization of the brain and thus the shaping of personality."[189] Earlier research found that London taxi drivers with advanced spatial and navigational skills had a larger posterior hippocampus[190]—I wonder if they also generated more neurons? New neurons and their incorporation into existing circuitry may help us meld new autobiographical memories into old ones, and allow us to separate new experiences from similar previous events.[191] Interestingly the hippocampus, with links to the hypothalamus, is also involved in affective processing, both positive (joy, compassion, empathy) and negative (fear, stress), and may play a role in social attachment and even in an individual's emotional personality.[192,193] Social interactions in experimental animals can enhance neurogenesis[184]—is the same true for *Homo sapiens*? Social attachment and interactions are important to us, throughout life, and it is therefore fascinating that at least two of the genes that differ between Neanderthals and humans make proteins essential for maintaining neurogenesis in the adult brain.[146]

It has been known for many years that, during cell division, parts of the genome (termed retrotransposons) copy themselves to RNA and then back to DNA, which is then integrated back into the genome in a different location, potentially changing "conventional" gene expression. In regions of the mammalian brain involved in learning (especially parts of the hippocampus), environmental stimuli influence these mobile elements of the genome, potentially contributing to plasticity, learning, and memory in adult brains.[176,194,195] Perhaps, then, the new neurons we now know to be born in our hippocampus have a genetic "hard drive" that is epigenetically altered by earlier life experiences? In animals, stress and mood may alter the levels of neurogenesis, and it is therefore intriguing that some have hypothesized that music, which influences steroid and cortisol levels,[196] may impact on neurogenesis.[197] We shall see in Chapter 8 that hippocampal volume in older humans is related to cardiovascular fitness, but also to exposure to music— does that mean more neurons are indeed being made and incorporated into hippocampal circuitry when we participate in social interactions driven by pleasurable musical activities, perhaps especially if dancing is involved?!

Genes, language, and intellect

So what do we know about our genetic history and loquacity? Bearing in mind all of the important provisos that I have discussed regarding the importance of non-coding mRNAs and epigenetic regulation of our brain DNA, an increasing number of genomic studies have nonetheless uncovered numerous intriguing human-specific micromutations of many protein-coding genes (the interested reader is referred to a recent review by Bae et al, 2015).[198] It is a tenuous link I know, but can any of these gene polymorphisms be related in any way to the evolution of speech and modern language behaviors, and perhaps more specifically to the evolution of a neural architecture that permits greater adaptability, enhanced vocal learning and articulate capability, a greater and more efficient memory and overall learning capacity, and, of course, greater reasoning power and intelligence?

There is rarely, if ever, a clear relationship between a gene and a complex behavioral or cognitive phenotype,[199] and in the following discussion we would do well to bear in mind these cautionary words: "Genes do not specify behaviours or cognitive processes; they make regulatory factors, signaling molecules, receptors, enzymes, and so on, that interact in highly complex networks, modulated by environmental influences, in order to build and maintain the brain."[48] A tangled web indeed, although numerous twin studies have revealed that there is a measurable genetic contribution not only to brain structure and plasticity, but also to working memory, cognitive ability, and "intelligence."[141,142,143,144,145,200,201] Even here there are issues however, because even in twins born in the USA, the extent to which intelligence (IQ measures) is heritable is influenced by the socioeconomic status of the home environment in which the children are raised.[202]

The term meta-analysis is a statistical approach that is used to combine and analyze all the results from a number of previous studies in order to uncover significant patterns or interactions in the data that may not have been evident in the original, individual studies. In a massive genome-wide association study involving a sample of over 100,000 individuals, several gene variants (SNPs) were identified that seem to be weakly associated with cognitive function, or at least with "educational attainment," which involves both heritable, environmental, and social factors.[203,204] Furthermore, genes do impact on individual differences in human intelligence (reasoning, problem-solving, acquired knowledge, etc), but in this case it appears that the heritable association is polygenic, "with many genes of small effects underlying the additive genetic influences on intelligence."[205] Importantly, in the context of human evolution, the genetic evidence suggests that intelligence is a selectable trait, even more so than personality or physical appearance.[206] There also appears to have been selection for alleles that afford at least some protection against cognitive decline in aging humans. Presumably, "such selection would operate by maximizing the contributions of postreproductive individuals to the fitness of younger kin,"[207] and I would argue that such selection would, in the long term, also benefit the social/cultural group as a whole.

With specific reference to genes and linguistic ability, earlier studies on "normal" adult human brains found no evidence of genes that were uniquely expressed in known language-related areas.[208] However, some possible candidates are now emerging, derived from studies of individuals or families with language-related disorders that cannot be explained by some other neurological cause such as mental retardation, autism, or hearing deficits.[209,210] As an example, specific language impairment (SLI) is a persistent impairment in language ability that is inherited through the family, and is known to affect as many as 5–8% of the English-speaking pre-school population.

Another intriguing and widely cited example of a heritable gene variant that affects language is the forkhead box P2 (FOXP2) gene.[48,199] The gene is located on human chromosome number 7 and codes for a transcription factor (see earlier). FOXP2 expression varies during development and is found in many tissues of the body, not just the brain. It is thought that the FOXP2 transcription factor may bind to, and presumably regulate, several hundred human gene promoters in the nervous system, often by repressing genes that are likely to be involved in molecular/cellular functions such as cell differentiation, axonal growth and guidance, signaling, plasticity, or synaptic function.[211,212,213] In the human brain, FOXP2 is expressed bilaterally in many regions, including the cerebral cortex, part of the basal ganglia known as the striatum, and the cerebellum, but the gene is only expressed by subsets of neurons within those regions.[209] Point mutations of the FOXP2 gene in humans have been linked to individuals who have problems with selecting and coordinating orofacial movements necessary for fluent speech production (verbal dyspraxia) and also lack several other language skills.[210] Recent work suggests that, in humans, the FOXP2 gene specifically affects aspects of neuronal morphology and the functionality of sensory and motor (sensorimotor) circuits between the cerebral cortex, cerebellum, and basal ganglia.[214] According to Enard, these circuits may not be needed for language processing per se but might be relevant in "the context of language acquisition," for example in learning complex motor sequences and more automated procedural tasks associated with vocal learning.

The gene is conserved in birds and mammals. In finches, for example, experimentally altered expression of FOXP2 affects learning and vocalization of "songs," effects mediated via dopamine-dependent pathways.[215] But there is also positive selection of this gene in birds that are not vocal learners, suggesting that "the selective pressure acting on FOXP2 in these birds is unrelated to vocal communication"[216]; this is a gene that can regulate many biological processes. In humans, there is evidence for the positive selection of specific mutations in the FOXP2 gene, suggesting that this version has functional importance in our species.[48] Against this, however, is the discovery that this same FOXP2 variant is also found in Neanderthals[217] and in another recently discovered archaic hominin, the Denisovan.[214,218] Apparently, the two amino-acid changes in FOXP2 common to all three hominins must have happened between 270,000 and 440,000 years ago.[46,214] More recently, another positively selected mutation in the human FOXP2 gene has been found that may have occurred as recently as 50,000–60,000 years ago.[219] The mutation is related to a binding site for a well-known transcription factor (POU3F2) that is active in the central nervous system and is itself, along with many other transcription factors, the subject of recent positive selection in humans.[159] It is suggested that earlier FOXP2 modifications allowed changes in plasticity and other qualities that were followed by "later regulatory changes that were unique to modern humans."[219] This is consistent with a relatively late advance in human language skills, and with the fact that our ancestral cousins did not possess articulate speech, a learned vocabulary and syntax, or our cognitive power.

Nonetheless, despite the clear link between FOXP2 gene mutations and aspects of speech and language dysfunction, it seems unlikely that this gene was the sole player in the changes that underlay the evolution of modern language capability in modern humans.[199] The gene is expressed bilaterally, yet cortical processing of speech and language is laterally biased, an issue raised earlier when discussing the primate mirror system. What else might have happened to take advantage of the FOXP2-enhanced forebrain circuitry in humans? There may have been additional evolutionary changes in genes transcriptionally regulated by FOXP2, genes that not only encode aspects of neural development and motor function but also other targets, including cartilage and connective tissue, "suggesting an important role for human FOXP2 in establishing both the neural circuitry and physical structures needed for spoken language."[213] Interestingly, FOXP2 regulates the transcription of a gene that encodes the protein MET, and mutations in the MET gene are a risk factor for autism, a developmental disorder that affects, among other aspects, social interaction and verbal communication (see Chapter 8).[220] Another downstream variant appears to be associated with SLI, and mutations in other candidate genes have also been implicated in language disorders.[209,210,221]

Language is built not only on grammar but also on the lexicon, the catalogue of learned words, and that library requires an efficient and high-quality memory and retrieval system in the human brain. As alluded to earlier, humans are fast learners; first words are often spoken by 9–12 months of age, with a vocabulary of up to 50 words, and three- to four-year-old children build a vocabulary by acquiring new words at an estimated rate of about ten words per day. As adults, we have a vocabulary that contains anywhere between 20,000 and 100,000 word families![41] All this learning first requires placement of new information into a short-term store, then presumably some form of implicit rehearsal is required to enable transfer into a long-term memory store. While the exact nature of the long-term memory trace (the engram) remains a mystery, new words are mapped in language areas in the temporal lobe, especially the left hemisphere, which has the "specific ability to store memory traces for familiar language elements regardless of their exact acoustic/phonological makeup."[222] The learning of new words is an incredibly rapid process involving the anterior superior-temporal areas of cortex, suggesting that "our brain may effectively form new neuronal circuits online as it gets exposed to novel patterns in the sensory input."[223]

What special features of the human brain give us this extraordinary learning capacity? As previously discussed, twin studies do suggest that heritable factors influence networks associated with working memory ability,[201] and a number of proteins and signaling pathways are now known to be involved in memory formation and consolidation.[224] Of particular interest is the small protein brain-derived neurotrophic factor (BDNF), one of many peptides that can promote the growth and plasticity of nerve processes. Expression and trafficking of the human BDNF gene is regulated by a variety of transcription factors[225] and the protein is widely expressed in the brain, especially in the hippocampus and cerebral cortex. Epigenetic modification of the histones surrounding the DNA also affects the BDNF gene, which in turn influences age-related changes in the structure and function of synapses via a number of mechanisms.[226,227,228] Overall, BDNF has important roles during brain development and is important in memory and for activity-dependent modification of neural circuits as we learn things throughout life, including interaction with excitatory neurotransmitter systems, themselves subject to evolutionary change in primates.[122] Importantly, the size of the hippocampus in older humans is correlated with circulating levels of BDNF,[229] possibly associated with increased production, maturation, and perhaps survival of new neurons in this memory-related structure throughout adult life.[188,230,231]

There are numerous small sequence differences or polymorphisms in the human BDNF gene.[232] One of these in particular—a single substitution of a nucleotide (SNP) at a particular point in the BDNF gene that produces a functional change in one amino acid (valine to methionine, termed "val66met")—results in altered processing, trafficking, and activity-dependent secretion of BDNF.[232] This single-nucleotide polymorphism in the DNA sequence of the human BDNF gene correlates with intriguing differences in activity-induced plasticity in the hippocampus.[233,234] Neuroimaging studies have also revealed that this methionine substitution affects the size of the hippocampus as well as the brain white matter (eg parts of the corpus callosum), and is associated with decreased volume of some cortical gray matter regions—including dorsolateral prefrontal cortex, which you may recall is associated with planning and higher level cognitive functions.[235] Parts of the temporal and occipital lobes are also smaller in humans carrying the val66met SNP. Differences in the connectivity and function of a number of distributed neural networks are already present in children and adolescents who carry the methionine allele.[236]

Individuals who carry the val66met polymorphism are more likely to have poorer memory of specific autobiographical events and may be more likely to have neurological problems such as schizophrenia and other psychiatric disorders, including bipolar disorder, depression, and anxiety.[232,235] If the mutated val66met form of BDNF is genetically engineered into mice, these animals generally learn new tasks less effectively, but are more likely to retain memories of aversive stimuli.[237] Such stressful/traumatic experiences are especially memorable owing to interactions between stress-related hormones and BDNF-dependent pathways.[238]

One other aspect of BDNF biology deserves mention here because this peptide has also been shown to modulate reward behaviors via the dopamine neuromodulator system.[239] Interestingly, polymorphisms of the BDNF gene interact with mutations in the gene encoding an enzyme (catechol-O-methyltransferase, COMT) that breaks down dopamine. These interactions affect cortical plasticity and, most interestingly for us in the present context, they affect an individual's ability to recognize and learn an artificial grammar.[240] As we shall see in Chapter 4, dopamine reward systems and musical appreciation are intimately linked, so it is unfortunate that musical ability was not tested in these subjects!

Variants of BDNF are not the only example of factors that impact either directly or indirectly on hippocampal structure and memory performance in *Homo sapiens*. Genetic variability in a serotonin receptor and a cluster of genes involved in memory-related signalling molecules have been correlated with episodic memory performance and reduced gray matter volume in the hippocampus and temporal lobe of human subjects.[241,242,243] SNPs in another growth factor known as fibroblast growth factor 20 are also associated with changes in the quality of verbal memory, the volume of the hippocampus, and how the hippocampus decreases in size with age.[244] There is also evidence that polymorphisms in receptors involved in the trafficking of lipids such as cholesterol impact on neuronal and synaptic plasticity, again with known links to neurodegenerative and neuropsychiatric disorders.[245] Physical exercise is now known to enhance hippocampal neurogenesis and have antidepressant effects, in part owing to secretion of a hormone called adiponectin, made in fat cells but also perhaps in the brain itself.[246]

KIBRA is a protein that interacts with a postsynaptic protein known as dendrin, as well as with other elements of the structural matrix within cells (the cytoskeleton).[247] These are all proteins associated with synapses, in particular on small processes on the dendrites called dendritic spines, where the great majority of excitatory synapses are found, especially in the cerebral cortex. These spines are the postsynaptic components of a synapse and are highly plastic during development. The greater the number of spines per neuron, the greater the number of excitatory contacts and potential combinations of activity, and it is therefore very interesting—from an evolutionary perspective—that neurons in the human cerebral cortex have a higher spine density than other species, including primates.[9] The shape and distribution of these spines on dendritic processes also differ between species, which will affect the strength of incoming signals on individual neurons. Neural activity can potentiate or depress signal transmission between neurons, and there are associated, usually more long-term, changes in the number and shape of dendritic spines.[248] This so-called "experience-dependent" functional plasticity alters the effectiveness of synapses between neurons, and thus potentially is the structural basis for the changes that occur in the pattern and weighting of circuits during learning and memory formation. If the protein synaptopodin is knocked out in mice for example, it results in decreased numbers of dendritic spines and impaired long-term potentiation of synaptic signaling. In addition, and potentially relevant to long-term memory capacity, KIBRA also interacts with a protein kinase that is known to be critically important to functional neural plasticity.[247]

One SNP (a T allele rather than a C allele polymorphism) of the human KIBRA gene has been reported to be associated with enhanced verbal and visual episodic memory performance[247,249,250,251]—but see Franks et al[252] for an alternate viewpoint. Initial storage of memories seems to be unaffected, but beyond about 24 hours there is enhanced memory performance in T-carriers, elevated hippocampal function, and better acquisition of long-term memory traces. This fits with data showing that T-carriers have a larger hippocampal volume, especially in sub-regions such as the dentate gyrus, which is known to be critical for memory.[253] Polymorphisms in another gene (SNAP-25) known to be involved in synaptic transmission and plasticity are associated with intelligence and cognitive ability to some degree,[254] and an SNP in another synaptic-related protein (CPEB3) is associated with performance in episodic memory tasks.[255] Because dendritic spines "may provide a structural basis for lifelong information storage, in addition to their well-established role in brain plasticity,"[256] SNPs in any of the plethora of genes that encode aspects of dendritic spine structure and function (neurotransmitter receptors, cytoskeleton, biochemistry, etc) could potentially alter processing power in the brain.[257] In fact, a very recent study found that genetic polymorphisms in a post-synaptic signalling complex involved in excitatory transmission and plasticity (the so-called "NMDA receptor complex") are associated with normal variation in human intelligence and cognitive ability,[258] emphasizing the importance of evolutionary changes in glutamatergic signaling in the primate lineage.[122]

Two other genes (ATP2C2 and CMIP) have some linkage to SLI,[259] with the former involved in calcium regulation and the latter in making a protein that forms part of the link between the external surface of the cell and the internal cytoskeleton. Potentially both may be involved in neuronal migration, synapse formation, and plasticity, and thus both may be linked to memory-related components of language acquisition and performance. Similarly, a recent analysis of the evolutionary history of ten genes implicated in SLI (and dyslexia) identified several genes (eg ROBO1) important in adhesion and axon guidance that may also be involved in hearing and speech.[216] Finally, to return to FOXP2, one gene that it regulates by suppressing transcription is the CNTNAP2 gene,[212] also on human chromosome 7. What is interesting about the CNTNAP2 gene is that it codes for a protein that "mediates interactions between neurons and glia during nervous system development."[209] A number of SNPs in this gene are associated with SLI, and especially language-related tasks that require a non-impaired short-term memory.[260]

Overall, together with the data on polymorphisms in genes that make growth factors and cytoskeletal proteins, I find the additional association of FOXP2 and various SLI-linked genes with neuron-glia interactions and plasticity especially exciting: a mélange of SNPs in the human genome influencing fine motor control, learning, and memory—all essential elements in the creation of new skill sets that surely must underpin the evolution of human language, with a vocabulary of thousands of words and the capacity to hear, learn, and then produce, articulate speech. But such SNPs are likely to have even more subtle and diverse effects on our species than that. As we shall see in Chapter 5, as well as micromutations that affect synaptic plasticity and cognitive performance, there is emerging evidence for genetic links to altruistic and prosocial behaviors, and in the more creative and/or emotional/empathic aspects of human behavior, including music and dance.

Finally, in addition to gene-driven, cell-intrinsic alterations in structure and function, other more global adaptive changes may also have occurred that led to subtly altered interconnections between different brain regions. Some unique characteristics of the cellular and connectional architecture of the human brain have already been discussed earlier in this chapter. Any change in the type and size of connections may have been driven by genetic micromutations, and/or existing cortical circuits could have been co-opted to perform different functions. Perhaps several such changes, together with altered neural processing capacity and plasticity, acted in a synergistic way to underpin our transition to a new hominin species. As Vilayanur Ramachandran has suggested, some additional cross-talk or cross-wiring may have emerged between existing brain regions, facilitating intermodal processing and "cross-modal abstraction."[261] We shall come back to this idea later on in this chapter when specifically discussing language evolution.

How old are we? Y chromosomes and mitochondria

While our immediate ancestors were surely capable of performing complex tasks and presumably possessed a cognitive architecture capable of reasonably sophisticated levels of thought and communication, the brains of *Homo sapiens* appear to possess an even more elaborate and flexible computational architecture, one that evolved in association with articulate language, sentience, enhanced social and cultural interactions, and a new awareness of "self." When did this happen, and where did we begin?

The general consensus is that we are perhaps 200,000 years old, at least in terms of modern skeletons, and that modern humans originated in the African continent. In his book *Lone Survivors*,[39] the paleoanthropologist Chris Stringer has summarized the skeletal features that characterize the species termed *Homo sapiens*. These include a large brain volume, a unique brain case morphology, a small and divided brow ridge, a bony chin, and changes to the auditory apparatus in the middle ear, as well as distinguishing features of the pelvis and thigh bones. There is evidence of what are thought to be early "anatomically modern humans" at the Omo site in Ethiopia, which have recently been dated to about 195,000 years,[262] and sporadic fossil and genetic evidence for the presence of *Homo sapiens* in the Middle East and Asia about 100,000–130,000 years ago.[263,264,265,266,267,268] These early migrations of *Homo sapiens* out of Africa may have been driven by a "megadrought" on the African continent dated at between 75,000 and 135,000 years ago, and by the presence of a more favorable humid environment further to the north.[267,269,270,271]

It is interesting to note that many of these fossils also appear to have some archaic hominin features as well.[272] For example, in Ethiopia 154,000- to 160,000-year-old skulls have human features yet they do not match living populations, and the famous human fossils found at Qafzeh and Skhull in the Levant (at the eastern end of the Mediterranean)— dated at about 90,000–120,000 years old—show considerable variability and are said to be more "robust" than modern humans. According to paleontologists, there is no doubt that these fossils have at least some morphological features that define them as skeletally "modern" humans, yet to my mind it seems unlikely that these individuals were entirely "modern" in terms of brains and brain power. Could there have been subsequent, critical evolution of the human brain into a much more aware and sophisticated structure, some tens of thousands of years later, that further improved the fitness and adaptability of the host species? The exact sequence of any such events must remain speculative, but numerous independent strands of evidence strongly suggest that something happened to *Homo sapiens* less than 100,000 years ago, perhaps in a relatively short period of time, that included the emergence of modern syntactic language and articulate speech,[273] increased memory capacity, new patterns of technology and social organization,[263] the evolution of a modern cortical interconnectional architecture, enhanced and more adaptable intercellular communication, and along with all of this, the origin of the modern human mind.

The term "archaic *Homo sapiens*" has sometimes been used to describe the early members of our fossil lineage, and the term *"Homo sapiens sapiens"* to define anatomically "modern" humans. The qualifying term "anatomically modern" is used to "identify our early ancestors that were physically much the same as living humans, but also to distinguish them from earlier hominins that could be called 'human' at some level based on features such as increased brain size relative to body size and the possession of material culture (including stone tools)."[274] The nomenclature *Homo sapiens sapiens* has also been used to distinguish us from *"Homo sapiens neanderthalensis"* because some anthropologists regard Neanderthals as a subspecies of *Homo sapiens* rather than an altogether separate species (ie *Homo neanderthalensis*). Our shared common ancestor—based on fossil evidence and genomic DNA studies, and acknowledging all the assumptions required for this kind of analysis—diverged from modern humans anywhere between about 450,000 and 700,000 years ago.[43,44,146,268,275,276,277,278,279] In the new binomial, taxonomic nomenclature devised in the eighteenth century by the great Carl Linnaeus in his now classic *Systema Naturae*, the term *Homo sapiens* was used to define modern humans. According to the *Oxford English Dictionary, Homo sapiens* is "the human species, the form of man represented by the surviving races and varieties," and the term made its English debut in the 1797 edition of *Encyclopaedia Britannica*.

But where does a 195,000-year-old fossil with an advanced skeletal form regarded as characteristic of *Homo sapiens*[262] fit into this, especially when I and many others take the view that modern language, articulate speech, and the modern sentient mind evolved some time later? With temerity, some years ago I suggested that the term *Homo sapientior* ("wiser" as opposed to "wise") might be more helpful in defining the beginning of this next (but not necessarily last?!) essentially neural and cognitive phase of human evolution. This term was subsequently taken up by my colleague Charles Oxnard in his book *The Scientific Bases of Human Anatomy*.[280] In the eighteenth century the alternative term *Homo loquens* ("having the power of speech, talking, articulate"—*Oxford Latin Dictionary*) was suggested by people such as the German philosopher J. G. Herder and the physician/anthropologist J. F. Blumenbach. More recently this term was again put forward by Chernigovskaya,[281] although as we shall see, language is not unimodal and can operate and be effectively used in the absence of speech. It could also be argued that you cannot describe a thing in a communicable way unless you think of it first.

We clearly have no evidence from the existing fossil record of when this new language-driven brain variant emerged in our species. This neurological revolution did not obviously reveal itself in the bones of *Homo sapiens*. This is not a new insight: papers on the origins of language were banned in 1866 by the Société de Linguistique de Paris because "fossil records could provide no evidence concerning linguistic competence."[282] To quote the anthropologist Ian Tattersall, there seems to be "no correlation whatever between the achievement in the human lineage of behavioral modernity and anatomical modernity."[283] As discussed later in Chapter 4, fossils provide some clues about our ancestors' capacity for breath control and production of complex vocalizations. But there are other more compelling markers of cognitive change over the past 100,000 years: we have artefacts and tools, and later on we find decorative art and symbolic figures. We have evidence of an apparent explosion of culture—clear indicators of modern human behavior, of recognizable intelligence.

As I have already argued, there must have been some positive selection of phenotype, underpinned by perhaps some relatively minor changes in genes such as those highlighted earlier in this chapter, changes that gave us a clear biological and intellectual superiority over closely related hominins, intelligence-related traits that were the subject of positive selection.[206] From that time onward we rapidly evolved and out-competed our relatives, and as a result one particular African-born subgroup of *Homo sapiens*, with a particular combination of genetic variants, became the dominant founder population from which all of us have now sprung.[39,45,271,284,285,286,287] What might have provided the impetus for this change, the selection and heritable success of this novel "*Homo sapientior*" genotype? And when might it have occurred?

Factors that impact on species survival and selection are usually multifactorial and are often interrelated. As again summarized by Chris Stringer, from a human perspective these forces could have been "climatic, dietary, social or even volcanic."[39] Members of such a group must have had some special attributes that provided a selective advantage during food shortages, climatic stresses, and so on, that allowed them to survive and continue to nourish, nurture, and perhaps clothe their slow-growing, highly dependent offspring, enabling members of the species to persist through adversity. It is reasonable to propose that these important attributes included not just a more diverse and nutrient-sufficient diet and better access and use of resources, but heightened social interactions and cooperative behaviors that were enhanced by a novel, highly sophisticated communication system that included language and articulate speech. Together with this advanced mode of communication, it is presumed, came the capacity to evolve a more complex and representational cognitive architecture that allowed newly acquired information to be transmitted within and, critically, *between* generations. As the eminent Cambridge archaeologist Paul Mellars wrote: "perhaps it was the emergence of more complex language and other forms of symbolic communication that gave the crucial adaptive advantage to fully modern populations and led to their subsequent dispersal across Asia and Europe ... ."[288] Importantly, our early founder members must also have possessed a neural architecture that produced and responded to the other uniquely human and universal communication stream, music.

In biology, the term "bottleneck" is used to describe adverse environmental events that put severe constraints on species and their ability to survive. We have seen that, within a species, there is often genetic drift, where there are a number of different populations with slight genetic differences. At some point a new environmental pressure suddenly appears, and members of one of these populations may have an advantage over all the others and therefore survive better or reproduce better. That population then moves ahead and the others may die out or become assimilated into the new, evolutionarily more viable group. Environmentally induced bottlenecks drastically reduce population size and usually reduce the amount of genetic variation in the surviving population. In turn, this may reduce adaptation potential to further environmental challenges—in other words, bottlenecks can be detrimental and reduce the opportunity for positive natural selection.

However, there is a special case of genetic drift termed the "founder effect," where a small group of individuals in a population separates from the original one and forms a new population, an event that can be precipitated by a bottleneck. Again, reduction in genetic diversity may be a disadvantage, but perhaps our ancestors actually carried a cohort of genes that proved to be of great survival value in a time of crisis. In fact, mathematical modeling suggests that mutants that arise from random genetic drift have an even greater chance of success when they are at the forefront of a rapidly expanding population that has a clear selective advantage, termed the "surfing effect."[52] There is evidence that serial founder effects have been an important influence on *Homo sapiens* populations since their expansion within, and their migration out of, Africa,[289] and there is also evidence that, at around this time, there were many small, geographically isolated and genetically varied populations of anatomically modern humans in sub-Saharan Africa.[290] Some of these populations survived—for example, the humans in southern and eastern Africa who speak click languages (clicks are used as consonants) appear to have separated from other modern human lineages some tens of thousands of years ago.[291,292] The size of founder populations is almost certainly quite small and the initial founder population from which our own species all derive may have contained as few as 2,000–10,000 individuals.[94,274,293,294] And we had a new type of brain....

In this context it is now appropriate to discuss an interesting but still highly controversial theory expounded by Professor Stanley Ambrose, concerning a catastrophic event that happened 74,000–76,000 years ago on the island of Sumatra.[295] This is the eruption of the mega-colossal volcano called Toba. The remnants of that explosion can still be seen as Lake Toba in Sumatra. Regarded as the biggest single eruption in the last million or so years, it has been estimated to have been anywhere between 1,000 and 5,000 times the size of Mount St Helens, the eruption cloud containing gases, ash, and rocks reaching a height of perhaps 30 km.

Researchers have studied climactic and biological changes that occurred as a result of the eruption. While recent studies suggest that global cooling effects were not as widespread or as dramatic as once thought,[296,297] there is a general consensus that the explosion would have resulted in an overall decrease in temperatures as well as a decrease in sea surface temperatures (and eventually sea levels). Some scientists believe the event may even have contributed to the coldest 1,000 years in the most recent ice age.[298] In the aftermath of this mega-colossal eruption there were widespread ash deposits of many centimeters in South Asia and the Indian sub-continent, and in parts of Malaysia and India these deposits were several meters deep.[299] Perhaps just as important as a temperature decline was the occurrence of devastating noxious (sulfuric) acid rain, and tsunamis, and because of massive quantities of dust and sulfuric aerosols in the atmosphere, there was relatively widespread loss of trees, plants, and, presumably, animals. Changes include a rapid decline in pollen counts in distant sites—such as the Grand Pile peat bog near Belfort in eastern France,[300] and a rapid decrease in the number of taxonomic groups of trees as far away as southern Italy. There may also have been a depletion of the ozone layer, which further compromised plant life.

These are changes that signal rapid environmental change, all presumably a consequence of this mega-colossal eruption. Ambrose has suggested that this catastrophic event created enormous and sudden environmental pressures and created a bottleneck that "*Homo sapientior*" somehow managed to squeeze through. One problem with this idea is evidence that Toba did not substantially lower the temperature in East Africa,[297] although there may have been other environmental changes that combined to threaten hominin existence. If Professor Ambrose and his colleagues are correct, and such a bold idea is—and should be—the subject of much debate and discussion, then the timing of this hypothetical bottleneck at about 74,000–76,000 years ago is very interesting because it is not long after the range of dates proposed for the origin of modern humans, dates that have been estimated using very different types of markers and analyses. These analyses are themselves not without controversy, and there is considerable latitude in the assumptions that are used, but I will attempt to lay out the essential caveats as I discuss the current thoughts on how old "*Homo sapientior*" really is.

Modern molecular genetics, and with it the development of new ways to handle and interpret the vast amount of data that is acquired with these techniques, have added important new information relating to the genealogy of *Homo sapiens*. As each generation produces the next, germline mutations in the DNA of sperm or eggs accumulate over time, theoretically providing a time-line of genetic change. There are various ways of measuring this change. One approach is to use so-called coalescence methodology, which allows researchers to work backwards from genetic markers (samples of DNA) from closely related living species (eg humans and chimpanzees) or from members of different human population groups in order to develop gene trees that identify the most likely common or shared ancestral population, and the possible geographical location from which all current individuals are derived (phylogenetic studies). Comparison of ancient DNA from fossil material in the human lineage is another important approach. Finally, recent high-powered molecular sequencing technology has permitted the analysis of germline mutations that occur in transmission from living parents to their offspring (pedigree studies). Obtaining and interpreting data from multiple DNA sites in different chromosomes and different human individuals require great care in handling any material (to prevent contamination), sophisticated molecular processing, immense data-processing power, and highly complex statistical and bioinformatic analysis capability.[301]

Essentially what scientists are looking at is the rate of change of DNA sequences over time—a molecular clock. So what are the assumptions that can affect such analyses? These have recently been nicely summarized in a number of articles,[292,301,302,303,304,305,306,307] and the interested reader can refer to these if he/she so desires. If I can summarize, the issues relate to a number of hard-to-quantify variables and depend on exactly what material is being analyzed. For example, fossil DNA is obtained not from the germline but almost always from bones. Similarly, in pedigree studies, DNA sampling of living people may not be from eggs or sperm; are mutations in somatic cells (the cells that make up the tissues of the body) necessarily the same as those in the germline? The basal mutation rate can also vary for different types of mutations, depending on exactly how the DNA is altered. Another potential confounder is that the mutation rate of DNA sequences is unlikely to be constant across evolutionary time. We know that rates vary between species—larger body size seems to be associated with decreased mutation rates—and in humans there is clear evidence that mutation rates increase with paternal age and may vary between different modern human populations. Furthermore, the rate of mutation also depends on generation time—at what age each generation produces the next—and this may also have varied across tens of thousands of years. Finally, the rate at which males generate sperm is not constant: we make less sperm than our living hominid relatives, and there is a decline in spermatogenesis in humans with age as well as a decreased sperm count in many young modern-day humans—some say due to wearing underwear and tight jeans!

Some sequence changes in a gene may *not* be the result of a frank mutation, but may be a consequence of DNA repair, the efficiency of which may vary across species and/or across evolutionary time. It is also possible that the same gene sequence may mutate more than once, affecting interpretation of results. Finally, only neutral mutations—those that do not compromise the species—are indicative of a mutation rate because deleterious genes would presumably be removed by natural selection. And any improved mate selection process that could well have occurred in "*Homo sapientior*" might have gradually removed lineages in which mutation rates tended to be higher.

So what do the data tell us—given the uncertainties briefly summarized above? Lineage information can be obtained from either paternal or maternal lines. The Y chromosome is required for the generation of males, and thus analysis of what is termed the non-recombining part of the Y chromosome genotype permits a study of paternal ancestry (patrilineage). The Y chromosome contains many regions that show little or no recombination, meaning that its DNA rarely breaks and rejoins with a different part of the DNA strand. This lack of paternal genetic change from generation to generation can help when researchers attempt to create an ancestral genetic tree across tens of thousands of years.[308] The other way of assessing genetic change comes from an analysis of maternal lineage relationships. In most nucleated cells in multicellular organisms DNA is also present in intracellular structures called mitochondria, organelles in the cytoplasm that may originally have been colonizing protobacteria and that are now essential for aerobic respiration, thus providing energy to each cell. This mitochondrial DNA (mtDNA) contains only about 16,000 base pairs, makes comparatively few proteins, and is found in large quantities in the female egg at the time of fertilization by a sperm. Sperm contain very little mtDNA, and any that is present seems to be destroyed or lost. Thus, mtDNA is passed down solely through the female line, and because there can be no intermixing of DNA from each gamete, there is minimal or no recombination, facilitating analysis and the generation of a maternal genetic tree. Note here that mutation rates appear to be slightly different depending on whether the DNA is sourced from the Y chromosome or from mitochondria.

There is general agreement that coalescence analysis of the sequence variability in Y-chromosome genes points to an African origin for our species.[263,285,294,309,310] The timing of this origin, our most recent common ancestor, is far more contentious. The confidence limits to these coalescence dates are very large, in part owing to a range of assumptions that need to be made.[302,305,307,308,311,312] These assumptions include estimates of the size of any founder population, and what happened to its offspring. Nevertheless, while still the subject of energetic debate,[39,305] estimates suggest that the ancestral founder population males—our most recent common ancestors, or "Adam" as the founder has sometimes been called(!)—who contributed some of their genome to all future human generations, were living anywhere between about 65,000 and 110,000 years ago. Carbon dating the exact age of fossils from which Y chromosomal DNA is obtained would help to reduce these uncertainties,[305] something recently performed for mtDNA (see below).

Initial studies strongly suggested that our most recent common maternal ancestor(s) ("Eve" or "mitochondrial Eve") was/were living in Africa in a relatively small population about 200,000 years ago.[274] Further analysis has suggested that our most recent common ancestor in our maternal lineage may have been around anywhere from 120,000 to 197,000 years ago.[292,313,314] Humans are remarkably similar in their genetic makeup, with much less variation than that found in the mtDNA of apes or chimpanzees, consistent with our species being relatively new in evolutionary terms, and perhaps also consistent with one (or more) bottleneck events. Nonetheless, owing to mutations there continues to be some variation in mtDNA sequences, and a close look at genetic diversity in mtDNA has revealed important information on the complex time-frame of modern human evolution.

Using a mathematical analysis called Bayesian coalescent inference, Atkinson et al described four major variants (termed haplotypes) of African mtDNA.[315] While there is increasing evidence that there were a number of periodic, sequential migrations out of Africa after skeletally modern *Homo sapiens* first emerged in the African continent,[268,271] of particular interest to me was the finding that there was a last and rapid expansion of the group carrying one of these four mtDNA haplotypes (L3) between 61,000 and 86,000 years ago. This L3 haplotype is the mitochondrial variant that is found in *all* humans outside Africa. Within Africa, L3-carrying populations originally in eastern Africa expanded rapidly, with migration into central and southern parts of the continent, perhaps driven by improved climactic conditions.[316]

Based on analysis of the L3 haplotype, one study put an upper time limit on the migration out of Africa of the founders of all non-African humans now alive at about 70,000 years (confidence limits 59,000–73,000).[316] This is consistent with a more recent report estimating the origin of *all* non-African (L3) mtDNA haplotypes at 72,000 years[278]—not long after the Toba eruption! These dates are similar to at least some of the Y chromosome date estimates for "Adam," meaning that a potential date of successful migration out of Africa derived from our small "uniparental" founding population could have been as early as 60,000–65,000 years ago.[284,285] Again consistent with all of this, a study examining potentially deleterious mutations in European versus African populations found less overall genetic diversity in Europeans, but a higher proportion of weakly deleterious versions of genes (alleles) in the European population, consistent with an "out of Africa" bottleneck, the emigrant "*Homo sapientior*" population eventually coming to differ somewhat from the population that stayed behind.[317]

A spanner was thrown into the works of the phylogenetic/paleontological dating of modern human evolution by a genomic study that measured mutations in living parents and their offspring which suggested that mutation rates were perhaps half as common as had previously been assumed, which would essentially double the date of origin of our most common human ancestors, and when we left Africa.[318] I have already discussed the uncertainties regarding mutation rates, yet these new data from pedigree studies were hard to fit with other paleontological and anthropological data. Then, the following year, Fu and colleagues analyzed mtDNA from ten carbon-dated fossils, spanning 40,000 years of human history.[292] Admittedly, mutation rates in mtDNA do not necessarily reflect mutation rates in germline DNA; nonetheless, analysis of carefully dated mtDNA suggested that perhaps the original date windows were about right. Examining the L3 mtDNA haplotype, the researchers concluded that the separation of non-Africans from closely related sub-Saharan Africans occurred between 62,000 and 95,000 years ago, with a mean of 78,300 years. As mentioned earlier, others have also recently estimated this separation and calculated/estimated a figure of 72,000 years ago.[278]

The jury is still out, and uncertainties remain. A recent report statistically analyzing mtDNA obtained from European hunter-gatherers spanning 35,000 years of prehistory has estimated that emigration of all non-African modern humans was as late as 55,000 years ago, with an additional major, climate-related bottleneck in Europe about 14,500 years ago.[319] Other research analyzing DNA from a 100-year-old lock of hair from an aboriginal Australian provides an independent estimate of divergence from the ancestral Eurasian population: between 62,000 and 75,000 years ago.[320] This work supports the notion of an early expansion wave but also suggests there may have been gene flow between hypothetical later dispersal waves. To quote from Atkinson et al: "The timing of the L3 expansion—8,000–12,000 years prior to the emergence of the first non-African lineages—together with high L3 diversity in eastern Africa, strongly suggests that the human exodus from Africa and subsequent colonization of the globe was prefaced by a major expansion within Africa, perhaps driven by some cultural innovation."[315] But, and it is a *big* but, even though Australian Aborigines seem to have separated spatially very early in our evolutionary history, and constitute "one of the oldest continuous populations outside Africa,"[320] yet they possess language, music, and dance—as clear an indication as there can possibly be that the universality of both music and language was there at our very beginning, in the founder population, a population able to thrive after the environmental stresses resulting from an event or series of events that might well be, or at least include, the Toba catastrophe.

Two further clues supporting this most recent expansion of modern humans out of Africa come from DNA analysis of the bacteria that cause stomach ulcers, and genetic comparison of human lice with lice found on chimpanzees/apes. The genetic diversity of Helicobacter pylori decreases with increasing distance from East Africa, and it is thought that this bacterium had already infected humans as our founders migrated away from this region about 55,000–60,000 years ago.[321,322] In fact, our modern human ancestors may have been infected with H. pylori as long as 116,000 years ago, and infection "may have been acquired via a single host jump from an unknown, non-human host."[322] These authors also found evidence consistent with another out-of-Africa migration that occurred 36,000–52,000 years ago. Based on their analysis of human and chimpanzee/ape lice, Reed et al suggested that there had been a wave of modern human migration out of Africa no more than 100,000 years ago, involving an initially small population that may have been reduced in size owing to a bottleneck of some kind.[323] Subsequent changes in global temperatures (ice ages) and associated changes in flora and fauna, changes in sea level, and so forth, then continued to influence the timing, direction, and viability of subsequent migrations.

Evidence of human cultural activity

What about evidence of human cultural activity? Pieces of red ochre possibly used for body painting/decoration have been dated at a remarkable 164,000 years of age.[324] As pointed out by Gillian Morriss-Kay in her review, a prerequisite for body painting is reduced hair coverage, and a hair-related gene functional in apes was inactivated in the human line within the last 240,000 years. More obvious items of material culture emerge, especially in southern Africa, in the Middle Stone Age 65,000–100,000 years ago.[325,326] Artefacts that are presumed to have had some symbolic or representational significance, for example perforated snail shells and decorative patterns on ostrich shells dated at about 80,000 years old, have been discovered at Blombos Cave in South Africa.[327,328] The shells appear to have holes pierced in them (presumably) by a bone awl. Marks around the holes suggest that they were strung together to make a necklace, bracelet, or anklet. Engraved patterns/designs on solid pieces of ochre have also been found from about that time. Similar ochre-colored perforated shell beads have also been found in a geographically dis-parate location—Morocco in northern Africa—dated at 82,000 years old.[329] What appears to be an ochre processing factory, with the processed dye stored in shells as containers, was recently identified at Blombos and dated at 100,000 years old.[330]

Archaeologists have also found beads, microliths (technologically more advanced stone tools), barbed points, tools made from bone, and other "advanced" implements dated at about 75,000–85,000 years old. Exciting evidence of the innovative manufacture of sophisticated ornaments and tools has recently been discovered in southern Africa at Still Bay and Howieson's Poort, dated to about 71,000–72,000 and 60,000–65,000 years old respectively.[331] By about 70,000 years ago, "*Homo sapientior*" had learned to manu-facture adhesives or plant resins to attach tools or weapons to a handle or somesuch.[326] Our ancestors had been making tools for at least a million years, with increasing sophis-tication, involving the evolution of new neural circuits in the cerebral cortex.[117,332] But at Blombos there are subtle varieties of bone tools, perhaps used for different purposes, leading experts to propose that "the differences in the technical procedures are probable indices of the different social roles of the users and of clearly distinct contexts of use of the two tool categories. It is logical to believe that in order to be passed from generation to generation, this difference in tool manufacturing must have been linguistically trans-mitted. Only a modern language, with its corollary of symbolic implications, can transmit a finishing technique that results in an almost imperceptible difference in appearance, to create meaning."[333] Similarly, subtle changes in the manufacture of string beads at Blombos about 75,000 years ago suggest a social influence on the design and production of symbolic material.[334] Whether this presumed language capability was truly modern has been questioned;[335] nonetheless, it seems clear that our ancestors were now able to coordi-nate and communicate within and across generations at an unprecedented cognitive level.

Overall then, such finds from prehistory 75,000–90,000 years ago provide evidence of a desire for personal ornamentation and the beginnings of a sophisticated, if sporadic, human culture with the capacity to plan and produce complex designs and conceptual symbols.[263,326] The apparent transience of many of these more complex decorative and tool-making technologies may just be due to a paucity of discovered archaeological mate-rial, or may be a genuine phenomenon. Perhaps in some groups there was no need for particular tools or implements, or perhaps cumulative technological advances were lost owing to changes in the size of sub-populations, skills being forgotten when populations moved or became less dense, with reduced sociality and inter-group interactions.[325,336,337] Human cognitive capacity and linguistic capability presumably continued to evolve to some extent, and by 45,000–40,000 years ago we find the emergence of a variety of indicators of modern symbolic human behavior,[336,337,338] including jewelry, representational figurines, improved tools, and cave paintings in Spain, France, and as far away as Indonesia.[339,340,341] In Steven Mithen's *The Prehistory of the Mind*,[342] he argues that this cultural revolution indicated a new cognitive architecture in our species, which he suggests evolved when separate domains or modules of the mind became accessible to each other—what he calls "cognitive fluidity." This resulted in an explosion of creativity and invention, with information and skills transferable from one domain to another. This interesting idea is in some ways not dissimilar to Ramachandran's "cross-modal abstraction" hypothesis involving the evolution of additional wiring and cross-talk between cortical regions.[261]

Musicality

A recent meta-analysis of many thousands of twin pairs found that the heritability of intelligence increases significantly between childhood and adulthood, a likely explanation being that "small genetic differences are magnified as children select, modify and create environments correlated with their genetic propensities."[206] In the same way, in a small founder population of "*Homo sapientior*," mate selection driven by cognitive/communication abilities might have been important in ensuring creativity and adaptability during times of environmental stress. This would have accelerated the selection of gene variants that underpinned, for example, enhanced planning skills, memory, vocabulary, and linguistic skills, in so doing guaranteeing the effective transfer of information within and across generations. And if it is true, as I argue in this book, that music acts (and has always acted) as one of the most powerful initiators of social/empathic behavior, was it also necessary to ensure a musical pedigree to foster prosocial, inter-individual cooperativity when critically needed? If this is the case, then when do we first see evidence of musicality in modern humans? This is tricky because until relatively recently there would have been little or no trace of music in our evolving human society. The voice leaves no trace (until the invention of recording technology of course), neither does dance, and it is only after the invention of non-wooden instruments or the survival of drawn or written evidence of music and notation that we can find evidence of musical activity/creativity. Perhaps the strings of shells and beads that have been found in Africa were rattled, or put around ankles to make a rhythmic noise when dancing?

A piece of bear thigh bone with two clear holes spaced in a similar fashion to holes in a flute was found in a Slovenian cave in Eastern Europe, dated at about 40,000–45,000 years old.[343] This artefact has been described as a Neanderthal flute because it was found amid other sorts of Neanderthal debris, but this conclusion remains highly controversial. Some argue that the holes were deliberately made by a hominin, but many others argue equally forcefully that it is far more likely that the holes were made by the teeth of a predator or scavenging animal.[333] Even if this artefact is a kind of primitive flute (which I think is unlikely), Neanderthals and *Homo sapiens* coexisted for many thousands of years in that part of the world, and it seems to me plausible that this cave site was shared, or more likely taken over, by modern humans (sometimes termed Cro-Magnon people). In other words our direct ancestors could have left the artefact behind, among the layers of Neanderthal detritus. As Bill Bryson wrote in his book *A Short History of Nearly Everything*,[344] when discussing the patchy nature of the fossil hominin record: "With so little to be certain about, scientists often have to make assumptions based on other objects found nearby, and these may be little more than valiant guesses. Or as Alan Walker and Pat Shipman have drily observed, if you correlate tool discovery with the species of creature most often found nearby, you would have to conclude that early hand tools were mostly made by antelopes."[345] Such are the inevitable imponderables of archaeology.

Very recently, a remarkable bone flute fashioned from a griffon vulture's wing has been found in a cave in south-western Germany—dated to be 35,000–40,000 years old, and assumed to be human in origin—relatively soon after their arrival in this part of Europe.[346] A flute made from the radius of a swan, and a great many other fragments of ivory flutes, have also now been discovered, some of these perhaps as old as 42,000–43,000 years.[347] These artefacts required complex manufacture and took time and care to produce, and must have been the "product of a long period of technological development."[348] They look (and sound) like the real thing, suggesting that a musical tradition involving more sophisticated motor performance, using instruments as well as vocalization, was well under way only some tens of thousands of years after the founders of our species first walked and danced in Africa. Pipes and other possible sound-producing instruments have also been found in France and elsewhere, and there is a suggestion that caves were deliberately used for their resonant properties. Conard et al elegantly described the likely importance of these finds at the end of their *Nature* paper in this way: "The presence of music in the lives of early Upper Palaeolithic peoples did not directly produce a more effective subsistence economy and greater reproductive fitness. Viewed, however, in a broader behavioural context, early Upper Palaeolithic music could have contributed to the maintenance of larger social networks, and thereby perhaps have helped facilitate the demographic and territorial expansion of modern humans relative to culturally more conservative and demographically more isolated Neanderthal populations,"[346] a conclusion that buttresses the belief that music has unique communal power, even in the twenty-first century.

Visual images such as cave paintings with ritual and symbolic significance were also presumably of great importance to the rapidly learning and adapting modern human species, and likely involved many individuals working as a team (painters, preparers of the surface and the pigments, etc). The art outlived its creators and must have remained relevant for many generations, whereas music and dance performance was ephemeral and required repeated and ongoing participation. While rock engravings depicting what seem to be dancers have been dated at about 16,000 years old, the earliest musical notations were not seen until about 5500 years ago, in Sumarian culture.[349]

An evolutionary synthesis (in for a penny …)

In summary, and when viewed as a whole—the Y chromosome and mitochondrial DNA data, the timing of climactic events such as droughts and mega volcanic eruptions, the onset of cultural symbolism and development of increasingly sophisticated technologies, and so on—it all seems to point to a founder population that gave rise to all modern humans perhaps as recently as 75,000–85,000 years ago. Seemingly, the evolution of our species happened in a comparatively short space of time, somewhere in East/southeast Africa. If we are indeed that recent, that means if we assume four or perhaps five generations per century,[44] there have been only about 4,000–4,500 generations of our new version of *Homo sapiens*. Quite coincidentally, this approximate number appears in the writing of the great biologist J. B. S. Haldane, quoted by Dennis Dutton in his book *The Art Instinct*.[350] Haldane calculated that "a variant that produces on average 1% more offspring than its alternative allele would increase in frequency from 0.1% to 99.9% of the population in just 4,000 generations." Haldane was also close to the mark about another of his suggestions—that there would be about 150 new mutations (most presumably neutral) in each of us.[351]

Long-term climactic and environmental changes such as drought likely provided the impetus for early emigrations of *Homo sapiens* out of Africa more than 100,000 years ago. The founder population—from whom all of us are derived—must also have survived various adverse environmental events, perhaps including Toba, and somewhere between 50,000 and 65,000 years ago began to move within and out of Africa,[284,285,319] a migration "characterized by rapid dispersal across Eurasia and Oceania and followed by subsequent pockets of isolation."[52] I have already mentioned that estimates of the size of our founder population are as low as 2,000–10,000 for individuals that were of reproductive age. Modern humans were to be found in the Middle East by 55,000–60,000 years ago,[286] in Australia by about 50,000 years ago,[352] in Europe by about 40,000–45,000 years ago, and in the Americas as recently as 15,000 years ago, *and presumably they ALL had language and music*.

It is important to emphasize here that there is now widespread agreement among anthropologists and geneticists that, while the ancestors of present-day *Homo sapiens* originated in East Africa, our current genetic makeup does not originate entirely from the founders who made up the last great migration out of that continent. In Asia, the Middle East, and Europe, there is increasingly convincing evidence of intermixing of hominin lineages over many thousands of years,[147,268,286,353] including limited interbreeding between newly arriving modern "*Homo sapientior*" and hominin populations such as Neanderthals and Denisovans, and perhaps also admixture with other more archaic or intermediate *Homo sapiens* groups[302,318,354,355] that remained viable in these regions following earlier waves of African emigration.

Occasional fossils have been found with skeletal features that seem to suggest a cross between *Homo neanderthalensis* and *Homo sapiens*. Genetic analysis of head lice suggests that there may have been contact and exchange of parasites between modern and archaic humans,[323] but the nature of that contact—sexual, accidental, combative—can never be known. Some earlier studies found no evidence of genetic overlap between the two species, and one modeling study suggested that the level of gene flow from Neanderthals to ancestors of current Europeans to be as little as 0.001% per generation.[276] However, more recent analysis calculates a higher gene flow between Neanderthals and humans outside Africa of 1.5–2.1%,[146] and perhaps even higher.[356] This admixture probably occurred over a period of time within about the last 60,000 years or so, and may have continued up until the extinction of the Neanderthals. Admixture with Denisovans was apparently even more prevalent in parts of Asia, with estimates of as much as 5% Denisovan DNA in some present-day humans, occurring perhaps 44,000–54,000 years ago![353] All this of course assumes that any common polymorphisms between modern humans and our extinct cousins are not merely a consequence of the retention of genetic information possessed by shared parental ancestors, before we split from each other.[267]

Gene variants beneficial to *Homo sapiens* may even have been passed on to us from "archaic" *Homo* lineages as a consequence of interbreeding with them,[357] most likely through the maternal line. There is no evidence for transmission via the Y chromosome.[279] This gene flow—from groups already adapted to particular environments, into newly arriving modern humans—may have had advantages, increasing the speed with which modern humans themselves adapted to new circumstances.[354] This may have been especially important in the adaptive immune system, admixture resulting in greater immune diversity in modern humans, who were now capable of functionally responding to a vast range of potential threats, including protection against novel infections.[358] The term for this type of inherited advantage is "adaptive introgression."[287] Far less Neanderthal and Denisovan ancestry is detectable on the X chromosome than on the non-sex chromosomes (autosomes), suggesting that male human/Neanderthal and male human/Denisovan hybrids were considerably less fertile,[353,359] perhaps even infertile.[279] Even if interbreeding between Neanderthals and modern humans was occasionally successful, what is surely clear is that the evolving *Homo sapiens* genotype, along with the presumed benefits of the resulting modern human phenotype, became relatively fixed and completely dominant.[288,354] Neanderthal and Denisovan genetic material seems to have been selectively removed over thousands of years of human breeding, especially in genes that are more highly expressed in testes than elsewhere in the body.[353,359]

Compared with modern humans, Neanderthals probably lived in smaller, more isolated, and less socially complex groups,[14] although a recent discovery in southwestern France suggests they were sufficiently organized to build "elaborate constructions" deep within caves. There is now evidence that, at about the time that "*Homo sapientior*" evolved, our cousins in Europe may have used ornamentation and begun to make some more specialized bone tools.[360] Nonetheless, compared with the subsequent rapid rise of the newly emerging hominin species, Neanderthals had been around for several hundreds of thousands of years and appear to have been in relative cognitive/cultural stasis. They were almost certainly smart enough, during their period of interaction with *Homo sapiens*, to assimilate some of their attributes and learn some new tricks,[361] and interbreeding with *Homo sapiens* may have led to the acquisition of a small fraction of "modernizing genes."[39] To quote the eminent philosopher/Jesuit priest/paleontologist Pierre Teilhard de Chardin, from his book *The Phenomenon of Man*, "Even to the more brutal Neanderthals, everyone is prepared to grant a flame of a genuine intelligence. Most of it, however, seems to have been used up in the sheer effort to survive and reproduce. If there was any left over, we see no signs of it or fail to recognise them."[362] This is, with the benefit of new data collected in the 60 years or so since then,[14] almost certainly an overly harsh assessment of the cognitive attributes of our cousins; nonetheless it is clear that Neanderthals lacked the blue touch paper that appeared in a small African group that rapidly came to dominate the global hominin landscape—a group that, in about 80,000 years and 4,000–4,500 generations, expanded exponentially from several thousand founder members to seven billion, and counting!

The language revolution

The eventual demise of the Neanderthals (and the Denisovans, and perhaps others) was likely accelerated by lack of intellectual and cultural flexibility, population fragmentation, and isolation, which may have affected their capacity to interact and learn from others and perhaps led to the adverse effects of inbreeding.[15,147,363] The blue touch paper that was lit— the engine that powered the unprecedented evolutionary acceleration in *Homo sapiens*— presumably involved the exaptation (new use of a pre-existing mechanism/structure)[364] of sensorimotor networks of great complexity that had slowly evolved in our *Homo* ancestors and had presumably been used for communication and other purposes,[98,348,365,366] as well as micromutations that permitted the development of modified neural architectures with enhanced plasticity and a more effective working memory,[367] and far greater processing capacity. Together, these formed the neural substrate that allowed for the development of modern language and articulate speech, and the evolution of the new-fashioned, inquisitive, sentient human—a feature that, in my view, was rapidly and positively selected for in the founder population.

Derek Bickerton, in an eminently readable review, put it this way: "The most stunning … aspect of human evolution is its suddenness. The emergence of our own species released a torrent of creativity that is still gathering speed. What caused the difference? Clearly, some startling increment in cognition. But what caused cognition to change so dramatically? The emergence of modern syntacticized language is the most plausible, indeed perhaps the only serious contender."[103] Bickerton believes that language, the rules of grammar/syntax, and "the linkage of symbolic units" evolved rapidly, abruptly—a view with which I concur: "If syntax confers enhanced cognition, and no enhanced cognition emerged prior to the appearance of our species, then syntax could not have developed gradually, period." Learning a language is enmeshed within our cultural background, and yet, as Henry Plotkin wrote in his book on evolutionary psychology,[42] its acquisition is universal and any human is able to learn any of the documented 5,500 languages. Furthermore, "the learning of language structure, that is the grammar and syntax that characterizes every language, occurs without the child ... having any idea what it is they have learned." We implicitly know the complicated rules, but not how we know them.

Presumably the creation of language in *Homo sapiens* must also have been closely linked to the shaping of what we describe (but not necessarily understand!) as conscious thought: "a dirty secret of modern science is that we have no way of explaining the fact that humans have conscious experience ... (in the sense of raw first-person subjective awareness) ... No one has adequately explained why it *feels like something* to be a hunk of neural tissue processing information in certain complex patterns."[368] Henry Plotkin summarizes various contentious views on what he describes as "the jewel in psychology's crown," and concludes that "consciousness, then, may well have evolved because of its adaptive advantages for us, both as an internalized device for testing possible future events, and for projecting onto others the capacity for such internalized testing and predicting the consequences for their behaviour."[42] Language, Theory of Mind, and an advanced frontal lobe are surely prerequisites for carrying out such sophisticated tasks.

Most importantly, with language comes the capacity to share information not just within, but now across, generations. "The emergence of language was the defining moment in the evolution of modern humans."[369] To quote Michael Corballis from a recent review: "My guess is that they (language and mental time travel) co-evolved to comprise the distinctive structure of the human mind."[99] In relation to "the evolution of foresight," there appears to be no convincing evidence for mental time travel in nonhuman species.[370] Rod Mengham enunciates a similar view about the significance of cognitive representations of time in his book *On Language: Descent from the Tower of Babel*[371]: "Without language with tenses that determine differences between past, present and future and without the means of defining the limits of personal agency, one cannot relate phenomena through time and in space." It is true that there are some languages that seem to lack tenses, but they may have other ways of defining events in time. Given how quickly languages change across generations, the presence now of some that lack overt constructions to express the passage of time may not necessarily reflect the original condition.

Human intelligence is inextricably associated with planning, foresight, and the development of multiple contingency plans ... we are chess players, strategists, dreamers ... we are an interactive narrative species that gossips and loves telling stories ... we can think and talk about events that are displaced from us in space and/or time. The famous linguist Noam Chomsky, who was perhaps most responsible for the concept of a universal grammar and the proposal that language is a completely new faculty, somehow genetically built into our brains, wrote: "to account for the normal use of language we must attribute to the speaker-hearer an intricate system of rules that involve mental operations of a very abstract nature, applying to representations that are quite remote from the physical signal."[372] As discussed more fully in Chapter 4, there are numerous points of concordance between animal communication and human language, such as sensorimotor processing similarities, vocal imitation, affective interactions between conspecifics, and occasional evidence of "cultural" or "dialectal" variation in vocalizations.[373] However, speculation about the evolution of modern linguistic capability based on other nonhuman communication systems may not be useful if, in fact, human language and articulate speech are based on different principles.

The extent to which particular components of language—eg grammar, semantics, and recursion—are unique core elements of language encoded in the brain of *Homo sapiens*, and the extent to which culture impacts on language acquisition and expression, remain a source of lively debate.[43,98,104,366,374,375,376,377] Speculations about the evolution of language—exactly how, when, and why it occurred—are also invariably controversial: "there are genuine problems in reconstructing how the language faculty might have evolved by natural selection."[1] The linguist Derek Bickerton has written a great deal on human language and whether it may have arisen from a protolanguage of some kind. Somewhat unpromisingly for a non-linguist like me, he states that: "the evolution of language is far too vast and complex (and vague) a concept for anyone to say anything sensible about it." He goes on to say: "it's a minefield out there, strewn with explosive charges of little-known fact ready to blow up the fanciest new theory."[103] But he does go on to point out that symbolism and syntax are essential elements of this uniquely human communication system, and suggests that symbolic units such as words evolved prior to the syntax and then linked these solitary units together into complex hierarchical and recursive structures, with concepts/phrases embedded inside concepts/sentences. Nonetheless, despite the manifest difficulties—difficulties that have engaged the greatest minds for centuries—it is just about impossible to think of the evolution of our modern cognitive architecture and intellectual power, our vivid sense of self and of others, in the absence of an associated evolution of syntactical language. Did one come before the other? Perhaps we will never know for certain, but I suspect the relationship between language and the modern mind is like the lyrics from the famous Frank Sinatra song: "Love and marriage, love and marriage, go together like a horse and carriage, this I tell you brother, you can't have one without the other."

Language is in some ways modality independent; it can be expressed and understood using non-aural means such as hand gestures (signing). However, the rapid and efficient transfer of ideas and plans, and the teaching of newly acquired specific and generic information and knowledge, particularly from one generation to the next, was presumably communicated mostly by word of mouth. "Language was the new and extraordinarily efficient means by which humans acquired and passed on from one generation to the next that flexible network of learned, rather than inherited, behaviour patterns and knowledge that allowed them to alter their environment and adapt to new ones. A simple culture now had a symbolic form that changed its whole nature."[378] Articulate speech must have been the primary vector for transmission of complex human thoughts, ideas, and aspirations—it is difficult for me to imagine evolving a neural architecture for grammar, syntax, and so forth, just in case it needed to be used by the occasional congenitally deaf members of the species. These circuitries and molecular foundations that underpin speech, and that continued to adapt and evolve, were superimposed on existing, already sophisticated aural communication systems that also utilized socially interactive modalities such as gesture, facial expression, and imitation.[379,380] And of course, writing and the invention of alphabets came much, much later in our history. It is interesting that while the grammatical principles of language seem to have been conserved through the millennia, there has been continued change in the number and type of symbols that are used to define the sounds of letters or words. In the book *Unweaving the Rainbow*,[381] Richard Dawkins accepts the idea that spoken language may have been the spark that began the self-reinforcing, rapid evolution of *Homo sapiens*, that started our evolutionary spiral. Dawkins talks about a self-feeding event where there was some co-evolution or co-adaptation of a software change and a hardware change that suddenly projected everything forward: "a social world in which there is language is a completely different kind of social world ... the selection pressures on genes will never be the same again."

In some ways Dawkins' insight is not that much different from Vilayanur Ramachandran's suggestion in his book *The Emerging Mind* that: "it is the fortuitous synergistic combination of a number of mechanisms which evolved for other purposes initially that later became assimilated into the mechanism that we call language."[261] We have already discussed some of the genetic polymorphisms that may have played a role in altering brain function, learning, and plasticity, and that may have improved attention mechanisms and memory storage. There may also have been subtle changes in circuitry between or within brain regions that perhaps slowly evolved for other purposes but were "hijacked" during the evolution of modern language and articulate speech. Could there also have been some impermanent or transient pathways that would normally have been eliminated during development that were somehow, perhaps accidentally, preserved in founder members of our new linguistic species? Were there some micromutations and novel interconnections between cortical regions in a small group of early, what I have cheekily termed, *"Homo sapientior?"*

In about 1–4% of the population, in response to one sensory input, people experience more than one sensation (eg music and color, sound and smell) at the same time—termed synesthesia. There are many forms of this cross-modality—usually unidirectional, perceptual interaction. Imaging and other studies suggest increased cross-activation and connectivity between cortical regions, and structural differences in the brains of synesthetes have been reported, involving changes in both gray matter and white matter. These changes have been reported to vary in cortical location depending on the type of synesthetic experience.[382,383,384,385] Sound-induced colors are associated with activity in the left inferior parietal cortex, a region important in integrating information from different sensory modalities,[386] and there is structural imaging evidence of increased connectivity between auditory and visual cortical regions and frontal cortex on the right side.[387] It should be noted here however that, similar to caveats discussed earlier in this book about the risks of over-interpretation of fMRI data when relatively few subjects are analyzed, a critical review of the neuroimaging literature of synesthesia "casts some doubts on whether any neural correlate of the synesthetic experience has been established yet."[388]

Viyalanur Ramachandran has a great interest in synesthesia, which, as he describes: "appears to be genetically transmitted (and) results in a mingling of the senses. For example, hearing a particular musical note might invoke a particular colour: C sharp is red, F sharp is blue, and so on. Visually perceived numbers can produce the same effect."[261] I can vouch for this: in 2010, there was a student in our third-year neuroscience class who saw particular letters and numbers in specific colors (color-graphemic synesthesia). An especially remarkable modern-day example of synesthesia was published in the journal *Nature* in 2005: a young Swiss musician tastes musical intervals—for example, a minor-second chord is sour, a major-third is sweet, a fifth is pure water, a major-sixth tastes like low-fat cream, and a minor-seventh is bitter![389] Ramachandran suggests that this cross-activation or "hyperconnectivity" in the brain may have selective advantages, such as enhancing cross-modal interactive networks,[390] enhancing abstract (modality-free) thought, and heightening the ability to link seemingly unrelated things—what I might call creativity or "inspiration," or perhaps what Steven Mithen called "cognitive fluidity."[342] Neurological links between the arts, creative cognition, and the synesthetic brain are becoming clearer,[391] and as a heritable condition[392] the linkage genetics of this remarkable phenomenon are just starting to be investigated.[393]

It seems to be a cross-cultural, innate phenomenon that humans do not arbitrarily attach sounds to shapes. The classic example of this is the kiki/bouba effect,[261] where subjects are asked to pick a word that most corresponds to a particular shape—and the word "kiki" is invariably attached to jagged shapes, and "bouba" to smooth, rounded shapes. This cross-modal abstraction is, in some ways, a type of synesthesia and seems to involve the left angular gyrus, "strategically placed to allow a convergence of different sensory modalities to create abstract, modality-free representations of things around us."[261] Interestingly, cross-modal interactions have even been reported within primary sensory processing areas in the human cerebral cortex of normal individuals,[394,395,396] and when one sensory modality is absent early in life, processing in the respective brain region can be reattributed to enhance perceptual processing in another modality,[397,398,399,400,401] a phenomenon discussed more fully in the following chapter. However, one fMRI study worth noting here confirmed activity in visual cortex in congenitally blind subjects when listening to sounds, but went on to show that occipital regions that normally process information about the location of an object in space were also activated by equivalent acoustic stimuli, and that these regions were connected to other brain areas known to be involved in spatial/motion detection. Thus, these regions seem to have an innate "computational role for processing space independently of sensory developmental experience."[402] These authors concluded: "We therefore postulate that cross-modal plasticity in congenitally blind allows nonvisual processes to find a 'neuronal niche' into a set of circuits that perform functions that are sufficiently close to the ones required by remaining senses."

In the context of language evolution, to again quote Professor Ramachandran from his excellent "Reith Lectures": "we have three things in place—first, hand to mouth, second, mouth in Broca's area to visual appearance in the fusiform and sound contours in auditory cortex, and third, auditory to visual … Acting together, these three have a synergistic bootstrapping effect—an avalanche culminating in the emergence of a primitive language." Similarly, W. H. Calvin[365] suggests that our immediate ancestors already had a core facility for stringing things together, perhaps common to utterance, hand movement, tool making, facial expression, and so on, and that the new language and articulate speech of *Homo sapiens* evolved and developed from, or was superimposed upon, these pre-existing neural structures. If there were shared circuitries between various complex behaviors, then the selection of any one of these might augment all aspects of the shared neural machinery. The emergent property of language meant that humans possessed new conceptual and representational capacity, differing from other species that lacked the "rich, expressive and open-ended power of human language."[366] Taken together, the result of these various evolutionary changes, as boldly suggested by Merlin Donald in his book *Origins of the Modern Mind*, is that: "if we compare the complex representational architecture of the modern mind with that of the ape, we must conclude that the Darwinian universe is too small to contain humanity. We are a different order."

At the beginning of the nineteenth century, Jean-Baptiste Lamarck proposed his theory of inheritance of acquired characteristics. An important element of this theory was that organisms adjust to the environment they encounter during their lifetime and, depending on use (or disuse) of particular characteristics, then pass these changes on to their offspring, which thus become more suited to that environment. Lamarck's theory has been battered from pillar to post since Darwin, but could it find some respite in relation to modern humans? In a recent short essay by David Deutsch, in a book critiquing the writings and thoughts of Richard Dawkins, he says Lamarckism is a mistake because "if, ahistorically, we express Lamarck's conception of the problem in terms of information flow, then he is asking how the knowledge of how to prosper in an environment gets from that environment into the organisms that live there. Since information does not and cannot flow in that manner, no way of answering that question could ever have explained anything."[403]

This seems to me to be undoubtedly true for almost all species, although some elements of cultural transmission are thought to occur in some non-human species.[404] But is it necessarily true for social and cultural "*Homo sapientior*," a species that can accumulate and transmit information from one (not necessarily related) generation to the next—that can teach and educate, and build alliances, each generation building on the intellectual knowledge, culture, and technological innovations of previous generations? "A common language connects the members of a community into an information-sharing network with formidable collective powers. Anyone can benefit from the stroke of genius, lucky accident, and trial-and-error wisdom accumulated by anyone else, present or past."[1] Acquiring information from, and actively changing, the social and physical environment in which we live is what we are really good (some might say really bad) at: "Cultural evolution has shown us that one word can be worth a thousand genes."[405] A similar type of view—human evolution having different properties to "traditional" biological evolution—was espoused by Sir Julian Huxley and also by Pierre Teilhard de Chardin, who wrote: "The consciousness of each of us is evolution looking at itself and reflecting upon itself."[362]

Because of the open-ended, generative, and symbolic nature of human language—the ability to intuit and express ideas, to create virtual realities and link independent strands of thought together, coupled with the capacity to assimilate and share data and knowledge of life's experiences with current and future generations—because of all of this we have rapidly moved on: culture is now helping to drive evolution. It has even been suggested that language is "the cultural replicator corresponding to the concept of the gene in biological evolution."[406] The links between genes and culture (gene-culture co-evolution) have received considerable attention in recent years. In this context, culture has been defined as "all of the information that individuals acquire from others by a variety of social learning processes including teaching and imitation. The fidelity of cultural transmission is often sufficiently high for culture to act as an inheritance system; however, cultural traditions also change with time, making culture a system of descent with modification."[407]

The issue of cultural and behavioral diversity within the extant human population is an important one that should be kept in mind from now on.[408] The vast majority of psychosocial, behavioral, and cognitive research and neuroimaging studies (including those described in Chapter 2) are carried out on people from "WEIRD" (western, educated, industrialized, rich, democratic) societies. But these people are by no means necessarily representative of all humanity, and when carefully tested, non-WEIRD populations can display quite different cognitive and behavioral attributes, such as differences in visual perception, fairness, cooperation, optimism, analytic and moral reasoning, memory, and heritability of IQ.[409] However, these are differences in degree, not absolutes, and socially driven cultural innovation and complexity remain common human characteristics.[337,408,410] Perhaps music and dance constitute the most universal behaviors of all—important proximate drivers of prosocial cooperativity in our species.[411,412,413] Recent inventions such as books and the worldwide web have overtaken oral traditions and accelerated information storage and transfer to an unimaginable extent, further influencing cultural differences.

The faithful accumulation, transmission, and sharing of cultural ideas, innovations, symbols, or practices from one generation to the next using speech, gesture, rituals, and so on, typical of our species as a whole are essentially enshrined in Richard Dawkins' memes, which he originally defined as a "noun which conveys the idea of a unit of cultural transmission, or a unit of imitation" (*The Selfish Gene*)—ideas and thoughts passed on to our children, and cultural traits that evolve by a form of natural selection. I especially like this passage from Chip Walter's book *Last Ape Standing*[45]: "Our special talent isn't simply that we can conjure symbols or even weave elaborate, illusory tapestries of them, but that we can share these with one another, roping together both our 'selves' and our imaginings, linking uncounted minds into rambunctious networks where thoughts and insights, feelings and emotions, breed still more ideas to be further shared. Creativity is contagious this way, and once a light emerged, it must have gone off like fireworks." And as ideas accumulated and cultural complexity evolved, better and increasingly sophisticated methods of teaching were needed to ensure faithful transmission within and between groups, and across generations.[414]

The meme idea has, as in all things associated with evolutionary biology, come under intense scrutiny and criticism. But, like others, I would argue that we have indeed entered an extended or neo-Darwinian world, with increasing emphasis on gene-environment and/or gene–culture interactions. In this world, language and culture permit a new type of knowledge transmission within and across generations, where individuals and groups in each generation share and accumulate information, and glean wisdom from their elders. These interactions do not necessarily respect gene lineage boundaries; large-scale networking with genetically unrelated individuals and with other socially compatible groups is also critically important in promoting "the evolution of cumulative culture."[258] In contrast to the frequently used term monogenesis—for example, the suggestion that all languages (and perhaps modern humans) originated from a single source—perhaps the term *polymemesis* could be used to describe the diverse epigenetic influences that impact on human evolution, resulting in the inherently changeable nature of human society and culture, including of course language and music. There is an inherent "state of inner restlessness" of language: "The simple truth is that all languages change, all the time—the only static languages are dead ones."[415]

Chiaroni et al wrote: "The increasing role of human creativity and the fast diffusion of inventions seem to have favoured cultural solutions for many of the problems encountered in expansion. We suggest that cultural evolution has been subrogating biologic evolution in providing natural selection advantages and reducing our dependence on genetic mutations, especially in the last phase of transition from food collection to food production."[52] And food availability, as discussed earlier in this chapter, along with the ability to utilize what is available, is critically important not just in adulthood but especially in children when building a healthy, metabolically expensive human brain,[36] and especially when late-developing cortical regions are so important for human cognition.[63] As reviewed by Christine Williams,[35] humans contain polymorphisms in genes involved in the processing of essential nutrients such as choline and folate. This genetic variation may affect how much of these nutrients we need to absorb to build and maintain normal brain function. Furthermore, lack of adequate nutrition during pregnancy and childhood can epigenetically affect gene expression,[416] cause DNA damage, and affect brain plasticity; thus, "food ingested early in life may have lifelong and potentially transgenerational effects."[35]

Our recent rate of adaptive evolution has been reported to be more than one hundred times higher than during earlier periods of our evolutionary history,[417] even though our actual genetic mutation rate may be slowing (see earlier). Of course, cultural transmission and "classical" gene selection and transmission are not entirely independent of each other; as Darwin understood, the creative and linguistically articulate human may have had (and continue to have) selective advantages when it comes to passing on genes. I mentioned earlier a review of many twin studies suggesting that intelligence is a positively selected trait,[206] but the evolutionary rate of change in our genes is clearly altered by cooperative behaviors and the influence of, and our interaction with, culture.[418] By comparing rates of technological change to changes in animal morphology, it has been concluded that the rate of cultural change is faster than that of biological change, allowing rapid evolutionary transitions in long-lived humans over short timescales.[419] "The human genome itself can be partly viewed as cultural creation."[407]

In discussing the work of the biologist Mary Jane West-Eberhard,[420] Petter Portin describes the concept of "social selection,"[406] a theory put forward to help explain the "ultrasociality" of modern humans. I consider in more detail the concepts of prosocial behaviors, empathy, and altruism, among others, in Chapter 5, but the principles of social selection are worth setting out here: "According to West-Eberhard, social selection can have an effect on the evolution of characteristics that make the individual more attractive as a social partner. These characteristics include, firstly, possessing resources such as good health and vitality, desirable personal capabilities, influential confederates and a powerful social status. Secondly, they include an inclination to distribute one's own resources faithfully and selectively with social companions. Thirdly, these characteristics also include the ability to have a feeling about what other individuals expect from a companion, and fourthly, a strong motivation to please companions and other members of the social group."[406] At the group level, cooperativity brings enhanced and rapid cultural adaptability, leading to social environments in which "natural selection favoured genes that gave rise to new, more pro-social motives."[421] Even the existence of prestige-based leadership of small groups can be predicted to foster cooperative cultural evolution and the selection of genes favoring prosocial behaviours.[422] Note here that the positive selection of alleles that protect the brain during aging would also permit a greater social and cultural contribution from extended families, including grandparents.[206]

Since our beginnings, the range of human cognitive skills must have continued to expand at ever-increasing rates on the back of our new and radical, linguistic-based framework. To borrow a phrase I heard used by Harvard Professor Jeff Lichtman at a meeting in Asilomar in 2009, we are obligate learners; we exhibit and transmit culture-based behaviors, and because of our inquisitiveness, language, and cognitive power, "*Homo sapientior*" is evolving via "intelligent design of hereditable traits."[423] Our recent evolutionary history is neo-Darwinian; it is also in some ways neo-Lamarckian in character, and I am not alone in espousing that view.[424,425,426,427] In the context of hominin evolution, we have entered a new epoch.

And yet, during this great and astonishingly rapid global radiation of *Homo sapiens*, this increasingly monopolistic take-over of planet Earth, we all of us continue to carry another seed of communication—the musical neural network. As Michael Thaut writes, music is "part of a comprehensive system of mental representations that function in the brain in different modalities. The brain thinks in multiple languages."[349] We must now ask, once again, the next key questions: how did musical communication evolve and from what precursor; what, if any, advantages did this musical network provide to "*Homo sapientior*"; how did it differ from language and articulate speech; why does the neural musical network persist; and why does music continue to be so fundamentally important to the welfare of our species in twenty-first century society?

Chapter 4

Why do we have Music as another Communication System?

If songs were lines in a conversation, the situation would be fine.
—Nick Drake, "Hazey Jane II"

This is primarily a book about music and its continued psychological, emotional, social, and therapeutic impact on our species. However, as I have alluded to several times, to get to the heart of the question as to why music is a human universal, we must confront the tricky, oft-debated issue of the evolutionary relationship between music and language. Put most simply, did music come before language, did language come before music, or did they co-evolve from some common progenitor? I have already discussed why I believe language as a communication system was an integral part of our recent evolution, but then how and why was music important to our early ancestors—that is, assuming it is not merely "auditory cheesecake?"

Darwin suggested that music may have preceded language; as quoted in Peter Kivy's essay about Charles Darwin on music: "As we have every reason to suppose that articulate speech is one of the latest, as it certainly is the highest, of the arts acquired by man, and as the instinctive power of producing musical notes and rhythms is developed low down in the animal series, it would be altogether opposed to the principle of evolution, if we were to admit that man's musical capacity has been developed from the tones used in impassioned speech. We must suppose that the rhythms and cadences of oratory are derived from previously developed musical powers."[1] Darwin believed that music was primarily concerned with mating calls and reproduction, similar to some of the functionality attributed to bird "song" for example. "The impassioned orator, bard, or musician, when with his varied tones and cadences he excites the strongest emotions in his hearers, little suspects that he uses the same means by which his half-human ancestors long ago aroused each other's ardent passions, during their courtship and rivalry."

I expect (somewhat salaciously I confess) that most rock (and some operatic) stars of today (male or female) in the prime of their reproductive years can attest to the sexual interest they arouse. Indeed, recent studies do indicate that women find males more attractive if the men are carrying a musical instrument such as a guitar, or even just a guitar case.[1,2,3] But how good-looking were these men, and how smart, and what about reciprocal attraction of males to musical females? Interestingly, the attractiveness of faces to the opposite sex is correlated with the genetic diversity of individuals, presumably helping in the selection of "high-quality mates,"[4] and as mentioned earlier, genome-wide studies indicate that intelligence, more than looks, is a key trait driven by natural selection in modern humans.[5] Nonetheless, a large-scale twin study found that genes that influence cognition or auditory function are positively correlated with musical aptitude,[6] supporting the idea that music has at least some role in sexual selection. But as to the "pheromonal" power of a guitar case, could this just be a modern-day phenomenon—women looking for the sensitive side to twenty-first century masculinity, or looking for a potential rock star with excellent financial prospects? As Tecumseh Fitch wrote: "A woman choosing a one-night fling with an itinerate musician today might have made quite different decisions knowing she might become pregnant with a bastard son in earlier times or other cultures!"[7]

The Swedish neurobiologist Björn Merker has argued that vocal learning, the ability to match vocal production to auditory models, first involved "songs" that, over many, many generations, became more and more analytically and semantically complex, with words and gestures evolving later: "language emerged as an inadvertent consequence of the inter-generational transmission of a rich repertoire of song."[8] According to Merker, this emergence would be a slow process ("hundreds and thousands of generations"). Perhaps the core syntactic and prosodic platforms took time to build, but as I have argued in the previous chapter, genetic and cultural evidence suggests that the final and critical piece of the jigsaw that led to the emergence of modern language and articulate speech, and with it the modern cognitive mind and "*Homo sapientior*," was a relatively rapid and recent event in our evolutionary history—at least within the last 100,000 years. Are musical humans as recent, or is music a much older phenomenon?

Vocalization in non-human species

Steven Mithen in his book *The Singing Neanderthals* has proposed that Neanderthals—who, as I mentioned earlier, separated from our own lineage 450,000–700,000 years ago[9,10,11,12,13,14]—were more "musical" than their *Homo sapiens* cousins. I put the word musical in inverted commas because to agree or disagree with this statement largely depends on how the term "music" is defined. The word "song" is frequently used to describe how, for example, birds, whales, dolphins, and gibbons vocalize, often in dazzlingly complex and sometimes (to our ears at least) enchantingly beautiful ways. But is it really song, or simply just a sophisticated means of communication—vocalizations motivated by emotional states and produced when animals are alarmed or involved in territorial disputes, or during requests/demands for sexual favors, pair-bonding, and so forth. By calling such communications song, are we being anthropomorphic, inappropriately ascribing to animal "song" similar attributes to the musical gestalt as *perceived* and created by modern humans?

Presumably, any type of biologically important vocalization that enhances interactions (competitive or attractive) with other members of the same species, or that results in scaring off other species, or warning predators, must necessarily have variable pitch, intensity, and rhythm components.[15] These vocalizations will have important "emotional" content;

they will be of overall survival value and will influence motivational states and "action readiness,"[16] and brains will have perceptual processing capabilities to match. Definitional difficulties in how to describe animal communication are perhaps exemplified by the language used in comparative reviews on animal and human acoustic communication. For example, in an excellent review focused on FOXP2 and language evolution, the authors state that: "animals are usually considered to have neither language nor music ...," yet the term "song" is consistently used to describe communication in birds, mice, bats, whales, and gibbons.[17,18]

Frequency, spectral content, intensity, and timing/temporal regularity are the essential elements processed by animal auditory sensory systems, and a few animals can respond in synchrony to a rhythmic beat, indicating early links between rhythmic auditory processing, perception, and motor activity.[19,20,21,22] In the laboratory, Rhesus monkeys do not synchronize tapping to a metronome but can be trained to remember the timing between two signals and tap this interval accordingly; humans are far better at it, and only humans are accurate during multiple interval trials, "a behavior that may be related to complex temporal cognition, such as speech and music execution."[23] More recent work suggests that the ability to accurately synchronize tapping to a beat is indeed linked to cognitive and articulate language skills.[24] In fact, the functional connections between motor planning and auditory regions in humans seem to be especially well developed, again thought to be "due to the evolution of vocal learning in our lineage."[25] And interestingly, the better the singer, the better the motor synchronization to a beat.[26]

While aspects of timing and rhythm are processed in the brainstem, including the cerebellum,[27,28,29] more sophisticated processing occurs at higher levels. Thus, when human subjects are asked to memorize, wait, and then recall with the use of finger tapping a seven-second rhythmic pattern presented either aurally or visually, regions active during this "rhythm working memory-related" task are often but not always bilateral, and involve not only the cerebellum but also inferior frontal cortex, inferior parietal cortex, and supplementary motor areas.[20] In addition to this remarkable neural convergence of processing rhythmic acoustic and visual stimuli, integration between auditory and cutaneous tactile inputs has also been found, which could help to explain why "we not only hear music but also have the experience of 'feeling' the music in our bodies."[30] This phenomenon, as discussed later in this chapter, is likely to be of vital importance to the deaf.

Of course, non-human visual and auditory communication systems have evolved over a long period of time and are often extremely sophisticated and versatile. Between members of the same species there can be a large repertoire of vocalized calls thought to convey complex information.[7,17,31,32] For example, monkeys encode pitch and harmonics in a similar way to humans,[33,34] and are able to recognize pitch sequences even when particular "melodies" are played an octave apart.[35] It is worth noting here that while monkeys can perceive so-called octave equivalence, humans are unique among primates in being able to vocally blend and imitate over this octave difference, to sing in harmony. In the natural environment, primates express and respond to a variety of sounds of different pitches, timbres, accents, rhythms, and sequences that accompany and presumably impact on social interactions.[15,36,37,38] Some monkeys also drum, perhaps as another form of communication between individuals.[39] There is evidence in primates for "preferential processing of vocalizations and voice-information that involves a large portion of the superior temporal lobe, often in both hemispheres,"[38] and the neural networks that process drumming and vocalizations appear to overlap, thought by some to support "the notion of a gestural origin for speech and music."[39] Importantly, however, and unlike non-human primates, even young children quickly learn to synchronize drumming speed with others, especially in a social context.[40] And group drumming is good for us—reducing feelings of anxiety and depression and improving our psychological and physiological well-being.[41]

There are numerous examples of animal vocalizations that are clearly expressive, which presumably reflect the "emotional" state of an individual and may influence the actions of others, such as the resolution of tensions between individuals. Specific short or somewhat longer species-specific vocalizations probably provide information about food and serve as an alarm to other members of the group about imminent danger from sources of threat such as snakes, carnivorous mammals, or birds of prey. Vocalizations and associated behaviors can be highly sophisticated; for example, there is self-identification as well as vocal copying of "distinctive signature whistles" in bottlenose dolphins, especially between mother–calf pairs and cooperative males, all indicative of a role in social bonding.[41,42,43] In primates, gibbons—which display very complex vocalization behaviors including duetting—have been found to alter their "song" structure when predators are around, the "syntactic" changes seemingly understood by others.[32] But are vocalizations of this type a specific reference to objects, or could they be a more generalized signal about the mode of escape?[44] In some circumstances primate vocal communication can be used to deliberately deceive others in the group, but there is only scant evidence that these non-human communications express or reflect virtual mind states such as beliefs, intentions, or reference to imagined objects. Despite the apparent semantic flexibility in gibbon calls that may have referential meaning to conspecifics,[32] gibbons do not learn their repertoire of vocalizations from their parents. The calls seem to be genetically programmed and perhaps therefore have minimal flexibility and adaptability.[45] For reasons such as this, Fitch, who defines "song" as "complex, learned vocalization," argues that gibbons—and all other primates except *Homo sapiens*—do not "sing."[7]

However, there is one new world primate species, the marmoset, that alters its vocal repertoire as a result of both maturation and social interaction with parents.[46] Takahashi and colleagues argue that this combination of morphological and neurological maturation, and influence of parental vocal feedback, is "consistent with preverbal vocal development in humans." Another research group also reported that "turn-taking" in marmoset vocalizations is a learned behavior, again influenced by cooperative parent–offspring interactions.[47] At the molecular level, various genes associated with disorders of human speech or reading show at least partially overlapping expression patterns in the visual, auditory, and motor systems of the marmoset.[48] The marmoset has many unique biological, social, and genetic characteristics, and separated from the human line about 40 million years ago.[49] Thus, any similarities between marmosets and humans in cooperative vocal turn-taking, probably linked to analogous prosocial behaviors, are almost certainly an example of convergent evolution.[50,51] Nonetheless, such phylogenetic studies may well provide fertile new ground for modeling how certain aspects of vocal interaction and speech may have evolved in *Homo sapiens*.[52]

In the context of the present discussion, however, it is interesting to note that marmoset vocalizations are referred to as "calls" and not "song," and are thought to be more analogous to human speech than to music. Marmosets generally live in dense jungle, and their vocal communications help—amongst other functions—to maintain contact with members of the group. These vocalizations can reduce stress and have a calming effect on conspecifics, reducing cortisol levels for example.[53] But we shall see that this is similar to the effects that music can have on humans. Is it the absence of a perception of melodic contour in marmoset calls that makes us think differently about them? I sense here again the difficulty in the anthropomorphic way we ascribe animal vocalizations to either a pseudo-linguistic or pseudo-musical domain.

Music in humans is special, and unique. My friend and colleague Nicholas Bannan has this to say about aural processing and vocalization involving pitch, duration, temporality, amplitude, and timbre: "While response to sound stimuli that exploits sensitivity to these parameters is widespread across a variety of unrelated species, a few of which also possess the capacity for imitation and vocal learning, the relationship between perception and production in humans that permits unison singing and precisely organised rhythmic-prosodic interaction is found in no other species. Above all, human exploitation of controlled exhalation in articulate vocalisation contrasts markedly with the relatively limited vocal repertoire of chimpanzees and gorillas."[54] In humans, auditory cortical regions in Heschl's gyrus that are sensitive to pitch compare and monitor voice production and "detect discrepancies between the intended and heard vocalization," aiding in error correction.[55] To be able to sing in tune is a remarkable feat for *Homo sapiens*, but singing different notes in harmony is even more remarkable, leading Bannan to suggest: "singing different notes that aggregate to make chords is equally something that only the later stages of the hominin line appear to have attained. Not only is this as astonishing an achievement as language itself: one explanation for the evolution of this ability is that it may have been a necessary condition for the development of the anatomical, aural and neural substrates on which language depends."[54]

Comparative research on vocalization in animals remains very important, and understanding neural and behavioral relationships between animal communication and human language/music will continue to be illuminating.[7,8,17,18,56,57,58,59] There are likely to be convergent structures and circuits involved in vocalization (see discussion in Chapter 3 on FOXP2 for example) and specific aspects of auditory processing that are specialized to process, among other things, tone-based contours, rhythm perception, and emotional encoding. Such comparisons may point to innate constraints on the mechanisms and neural architecture involved in the production of, and response to, patterned vocalizations, perhaps a necessary foundation for music and human song. As Hauser and McDermott wrote: "Human and nonhuman animals thus encode emotional information in their vocalizations and have perceptual systems that are designed to respond appropriately to such signals. Given its evolutionary ancestry, our music faculty may well have co-opted this mechanism for use in music, even if it did not evolve for this function."[15]

More recently, similarities have emerged in the transcriptomes obtained from brain regions in "song"-learning birds and humans known to be involved in learning and motor control of vocalization.[58,60] There is also, in a somewhat similar way to humans, a left-sided dominance for vocal learning in juvenile (but not adult) male songbirds,[61] and a neural reward system similar to that found in humans listening to music that is activated in the limbic system of female (but *not* male) birds listening to male "song" bird vocalizations.[62] The responses varied depending on whether or not the females were in a breeding state, and in males the responses were different, only driving regions thought to be associated with sexual behavior and aggression. Note that only some birds (usually males), and even fewer mammals, have the "capacity to reproduce by means of the voice that which has been heard by ear"—vocal production learning, a competence obviously found in us, but importantly not in any other primate.[8] Merker suggests that this ability, which is essential for song learning in birds, "played a crucial role in the genesis of central human traits such as imitation, ritual culture and brain expansion, besides being an essential prerequisite for our singing and speaking."

This is a big call. However, in my view, attempts to find in other, evolutionarily distant species the precursors of our own communication systems can perhaps be taken too far. I pointed out in Chapter 3 that most of these species have had many millions of years to independently evolve their own communication systems in parallel to our *Homo* lineage. As Silvia Bencivelli commented in her excellent book *Why We Like Music*[63]: "the observation that, from the behavioral and neurological point of view, people and apes respond to certain acoustic stimuli in the same way might mean that the structures that give us our perception of sound are much older than we are." I would take out the word "might" from that sentence; surely when a sophisticated conspecific vocalization system evolved in a particular species, one would expect the neural circuitries needed to receive, process, and then assess the biological relevance of complex sounds to co-evolve,[62] and, as others have argued, we would expect such vocalizations to profoundly influence the affective/emotional state of self as well as other members of the species.[15,64,65] Otherwise, the communication system would be behaviorally redundant, and probably would not have evolved in the first place?

It is certainly interesting that the circuits in male "song" birds are similar in principle to at least some of the circuits in the human brain that are active when listening to music. From the perspective of language, the finding that, in juvenile finches, the circuits active during vocal learning are left-lateralized, similar to the lateral bias for speech and language in humans, is intriguing. As in many primates, in the vervet monkey there is also lateralization of response to vocalizations by other vervets, but this processing occurs on the right-hand side![66] Taken together, it seems likely that some form of unilateral dominance is needed for auditory-vocal learning for at least some form of communication between members of a species.[61] But is bird "song" a language or is it music, or is it a mixture of the two?—I sense confusion here in the parallels drawn with human communication systems.

If it were truly "song", then shouldn't the lateralization be more on the right side of male songbird brains? And in the transcriptome analysis discussed earlier, the mRNA similarities between "song"-learning birds and humans were strongest in "human laryngeal motor cortex and parts of the striatum that control *speech* [my emphasis] production and learning."[58]

In summary then, despite the vast array of excellent and important work focused on animal vocalization and communication, I prefer not to think of these animal communication systems as "song", as being "musical". We have seen that different animal species use communication systems that contain certain sonic elements (discrete pitch, short "melodic" phrases, rhythmic entrainment, drumming, etc) that are also characteristic of human music, but "it is the combination of these features as a package that seems unique to humans."[67] Moreover, as we shall see later in this and the following chapter, music as perceived by humans activates areas in prefrontal cortex that overlap with areas involved in the processing of prosocial, cooperative behaviors, regions that have no obvious parallel in other "singing" species. According to Hauser and McDermott: "animal songs are neither homologous nor analogous with human music ... none of the great apes sing, indicating that our last common ancestor did not sing."[15] Of course the opposite *could* also be true, though I think it highly unlikely—that many millions of years ago the last ancestor common to both humans and the great apes could in fact sing, but our lineage was the only one to retain that ability.

Complex animal vocalizations convey, primarily, life-relevant information. Music to some extent does so too of course (why else write this book?!), and it may well be that animals feel some type of reward when "singing", just as we do. But in humans it is language (usually speech) that is the main mode of information transfer, of structuring thought and conveying meaning; music in "*Homo sapientior*" is essentially a parallel communication stream. I do not mean to be "homocentric" about this, but in my view over-use of the term "song" has the potential to confuse and blur arguments about the origins and unique meaning of music and its place alongside language as a vital communicative resource for *Homo sapiens*. It may seem like mere semantics, but words do have the capacity to influence thought processes, channel ideas, and lead to constraints or boundaries on analysis. Interestingly, the linguist David Crystal has similar concerns about the use of the word "language." In his book "*How Language Works*" he writes: "Despite some superficial similarities, so-called 'body language' and 'animal language' are very different from what happens in language, in the sense of this book. I find it clearer to avoid the use of the term *language* altogether, in fact, and to describe these phenomena in more general terms—as *body communication* and *animal communication*. There is nothing wrong with the 'language' metaphor, of course, as long as we realize that that is what it is—no more than a vague approximation to the structurally complex and multifunctional behaviour we find whenever we speak, write, or sign."[68] Lack of a clear definition of "language" may also contribute to disagreements in the literature about whether it evolved slowly over hundreds of thousands of years,[69] or whether it is a recent, rapidly evolved communication system, unique to our species.[70]

Music and *"Homo sapientior"*

I recall that the *Oxford English Dictionary* definition of music is: "That one of the fine arts which is concerned with the combination of sounds with a view to beauty of form and the expression of emotions." While the great Russian composer Igor Stravinsky did not believe that music has the inherent capacity to express anything at all—it is "by no means the purpose of its existence"[71]—he agreed that in addition to coordinating "man and time," it can yet express things through illusion, through cultural attribution. But surely these are exactly the types of things music can do—why music remains a core communication stream for our species. With rare insight, the composer Paul Hindemith wrote that "music is meaningless noise unless it touches a receiving mind" (quoted in Shapiro,[72] p 14). If Hindemith was referring to the *human* mind in this statement, then whale "song," bird "song," gibbon "song," and so on, represent patterned and highly sophisticated modes of communication that strongly influence individual and group behaviors, and may elicit affective responses, but by this refined definition they are not what we, as humans, implicitly understand to be "music." In a similar vein, Michael Arbib, in his introduction to a recent multi-authored book on the "mysterious relationship" between language and music wrote: "… it can be argued that the song of a nightingale is not music until heard by a musician who reinterprets it,"[73] and as Israel Nelken wrote, "while music has to do with sounds, not all sound is music."[74]

Music requires spatio-temporal organization of sound streams, not just sound per se. The music we humans like and respond to is an entirely individual percept and unique to each of us, dependent as it is on emotional context, and the time and place we first experienced that music, and with whom. And there needs to be cultural and social agreement about what is perceived as music, otherwise we cannot sing and dance together and "there can be neither music nor musical communication."[75] That is why no one should ever patronize or criticize another person for the music that rocks (or soothes) their particular boat. To again quote John Blacking from his book *How Musical Is Man*: "What turns one man off may turn another man on, not because of any absolute quality in the music itself but because of what the music has come to mean to him as a member of a particular society or social group."[75] In fact, with culturally familiar music we develop specific rules, expectations, and learning strategies that make the music easier to remember, but when listening to, and recalling, culturally unfamiliar music there is greater activity in a broad range of brain areas, mostly in the right hemisphere, consistent with the task being more cognitively challenging and the need to process these novel musical stimuli.[76]

The proposal, then, is that music does not exist unless it is perceived by a modern human mind. The great variety of sounds emitted by other species, including, I suggest, our *Homo* ancestors, constitute complex types of vocal communication—often amazingly beautiful and sophisticated, but they should not be regarded as "music." I argue that the term is only truly appropriate when there is a need to differentiate this mode of expression, and the impact it has on our behavior and our state of mind, from the other communication system that we possess, ie language. To my knowledge, this duality exists in only one species, *"Homo sapientior."* To quote the great French philosopher Jean-Jacques Rousseau from his *Oeuvres complètes*: "Birds whistle, only man sings, and one cannot hear a song or a symphony without immediately saying: another sentient being is here." Or as John Blacking wrote: "There is so much music in the world that it is reasonable to suppose that music, like language and possibly religion, is a species-specific trait of man."[75] The psychologist and musicologist John Sloboda concurs: "it is clear that the functions of music for man find no parallel in the animal world" (Sloboda, 1985, cited by Silvia Bencivelli[63]). Humans are thought to be the only mammalian species that can truly synchronize and coordinate sound production with others—as we do in choirs for example—as well as synchronize movement (dance) in a social/group context,[67,77] a sensorimotor interaction that is at the heart of the effect of music on our species. The relationship between music and movement and the emotion that goes with it is universal, with common responses within and across cultures.[78]

We can only guess at the nature of the communication systems used by our immediate ancestors, but the question as to whether it was music or speech/language that came first may in fact not be the correct question to ask. There is an additional possibility, discussed by a number of scholars over recent years. Given the cumulative and generally conservative nature of evolutionary progress, using and building on pre-existing structures and processes, it is probable that neither music nor language evolved de novo in modern humans, neither system was an entirely new creation. The proposal that modern language, with its hierarchical syntactic organization, emerged and evolved from preexisting networks, from some form of protolanguage, was discussed towards the end of Chapter 3. This precursor may in fact have been the common progenitor that spawned *both* music and language, a precursor that was perhaps mostly prosodic in nature that somehow separated into two complementary strands when *"Homo sapientior"* evolved, with both resultant types of communication universally retained: music with its social rewards, emotive content, and links to movement and dance, and language with its new intellectual, generative, and open-ended symbolic power, but also containing prosodic elements of altered pitch, rhythm, and intensity, incorporating gesture and the careful monitoring of facial expression, eye position, and so on. Iain Morley has proposed something similar: "the culturally shaped melodic, rhythmic behaviours that we call music, and semantic, lexical linguistic abilities ... emerged as specialised behaviours building upon the foundations of this system of vocal and kinaesthetic communication of emotion."[79] Affective vocal expression is common to both streams, with—according to the psychologist Klaus Scherer—the aroused emotions separable into primarily utilitarian for speech, and aesthetic for music.[16]

Twenty-first century evidence supporting the existence of such a precursor can in fact be gleaned from recent neuroimaging and other studies, and is discussed in more detail later. So, for me, the appropriate questions are: when did language and music diverge, and why did we, *"Homo sapientior,"* retain both forms of communication? Why did we keep music? Why, when language became the dominant means of communication and information transfer, linked to the evolution of the modern mind and new cognitive power,

did we not lose music as a consequence—why did it not just disappear over the generations? Why does music—about 3,000 generations after our globe-filling journey out of
Africa—remain a much-loved and much-needed universal phenomenon?

In the previous chapter I put forward some ideas about the types of small, but perhaps
relatively rapid, evolutionary changes that may have been positively selected, resulting
in a transformation of the neural circuitry of "archaic" *Homo sapiens* into the functional
architecture typical of modern human brains, in other words the evolution of *"Homo
sapientior."* Some further examples of genetic micromutations that may have influenced
the development of human social and empathic behaviors are provided in Chapter 5.
Assuming there was indeed a critical evolutionary change in certain aspects of *Homo*
brain function and organization, we almost certainly cannot tell when this occurred from
fossil skeletal evidence. As discussed in Chapter 3, we have no brain material from our
immediate ancestors or from our contemporaneous "cousins" such as the Neanderthals—
a missing and crucial part of the puzzle. Anthropologists and linguists have therefore
attempted to shed at least some light on the evolution of language (and perhaps also
music) by examining other parts of the anatomy, including the hominin upper respiratory
tract (larynx and pharynx) (Figure 4.1), where vocal sounds are produced.[80,81,82]

From a sensory perspective, as pointed out by Iain Morley, it is important to examine
the middle and inner ear anatomy of closely related hominins to gain some insight into
their peripheral auditory processing abilities.[79] The cochlea itself seems to be of similar dimensions in Neanderthals and anatomically modern humans, but a recent very
detailed comparison of fossilized middle ear ossicles between the two species revealed
"striking morphological differences".[83] Nonetheless, computer modeling revealed that
the *functional* properties of the middle ear in Neanderthals and anatomically modern
humans were likely to be similar, suggesting a similar level of auditory sensitivity, at
least at lower sound frequencies.[83] On the motor side, the anatomy of the Neanderthal
hyoid bone (a horseshoe-shaped bone in the neck that aids tongue movement and
swallowing), presumed vocal apparatus, and upper respiratory tract is said to resemble
that of a young human. Much has been made of the morphology of the hyoid bone
in Neanderthals, and while by no means a definitive indicator of speech and modern language capability,[70] at the very least its structure suggests a capacity for complex
vocalizations.[84] The epiglottis is a small flap of elastic cartilage attached to the larynx
(Figure 4.1) that, in adults, closes over the trachea when swallowing. Compared with its
position in adults, in human infants the epiglottis is located higher up so that they can
breathe and swallow at the same time—very useful when suckling. The adult larynx lies
further down the throat, lengthening the flexible pharynx (which is above the larynx),
and thus increasing the potential for sound modification and modulation. There is a
cost to this; humans cannot breathe and swallow at the same time, and there is always
the potential for choking, perhaps resulting in death but at the very least disrupting
normal communication and often causing significant embarrassment. In fossil hominins the position of the larynx is much higher than in modern humans, and the pharynx and oral-nasal cavities differ in their structure too.[80,81,85]

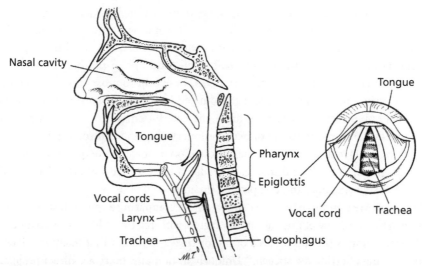

Figure 4.1 The anatomical organization of the human pharynx, larynx, and vocal cords.
© Martin Thompson, 2016.

Articulate speech requires exhalation of air of extended duration and rapid alteration in the structure of the vocal cords (or vocal folds), which are located in the larynx (Figure 4.1). Fine respiratory control and precise movement of the tongue within the oral cavity are, of course, also a necessary prerequisite for vocalization when singing.[7] Based on an examination of fossil thoracic vertebrae it has been suggested that our immediate ancestors and close cousins evolved better control over air exhalation;[79,86] the general view is that Neanderthals, for example, possessed good vocal control and could utter some consonant- and vowel-type sounds, requiring coordination between lungs (in turn controlled by the diaphragm and abdominal/thoracic musculature), vocal cords in the larynx, the pharynx, and muscles controlling the jaw, soft palate, lips, and tongue.[87] Receptors are also needed to convey sophisticated sensory feedback in order to monitor, and if necessary modify, the complex machinery used for vocalizations.[88] According to Chip Walter in his book *Last Ape Standing*,[89] Neanderthals probably could not make certain vowel sounds, compromising potential speech capacity. Perhaps they used tones more, a vocal communication with a limited type of vocabulary "based more on inflection and context."[89] The canal in the floor of the cranium that carries the motor nerve innervating the tongue (the hypoglossal nerve) is similar in size in Neanderthals to that in modern humans; however, it is now clear that the size of this canal does not correlate with the size of the nerve itself, and the "size of the hypoglossal canal does not reflect vocal capabilities or language usage."[90]

Of course, the ability to generate (and understand) human-like language requires more than just mechanics and the appropriate physical apparatus; it requires the internal, complex neural architecture to drive, coordinate, process, interpret, and remember it.[82] The vocal cords themselves are subtly controlled by a number of muscles that are innervated by motor output via the 10th cranial (vagal) nerve from a nucleus delightfully called the "nucleus ambiguus" in the brainstem. Altered cord vibration affects pitch and loudness, and the stream of air is also then modified in what is termed the vocal tract (pharynx, oral, and nasal cavities) by the tongue, soft palate, and lips to produce different resonating frequencies (called formants), harmonics, and vocal sounds. This whole complex, interactive apparatus is controlled and coordinated by neural structures including parts of motor and premotor cortex (Broca's area), the anterior cingulate cortex, basal ganglia, cerebellum, and the brainstem motor neurons innervating and controlling the peripheral musculature.[88,91] Dynamic and volitional modulation of voice frequency and timbre contributes to speech prosody and may have predated the evolution of articulate speech— important in social, sexual, and competitive situations.[92]

In humans, fMRI studies have revealed that, when comparing a speech task with tongue or lip movement, or vowel phonation, the region with relatively highest activity during speech production is the larynx area of motor cortex, a region that likely mediates the melodic voicing of articulate speech.[93] Uniquely in humans, there are direct projections from this "phonatory region" of primary motor cortex to the brainstem motor neurons that control voluntary vocalizations.[88] In addition, imaging analysis of human white matter tracts has revealed that, compared with monkeys, there are far more extensive connections between the human laryngeal motor cortex and somatosensory and inferior parietal cortices, increasing the capacity for sensorimotor integration, and allowing for "more complex synchrony of higher-order sensorimotor coordination, proprioceptive and tactile feedback, and modulation of learned voice for speech production."[91] The part of the motor cortex that voluntarily controls the larynx is bilaterally activated during breathing, but is more functionally lateralized to the left side during the voiced production of syllables.[94] Lastly, from an auditory perspective we perceive sounds in and around the frequencies most useful for hearing speech.[95]

Taken together, it is clear that general knowledge about gross anatomy does not necessarily reveal how a structure is controlled, nor does it reveal its neurological and behavioral function. To emphasize again, we need to study the living, functional brain to know exactly what is processed where, and we cannot do that with fossils. Of course it would be seriously helpful to obtain some neural, as well as other soft tissue, samples from both *Homo neanderthalensis* and ancestral *Homo sapiens* 100,000 and 60,000 years ago; perhaps specimens are frozen somewhere to be revealed as the planet warms? But in the meantime we can only make intelligent assumptions about what sort of communication system was used by our cousins and immediate ancestors, and where and how this was processed in their brains.

Similarly, although we know of the existence of a very primitive form of notation (proto-writing?) in the Middle East about 10,000 years ago, there is no corroborative evidence from fossils that this critically important cultural and cognitive development was accompanied by a change in the external morphology of the cerebral cortex. Writing appears to have developed independently in the Middle East and in South America, and perhaps also in China. In the Middle East, written symbols on clay tablets date from about 5500–6500 years ago, and in China different types of symbol were carved into tortoise shells and bone found in graves dated at about 8600 years old.[96] The forerunner of our own alphabet seems to have been invented only about 4000 years ago, but of course other types of writing also exist.[68] Presumably the human cortex already had most of the capacity to read and write owing to the presence of language networks pre-adapted for oral communication, but the potentiality was not harnessed until there was a demand for inventing a new way of storing and transmitting data. After the last ice age, in the transition in Eurasia from hunter-gatherer to farmer, perhaps there was a need to begin to keep track of the production and trade of a range of agricultural goods and services?

Although not entirely clear, it seems that *Homo sapiens* may have first arrived in Australia somewhere between 50,000 and 60,000 years ago,[97] but while further immigration and admixture with other hominins would likely have occurred over the following millennia, there is no evidence of phonetic writing in Australia until the arrival of Europeans, at which point indigenous Australians learned the knack within one generation. Thus, for tens of thousands of years this ancient, linguistic hunter-gatherer population had evolved a complex social culture, celebrated life with music and dance, used symbolism in their art, possessed sophisticated spiritual beliefs, and possessed a brain with visuomotor and cognitive capabilities sufficient to develop alphabets and intuit the semantic leaps required. Yet there was no emergence, as far as we can tell, of writing and reading in any of their diverse languages; presumably the need was not there? As suggested above, such emergent properties may only occur when human populations become sedentary, whereas with agriculture and livestock there is a need for trade, more sophisticated technologies, and the ownership (and value) of property.[98] "Materiality, cultural practices, and social interaction" play a crucial role in shaping what the human brain and mind can (will?) do.[99] The neural architecture, including the complex connectivity now known to be needed between particular cortical regions,[100] was clearly present in indigenous Australians because the famous Woollarawarre Bennelong, who was captured near Sydney in 1789, astonishingly wrote the first letter by an indigenous Australian in English text in 1796, just seven years after his first interaction with the rest of the world.

"Musilanguage" or "protolanguage"

The idea of an ancient communication system that spawned both music and language in "*Homo sapientior*" has been proposed by a number of scholars. The thirteenth-century philosopher Roger Bacon considered music to be a part of mathematics, but he also suggested that music constituted the "theoretical foundation upon which language itself is built."[101] Rousseau, who wrote a great deal about the origins and meaning of language and music,[102] thought there must initially have been primeval sounds with both musical and linguistic content. Such a precursor has been termed a protolanguage or musilanguage (to use Steven Brown's term[103]), or prosodic protolanguage.[104] People with congenital amusia have more trouble in interpreting emotional content in speech, "supporting speculations that music and language share mechanisms that trigger emotional responses to acoustic attributes, as predicted by theories that propose a common evolutionary link between these domains."[105]

The late Bruce Richman pointed out[37] that the ability to repeat long, meaningful, and memorable sequences of sounds during interpersonal communication is common to both music and speech, and thus proposed that in early *Homo sapiens* there was no distinction between them: "speech and music-making were one and the same: they were collective, real-time repetitions of formulaic sequences." Recursion (embedding phrases within phrases) is a structural property of syntax that seems to be common to both language and music, although of course in language we take turns to speak while music is much more about coordinated behavior and togetherness. But because both of these universal communication streams also contain prosodic elements and involve learning and cultural transmission, "any theory of the evolution of language will have implications for the evolution of music, and vice versa."[104] And as we shall see later on in this chapter, the existence of at least some common elements in the neural networks that process music or language is not inconsistent with the derivation of these two communication systems from a single precursor of some kind.

Steven Mithen has put forward some stimulating ideas about the nature of this hypothetical precursor. He uses the term "hmmmm," which stands for holistic, manipulative, multimodal, musical, and mimetic. In essence, Mithen envisaged "hmmmm" to have "a large number of whole meaning utterances, each functioning as a complete message in itself rather than as words that could be combined to generate new meanings." In "*The Singing Neanderthals*"[106] he hypothesized that "hmmmm" was an elaborate, versatile communication system that used not only gesture but also dance, and incorporated rhythm, melody, timbre, and pitch, especially when conveying emotion, and especially when communicating with offspring. Like many others, including Ellen Dissanayake and Sandra Trehub, Steven Mithen sees links between "language" in prehistory and the infant-directed nonverbal communication that is now used between mothers and their babies in all cultures across the globe, a topic I will return to later in this chapter. "Hmmmm" would also have had a role in mate attraction, perhaps also in emotional manipulation and the fostering of cooperative group behavior. In Chapter 2, I briefly discussed the remarkable case of two Indian girls who had been raised by wolves, and commented about the surviving girl who never acquired language skills. In thinking about the possible existence and constituent elements of a protolanguage, I wonder if such an individual responded to rhythm, to music? It would be fascinating to know the answer.

The mimesis idea has some historical precedence. In the eighteenth century, music was "considered to be both an art dependent on mimesis and a science that dealt with the realm of sensory impressions."[107] Mimesis, to paraphrase Merlin Donald in "*Origins of the Modern Mind*," describes the ability to produce conscious, self-initiated acts that are intentional but not linguistic in nature. They are defined primarily in terms of their representational function and include gestures such as bowing the head, putting your hand over your heart to show love, covering your face to show embarrassment or shame, shrugging the shoulders, or raising two fingers (Churchillian style of course). Humans still do this: just think of the great mime artists such as Marcel Marceau and Charlie Chaplin, who were able to nonverbally express and communicate a particular, sometimes subtle, emotional state by body movement and facial expression alone. In everyday life we do this as conscious, self-initiated, nonverbal acts of communication, almost always involving changes in facial expression and the creative use of the hands, with some nationalities using their hands far more than others when gesturing during speech. In addition, eye contact forms a major part of interpersonal communication and recognition, with recent imaging studies revealing strong interconnections between voice- and face-recognition areas in the human brain.[108]

Have you ever watched someone's mouth and tongue as he/she tries to thread a needle—the orofacial musculature seems to be attached by invisible pulleys to the hands as they move? Such intimate interactions imply proximal or shared neural circuitries of some kind, and it is therefore fascinating to note, as mentioned in the previous chapter, that Broca's area is not only a motor speech area but also participates in gesture and the processing and sequencing of structured, complex hand movements (sometimes called motor syntax[109]). Recent neuroimaging studies of subjects producing words or gestures have confirmed that overt speech production and the motor control of gesture share a functional network—largely but by no means entirely left-lateralized—that is connected to this area in the inferotemporal cortex.[110] Not inconsistent with this, there is evidence that Neanderthals were predominantly right-handed,[111,112] so perhaps our immediate ancestors were as well? Is this the left-biased motor network that was hijacked by articulate spoken language tens of thousands of years ago? Was this distributed network, which includes areas involved in cognitive and sensory processing, also in some way associated with the planning and sequencing of complex eye–hand coordinated activities? Was it needed for tool-making for example? This is not a new idea by any means, but one that cognitive neuroscientists have intensively investigated in recent years.[113]

When making a tool, one action sometimes has to be performed before another, and embedded in that action is another structured motor activity that allows the second action to be completed (a form of recursion), and so on. It has been proposed that the intentional acts of demonstrating, observing, and then learning and performing such structured, hierarchical tasks "could have provided an adequate scaffold for the evolution of intentional vocal communication."[113] Watching hand gestures when listening to speech increases activity in auditory regions of the left superior temporal gyrus and elsewhere, especially when the speech is difficult to understand,[114,115] providing additional integrative information that boosts verbal language performance and comprehension[116,117] and enhances memory performance.[118] In humans there are, in fact, close and intimate links between manual gestures, gaze, and speech, and the complex processing of these differing modalities is undertaken within a common, diverse network that includes language-related areas such as parts of temporal cortex and the inferior frontal gyrus.[119]

Although we mostly associate human language with speech and hearing, as many others have pointed out, and as I briefly discussed in Chapter 2, our language ability is remarkable in that its expression and reception are not restricted to the auditory modality.

Deaf people communicate using syntax and so forth, but they can do this by lip-reading, using their hands to sign, for example, words and sentences. Sign "language" (of which there are a number of types) has a complex structure that can substitute for spoken language, fulfilling similar roles. The deaf can also respond to, and participate in, music using vibrotactile as well as visual signals.[30,120] Similarly, congenitally and early-blind people also have enhanced tactile discriminative abilities[121] and read by using the somatosensory system and their fingertips—Braille. In the congenitally blind, some "visual" areas appear to become responsive to aspects of language processing and comprehension,[122] a responsiveness that emerges early in life,[123] consistent with the idea that "there are areas that are selective for language tasks regardless of modality, and as such 'universal.'"[124] However, it is important to point out here that, even in normal brains, visual stimulation modulates activity in parts of auditory cortex in the temporal lobe.[125,126] Such integration is likely to be important in voice and face identification.[127] In other words, altered processing due to a specific sensory loss may be a matter of altered emphasis within existing systems rather than the creation of an entirely new processing network.

Given the links between hand movements, gesture, and language, it seems clear why sign language works so well; its production and interpretation are part of an overlapping neural network, a combination of speech and gesture.[128] Imaging studies using positron emission tomography (PET) to measure cerebral blood flow showed that sign language in deaf people, which involves different modes of communication (hands vs sound production) and different receivers (eyes vs ears), involves activation of what were traditionally thought of as verbal linguistic regions—in the left hemisphere for right-handers.[124,129,130] As in aural–oral language processing, semantic versus syntactic elements are processed in different regions in deaf "signers."[131] The major auditory cortical regions (Heschl's gyrus and planum temporale) are structurally similar in deaf and hearing people, even down to the characteristic left–right asymmetries, features that are already seen at birth;[132,133] however, there is increased gray matter density in the left motor cortex[134] and parts of the insula cortex[135] that may relate to use of the dominant right hand in signing and lip-reading respectively. Interestingly, there may be some sexual dimorphism in all of this. In females but not males, the left primary auditory cortex is active during silent lip-reading;[136] females appear to transfer visual speech information across to auditory processing areas, but males interpret lip movements more by using the visual input itself. Whether this has anything to do with the reported increase in gray matter volume of the left superior temporal sulcus, and right Heschl's gyrus and planum temporale in females vs males,[137] is a matter of interesting conjecture.

In his book *A Commonsense View of All Music*, John Blacking suggests that our Homo ancestors were able to dance and "sing" well before language and speech evolved.[138] The notion of a pre-linguistic, sophisticated, multimodal communication prototype, whatever it is called, seems completely reasonable to me—but as I intimated earlier in this chapter I am not convinced that the term "musical" need necessarily be used to describe a type of communication just because it involves patterned changes in pitch, tone, volume, and rhythm. What is almost certain—and I think Steven Mithen and others are absolutely right—is that our immediate ancestors, as well as hominins such as the Neanderthals, had a very sophisticated way of communicating with others and must have evolved effective social systems and networks. There is evidence from the fossil record of some form of social care, of looking after injured individuals,[139] perhaps genetically related. Evidence has also been found in Europe of large, delineated circular spaces that may just have been performance areas, dated at about 300,000 years old,[140] and underground constructions, dated at about 176,000 years old.[141] More recently, in southwest France there is evidence of continuous occupation for perhaps 50,000 years, and even evidence of post holes suggestive of shelters and communal living spaces (Klein 1999, quoted in Freeman 2000[142]). But if indeed, in Mithen's phraseology, Neanderthals had "Hmmmm" it didn't seem to advance their cognitive thinking very much. Their gesture and vocal communication systems had great emotional power, but these systems had significant limitations; Neanderthals hummed along for several hundred thousand years without any clear-cut cognitive advances. It seems, as Steve Olson wrote, that they were "living in the moment."[143] Perhaps, as has recently been found in monkeys,[144] our ancestors had a comparatively limited auditory short-term (or working) memory capacity,[145] and memory—as discussed in Chapter 3—is a critical element in evolving complex communication systems such as language, and music.

In contrast, in *Homo sapiens* some explosion happened that advanced our cognitive and rational powers, that permitted a new awareness and a unique sense of self, a capacity for objective planning and abstract thought, a capacity for mental imagery and setting goals well beyond the here and now—what Daniele Amati and Tim Shallice call "abstract projectuality."[146] As described in the previous chapter, the evolution of human language must surely have involved at least some alterations in neural circuitry and a heightened ability to coordinate, encode, and remember patterns of neural activity. We have seen that the human cerebral architecture specialized for language functions is not exclusively driven by speech and linguistic sounds, and that articulate language was almost certainly an extension of, and built onto, pre-existing vocal and gestural communication systems. Again quoting Derek Bickerton from his book on the evolution of language: "My own preference, for what it's worth, is that language (or should I say protolanguage) began as a free-for-all, catch-as-catch can mode that utilized sounds, signs, pantomime and any other available mechanisms that would carry intention and meaning, and that it only gradually focused on the vocal mode, due to the latter's greater utility."[147]

Music and language share a number of features; we know that music contains an organized structure, viewed by many as a type of syntax, and has common prosodic elements with language and articulate speech. We shall see soon that, at least for a number of basic components, the evidence points to a degree of overlap in neural processing architectures for the two communication streams. But exactly how music and speech/language separated from a presumed common precursor is, for me, the real question; the answer must lie in elements of this precursor being carried forward into each stream, but with the addition of computational elements that underpin the cognitive architecture of each system, including a much greater learning capacity and a super-enhanced storage and retrieval capacity. A similar but more radical hypothesis has been put forward by Leonid Perlovsky,[148] where he suggests that there was a "split in the vocalizations of proto-humans into two types: one less emotional and more concretely-semantic evolving into language, and the other preserving emotional connections along with semantic ambiguity, evolving into music." A divergence perhaps, but in my view there are too many commonalities in prosodic and some syntactic elements of each communication stream to warrant the suggestion of a complete split. Older multimodal, mimetic communication systems continue to contribute essential elements to language and human communication, but the prosodic elements of this pre-verbal system probably also provide the foundation of what we today understand as music. What this parallel, nonlinguistic communication system sounded like early in the history of "*Homo sapientior*" is unknowable, but it must be remembered that, as with speech, our musical brain has had perhaps 4000–4500 generations to evolve its own, to some extent independent, processing requirements and assembly of rules and conventions.

Neural networks for music and/or language

In Chapter 2, I presented the various types of evidence that emphasized the differences in circuitries and areas of the modern human brain that are activated by music or language. In particular, acquired brain injury studies of amusia and aphasia, so eloquently described by Oliver Sacks in his book *Musicophelia,*[149] consistently point to differences in the neural networks involved in the higher level, syntactic, and contextual processing of music versus language. Music tends to be right hemisphere biased, and in right-handed individuals language is biased towards the left-hand side. Modern neuroimaging studies of normal subjects lend some weight to this idea of hemispheric specialization, although when activity is visualized with these techniques the left–right distinction is less clear-cut. Overall, music and language "networks" are generally associated with greater activation and increased inter-regional connectivity in right and left cerebral cortices respectively.[150,151,152,153,154,155,156,157,158,159,160,161] There are also hemispheric differences in how these two networks code for pitch intervals (spectral resolution) and the "dynamic temporal structure" of speech versus music, in other words how components of language and music are ordered and modulated over time.[160,162,163,164] The right auditory cortex is "more specialized for resolving smaller frequency differences," needed for processing musical information, while the left has better temporal resolution, needed for analysis of the rapid transients so important in speech.[165]

I have also briefly discussed the white matter tracts that interlink auditory regions in the superior temporal gyrus, and other regions in the temporal lobe, with specific zones in other cortical lobes—frontal, parietal, and occipital (see Figure 2.8). Many of these fiber tracts, which include the arcuate and superior longitudinal fasciculi, have typically been linked to language and speech,[156] but it is increasingly being appreciated that they are also important in music processing and singing. To recapitulate the situation for language and speech, and as summarized by Josef Rauschecker:[156] the ventral pathways are involved in the "decoding of spectrally complex sounds" (a form of object recognition, eg lexical and semantic information), important in the perception and processing of speech, while the dorsal streams are more involved with "sensorimotor integration and control" (a "how-to-do" function)—that is, the analysis and production of coherent and semantically correct segments of speech. In right-handed people the relevant language-related pathways tend to be left-hemisphere biased. But similar ventral and dorsal tracts exist in the right hemisphere, and on this side the dorsal stream is biased towards integrating sensory feedback with vocalization in the musical context, in particular: "higher order processing of musical stimuli, apart from pitch and melodic contour extraction, engages regions within the dorsal auditory stream."[165] The processing of certain structural aspects of music, such as pitch categorization and pitch contour (melody) in prefrontal and inferior cortical regions, is thought to be mediated by the ventral stream.

When vocalizing, there are of course common elements in the production of complex sounds (phonology) and the generation of phrases in music (singing) and language (speech). An account of these interrelationships is provided by Aniruddh Patel in his book *Music, Language, and the Brain*.[166] Nonetheless, while it is increasingly clear that there is "a general functional network for human vocalization,"[88] differences between overt singing and speech have also emerged. For example, an early study found that singing is associated with an additional region of activity in right superior temporal gyrus (Heschl's gyrus) and parts of the basal ganglia, in experienced singers perhaps related to pitch perception and analysis of the singer's own voice for "feedback-guided modulation" and improved accuracy of intonation.[167,168] Other neuroimaging studies have reported bilateral activation of cortical areas but with greater activation on the left-hand side when linguistic elements were discriminated for, and greater activation in the right hemisphere when subjects sang, either covertly or overtly.[150,169] The general consensus now is that, via the dorsal stream in the right hemisphere, auditory and parietal cortex monitor pitch information and send this through to premotor cortex for vocal correction—input and output circuits that are especially sensitive to vocal training.[88,170,171]

Note that when simple singing involves the introduction of rhythmic complexity, a relative increase in activity is also noted in various cortical regions in the left hemisphere,[172] and non-expert singers seem to use more of the language network during singing, "likely accounting for their less tuneful performance."[56] Similarly, if both melody and lyrics of a song are learned together there is associated activity biased to the left, typical of linguistic processing, but learning the melody to "la" results in a wider network of activity including the right hippocampus, right inferior frontal gyrus, basal ganglia, and cerebellum.[173] The choral director of the amateur choir in which I sing, Margaret Pride OAM, was most pleased to hear of these studies because she has always believed that learning new music is easier if initially sung to "da"—reading new lyrics at the same time has a negative impact on our ability to learn the notes! The ability to monitor and adjust musical vocalization in terms of both pitch and rhythm is obviously a special human trait, evidenced by our unique ability to sing together in time and in harmony, an ability again suggestive of the positive selection of circuitries associated with musical aptitude, lineage, and group inter-actions in "*Homo sapientior*"[174] (see also Chapter 5).

The foregoing examples, especially when taking into account the wealth of information from acquired amusia studies described in Chapter 2, generally emphasize differences in linguistic and musical processing networks. However, there is increasing evidence—particularly from neuroimaging and other physiological studies—that there is considerable overlap in the neural architecture that is activated during the processing of music and language. The nature and extent of this overlap appear to depend on what features (simple or complex) are being tested, whether they are perceptual or motor, and how particular tests and analyses are carried out. In an early PET study that measured cerebral blood flow in a group of neurologically healthy amateur musicians, it was found that blood flow to some cortical areas was increased only by melody or sentence generation, but there were some regions of cortex and other regions of the brain (eg basal ganglia, ventral thalamus, poste-rior cerebellum) in which cerebral blood flow, and thus by association neural activity, was increased when performing either task.[175] In cerebral cortex, overlap in activity was seen in areas such as supplementary motor cortex, auditory cortex, the insula, and Broca's area. The authors concluded that music and language utilize neural systems with parallel and distinc-tive, but also shared, features. Similarly, comparison of cortical activation when listening to real versus scrambled music revealed processing in the left and right inferior frontal corti-ces, the left side corresponding to a region also implicated in linguistic processing.[176]

Because pitch is a core component of both language and music, it is perhaps not surpris-ing that in this particular domain there seems to be extensive overlap in neural processing machinery: "the persistent relationship between participants' ability to discriminate dif-ferences in linguistic pitch (sentence prosody) and musical pitch (melodies) is consistent with the hypothesis that cognitive mechanisms for pitch processing in language and music are shared beyond simple reliance on overlapping auditory sensory pathways or domain-general working memory and attention. There exists a significant and strong relationship between individuals' pitch processing abilities in music and language."[177] In fact, areas of the brain activated by the prosodic and affective elements of speech, which involve alterations in emphasis as well as pitch, have been delineated. For example, Rogalsky et al described overlap in neural activity when processing melodic contour and the prosodic elements of language in the anterior temporal lobe.[178] No language is delivered entirely in a monotone, and changes in pitch help define emotional content, although some so-called tone or tonal languages (eg Mandarin and Cantonese) are more dependent on pitch changes than others, and different languages have different rhythmic patterns. Cantonese speakers perform better than English-speaking subjects—and as well as musicians—in a test designed to measure aptitude for pitch acuity, music perception, and general cogni-tive ability, including aspects of memory performance.[179] A study on Mandarin-speaking musicians found considerable overlap in bilateral brain regions processing pitch informa-tion in either music or the Mandarin language, primarily in pars triangularis in Broca's area and parts of the temporal lobe, although some aspects of pitch perception in music induced greater activation in the right superior temporal gyrus.[158]

According to the ethnomusicologist Curt Sachs, in some languages and "primitive" cultures, music and singing can sometimes be far less emotional than the exuberance and passion that is exhibited in linguistic speech. In western culture and western languages this is perhaps most obvious when giving an oration to a crowd of people, or when reading or listening to poetry. In tonal languages the nature of the pitch-change, or whether the pitch is high or low, can completely alter the meaning of a particular word or phrase. Consider, for example, the use of the word O-K-O in African Guinea:[180] in middle pitch o-k-o means husband, and in low pitch o-k-o means spear, while o-k-o (rising at the end) means "hoe" and o-k-o (falling at the end) means canoe … so in languages like this, one must be careful how things are said, and listen carefully, or you might get a nasty surprise! In our own language, pitch and phrasing also matter; thus, for example, there is more than one way to phrase and interpret: "What is this thing called love?"

Individuals with congenital amusia or tone deafness are also of relevance here. As described in Chapter 2, this type of amusia is associated with some very specific neuroanatomical changes in cortical thickness and loss of connectivity in white matter, but importantly these changes are only evident on the right-hand side of the brain. Despite this apparent right-sided emphasis, as mentioned earlier, individuals with congenital amusia have problems with interpreting intonation contours in speech,[181] especially those who speak tonal languages such as Mandarin.[182,183,184,185] Once again, the inability to interpret emotional/prosodic content adversely affects both linguistic and musical communication systems.[105,186]

Of course, vocal communication can convey even greater meaning through the combination of words and music. By combining presentations of musical excerpts and words it has been shown that music is just as good at enhancing word recognition (priming) as language, suggesting close interrelationships between mnemonic and semantic memory processing and perception in music and language.[151,187,188,189,190] Consistent with this, alignment of musical and linguistic rhythm and meter significantly enhances neural activity.[191] fMRI analysis has revealed that the processing of lyrics and tunes (in this case both initially *unfamiliar* to the listener) is to some extent integrated in the left superior temporal region of the human brain, but more anteriorly in the temporal lobe there is a region where lyrics seem to be processed independently.[192] Only tunes activated the superior temporal cortex in the right hemisphere. Another study,[193] using the magnetoencephalography (MEG) technique (see Chapter 2), found that signal responses to errors in the expected sequence of lyrics or melodies of *familiar* songs were greatest in the left and right hemispheres respectively, leading these authors to state: "It is thus intriguing to note that these different aspects of speech processing (syntax vs prosody), or of music processing (lyrics vs melody), correspond to the dominance of left and right brains." A more recent fMRI study also found that: "while the left inferior frontal gyrus (IFG) coded for spoken words and showed predominance over the right IFG in prosodic pitch processing, an opposite lateralization was found for pitch in song."[155]

Morse code is pure rhythm, but with training it is perceived as a language, not music. Rap is essentially rhythmic language, but is regarded as music, yet poetry is not. In Africa there are "talking drums" that mimic and therefore communicate essentially linguistic messages, allowing transmission of information across great distances.[166] Whistling is usually associated with music, but it can be used to express feelings—for example the wolf whistle! There are even so-called whistle languages[68] where the communicative elements of whistling reach their zenith. Communication between individuals over a distance seems important here.[194] According to David Crystal, whistling dialogue follows the tonal and rhythmic changes of the whistlers' normal spoken language and can convey quite sophisticated cognitive information by recoding vowels and consonants into whistles, but conversations are succinct and whistling speech "does not really correspond to the complexity and functional breadth of spoken language."[68] Interestingly, the human brain processes this unique communication mode in a way that is very like spoken language.[194] I presume this is because whistling speech is used by individuals who have already acquired spoken language—it is a second language, if you will.

Particularly interesting from an evolutionary perspective is the suggestion that musical structure or "syntax" is processed, at least in part, in classical expressive speech areas in the inferior frontal lobe—a sharing of cognitive resources.[195] To remind you, syntax refers to the rules governing the arrangement of specific elements into sequences within a systematic, orderly, and predictable structure, and both language and music do have an organized hierarchical structure. In music, these elements may be tones, intervals, or harmonic progressions, and the storage and recall of this information require excellent acoustic memory.[196] Using MEG to study brain function, Maess and colleagues found that the region activated when imagining and processing a series of chords with a regular and predictable sequence was Broca's area.[197] Based on this result, the authors suggested that "the source of activity was localized in Broca's area and its right-hemisphere homologue. We find that these areas are also responsible for an analysis of incoming harmonic sequences, indicating that these regions process syntactic information that is less language-specific than previously believed."

Because the overall pattern of activity appears to be present in musicians and non-musicians, the neural networks for so-called musical syntax, which involve the inferior frontal gyrus (hierarchical relationships), anterior superior temporal gyrus (acoustic processing), and lateral premotor cortex (prediction of what is to come), may be intrinsic and not dependent on experience.[198,199,200,201] We have already discussed the mirror neuron network and the links between hand movement, gesture, and language. It is therefore of note that activity in Broca's area is especially evident in trained musicians who are watching hands playing unfamiliar versus familiar melodies, a finding consistent with involvement of this region in the broader, generalized context of "hierarchical processing of observed action."[202] In a different type of study, stroke patients with injury to the left Broca's area, but not the left anterior superior temporal gyrus, showed deficits in processing musical syntax,[192] and an EEG study using electrodes placed beneath the thick membrane surrounding the brain (the dura mater) also found evidence for co-localization of processing violations of musical and linguistic syntax in the temporal lobe, at least for early levels of processing.[159] Even more recently, a study using multiple neuroimaging techniques identified cortical networks that were mutually activated during the recognition and integration of words or chords that deviated "from the universal principles of grammar and tonal relatedness."[203] Again, the left inferior frontal gyrus was a core component, but with interactions with temporo-parietal regions as well. Interestingly however, the authors of this study also observed additional activation of areas when processing language or music that were biased to the left and right hemispheres respectively. Finally, an fMRI study using a different experimental paradigm provided additional evidence to support the proposal that there is an interaction between the syntactic processing of music and language in Broca's area.[204]

Differences in brain activity have even been documented when subjects listen to unexpected or expected chords at the end of a harmonic sequence,[205] rated by the listeners as unpleasant or pleasant respectively. When a chord sequence ended on an irregular chord rather than a "music-syntactically" regular tonic chord, activity was increased in the amygdala and caudate nucleus on both sides of the brain. Responses to irregularities in musical sequences are also seen in newborn infants[206] and in musically naïve children,[200] suggesting there may be a degree of in-built musical short-term memory in the brain of *Homo sapiens*. Similarly, human brains can detect violations of syntax in language even though this may not be conscious, suggesting that "at least part of the mental computations necessary for language processing take place outside of awareness, leaving only a subset of processes for the conscious mind to manage."[207] If the same is true for detecting syntactic errors in music, this might provide further evidence that music and modern language originated from a common precursor.

Importantly, however, not all imaging studies support this idea of shared processing networks for structure (syntax) in language and music,[152,178] and the stroke literature contains examples of individuals who can still process and interpret harmonic structure in music but not linguistic syntax, and vice versa.[208] For example, one fMRI study used a different way of analyzing structure in music and language, and concluded that there was little evidence for overlap in patterns of activation elicited by speech (sentences) and music (simple melodies), and little activation of Broca's area in either case.[178] These authors temporally modulated the overall acoustic envelope (the overall structure of the sound) of coherent sequences of speech or music and concluded that "neural systems involved in processing higher-order aspects of language and music are largely distinct" and that previous studies may have been looking primarily at common computational operations and/or working memory involved in detecting and processing errors—structural irregularities in the tasks used to assess function. These results should also be viewed in light of the suggestion, discussed earlier, that musical syntax is mostly related to auditory short-term memory capacity, whereas syntax in language involves the processing of higher-level conceptual information.[196]

One possible reason for such discrepancies, alluded to at the beginning of this section, may be that different groups use different tasks, and different ways of controlling multimodal sensory cues, when activating neural circuitries in the brain. The presence or absence of pleasurable thoughts related to movement or vocalization may also be important (see also below). A recent meta-analysis of 80 music and 91 speech neuroimaging studies,[209] the first study of its kind in the field, found that the musical tasks used by researchers essentially fall into four categories: music passive listening, music discrimination, music error detection, and music memory. The authors also included studies on passive listening to speech. To summarize their findings: "We found that listening to music and to speech preferentially activates distinct temporo-parietal bilateral cortical networks. We also found music and speech to have shared resources in the left pars opercularis but speech-specific resources in the left pars triangularis. The extent to which music recruited speech-activated frontal resources was modulated by task. While there are certainly limitations to meta-analysis techniques particularly regarding sensitivity, this work suggests that the extent of shared resources between speech and music may be task-dependent and highlights the need to consider how task effects may be affecting conclusions regarding the neurobiology of speech and music."[209] A reminder here that the pars opercularis and pars triangularis are small lobes within the inferior frontal lobe, generally regarded as co-existent with Broca's area (see Figure 2.8). Others have found that language-specific effects only become obvious "under conditions of increased demands on shared neural resources."[204] LaCroix and colleagues cite others[195,210] in arguing that any shared music–language circuitry revealed in experiments may be a reflection of generic executive control of cognitive function. Such cognitive control is needed for working memory and analysis of hierarchical structures, when there is a need to "detect and resolve conflict that occurs when expectations are violated and interpretations must be revised."[208]

How the nature of a task chosen by an experimenter affects a read-out from the brain is exemplified by recent work imaging neural activity while subjects listened to highly complex acoustic stimuli or natural sounds.[164,211,212,213] Supporting earlier amusia and aphasia observations after acquired brain injury, these imaging studies identified music and speech-specific regions in the human brain, specifically in secondary auditory cortex in the superior temporal gyrus. In one study,[164] complex and sophisticated algorithms were used to discern sub-populations of neurons that showed preferential, statistically weighted responses to 165 different *natural* sounds. Six different population "components" were identified, four responding selectively to acoustic features such as pitch and frequency, and the remaining two in nonprimary auditory cortex showing preference for either music or speech. These two regions were spatially distinct. As the authors point out, previous work attempting to discern differences in music and speech-processing networks has been, to some extent, hampered by the fact that in almost all studies: (i) there has been some inherent bias because specific acoustic stimuli are chosen to test a particular hypothesis, and (ii) fMRI has relatively coarse spatial resolution, meaning that selective responses might remain unrecognized owing to overlapping activity, as measured by standard voxel analysis. Better to get the neuronal population itself to "infer response dimensions from structure in the data, rather than test particular features hypothesized to drive neural responses." In fact, a similar type of approach was pioneered many decades ago by a Dutch group, the ensemble of natural stimuli used to correlate with neural events called the "acoustic biotope,"[214,215] a phrase that perhaps should regain some currency.

To summarize this section, recent research has reinforced the long-held view that certain discrete regions exist in the human brain that are biased towards the processing of either language or music. Left–right differences in the cerebral cortex in particular are most evident when examining cases of acquired amusia, and there are numerous subtle morphological differences, although the extent of this functional lateralization of language/speech versus music/song is not always as clear-cut when recording from, or imaging, normal human brains. Overall, I view the presence of at least some disparity in the networks that underpin language versus music processing as support for the evolution and positive selection of both modes of human communication. These networks are built upon shared systems that process prosody and many of the core elements of both speech and music, which, in addition to basic auditory information such as pitch, timing, rhythm, and timbre, include short-term storage of acoustic information, self-monitoring and production of vocalizations, and facets of syntactic processing.[88,201,209,216]

With regard to lateralization of function, perhaps there was less need for hemispheric specialization in our immediate ancestors' musilanguage or protolanguage networks. However, during the emergence of our two communication systems, language and music, with subtly different processing requirements it became necessary to separate out some distinct circuitries for each mode of communication. Because the overall cellular and connectional organization of the two cerebral hemispheres is relatively similar, perhaps some left–right parcellation of function was the simplest and most conservative option in evolutionary terms. Highly speculative it may well be, but the links between handedness, tool use, gesture, and emergent language may have contributed to a left-sided bias for articulate speech, while the right—with its "greater global connectedness" and role in longer-duration "large scale spatio-temporal and/or conceptual integration of behaviour"[113]—may have been more suited to specializations associated with the development of interactive musical capability.

According to Cross and co-authors, a key attribute that distinguishes language from music is "propositionality"—"a way of sharing information about states of affairs by means of truth-conditional propositions and thus coordination of action. It enables mapping between worlds, thoughts, and selves."[217] But if the lexical, semantic, syntactic elements of human language rapidly evolved hand in hand with the evolution of the modern, representational mind, if it was the primary driver of evolutionary change that led to the newly creative, curious, and imaginative "*Homo sapientior*," then the question remains: *Why music?* What was the value, if any, of maintaining and perhaps continuing to evolve this additional communication stream? What was its worth?

Music, emotion, and reward

Music can stir the soul; listening to music you enjoy is a highly rewarding experience. Given the emotional impact of music[16,218,219,220] it is perhaps not surprising that modern neuroscience has discovered that there are close associations between aspects of musical processing and areas of the human brain known to be involved in subjective or affective experiences. To quote Stefan Koelsch from his review on this topic: "These structures are crucially involved in the initiation, generation, detection, maintenance, regulation, and termination of emotions that have survival value for the individual and the species. Therefore, at least some music-evoked emotions involve the very core of evolutionarily adaptive neuroaffective mechanisms."[221] Steven Rose, in his book *The 21st Century Brain*[222], goes so far as to argue that, along with self-awareness and consciousness, human emotions are adaptive, evolved properties, and he somewhat provocatively rewrites Descartes thus: "*Emotio ergo sum!*"

As mentioned earlier, initial research on music processing and human brain imaging was often reductionist and academic, not involving natural sounds and not taking into account the accessible, emotional core of music.[223] But, both experimentally and therapeutically, getting the subjects/patients to subjectively choose the music they wish to listen to has revealed crucial new information about the power of music, and how it affects the human brain. Listening to music can sometimes give a listener the sensation of chills; to quote the author Nick Hornby: "At certain spine chilling shivering moments—and you will have your own, inevitably—it becomes difficult to remain a literalist."[224] How much we experience pleasurable chills when listening to music is related to the degree of emotional arousal,[221,225,226] a relationship probably mediated by the amygdala and associated circuitry.[227] Thus, music is not only capable of mentally transporting us into another dimension, another place, and another time, its emotional impact also has overt physical and psychological manifestations. These include not just chills, but also tears, shivers, and goose bumps; it can even cause our hair to stand on end![226] These responses to music are associated with a number of measurable physiological changes including, for example, changes in heart rate, respiration, body temperature, and blood pressure—physical manifestations presumably driven by altered activity in the autonomic nervous system.

But before I discuss what we know about the brain circuits that specifically underlie the emotional impact of music on "*Homo sapientior*," a reminder about some of the possible difficulties in interpreting fMRI data, especially when subjective behaviors are under scrutiny. As discussed in Chapter 2, the search for neural processing correlates of a particular behavior or stimulus requires a great deal of technical, biological, and medical know-how, and scientists must necessarily make a number of assumptions along the way. When imaging, great care must be taken with the choice of test controls to (hopefully) permit the elimination of any extraneous signals and the removal of nonspecific background activity. In addition, sufficient numbers of subjects in each experimental group are needed to gain sufficient statistical power to interpret the results appropriately.[228]

Attempts have been made to map the prosodic and affective elements of speech,[229] but when we study our qualitative emotional responses to music (do we like it or hate it? is it nostalgic or uplifting?), can we really monitor and analyze these inner subjective feelings satisfactorily? MRI machines can be claustrophobic and are very noisy, with clicks and clunks and beeps. In some machines the noise levels can be almost as loud as a jet engine! Having been in a noisy and somewhat claustrophobic MRI machine myself, I find it difficult to imagine how subjects are able to stay emotionally neutral and ignore background issues, and how they comfortably maintain focus and attention when listening to various sound presentations. Indeed, as I pointed out in Chapter 2, scanner noise can significantly influence activity in widespread neural networks[230,231] and it is now known that the amount of scanning noise that is present when subjects are asked to listen to music that is fearful, neutral, or joyful alters the fMRI signal in several cortical regions.[232] Emotional responses to music are complex and multifaceted. Nevertheless, numerous research groups have published useful and intriguing functional imaging data on the way the adult human brain processes music that is subjectively perceived with different amounts of valence and different emotional content.

Early and ground-breaking studies, using PET to measure changes in local blood flow to different parts of the brain, showed that there was increased flow to particular areas of the brain that positively correlated with "chills intensity ratings" in subjects listening to music.[233,234] Regions activated by these intensely pleasurable responses to music included parts of the anterior cingulate cortex, the insula (both sides), right orbitofrontal cortex, the supplementary motor area, regions around the thalamus and left ventral striatum, and the dorsomedial midbrain and cerebellum. Brain areas with reduced blood flow that were negatively correlated with chills included another part of frontal cortex (the ventromedial part), the amygdala, and the left hippocampal region.

In another important early study, a correlation was found between changes in cerebral blood flow and brain activity in different areas, dependent on whether the music had positive or negative attributes for the listener.[235] These researchers visualized areas of the brain that were active when subjects listened to musical stimuli versus scrambled music. Various areas on both sides of the brain showed selectively increased neural activity, including within a structure called the nucleus accumbens. The nucleus accumbens forms part of the ventral striatum, which in turn constitutes part of the complex of bilateral subcortical nuclei described earlier in this book—the basal ganglia (Figure 4.2). The nucleus accumbens receives inputs from prefrontal cortex, amygdala, hippocampus and ventral brainstem, and sends axons out to other parts of the basal ganglia, which in turn project

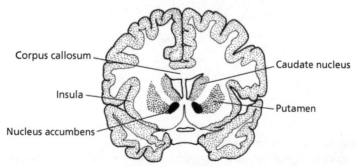

Figure 4.2 A cross-section through the human brain at the level of the basal ganglia, showing the location of the bilateral nucleus accumbens (NA) and its relation to other parts of the striatum (caudate nucleus and putamen).
© Martin Thompson, 2016.

to the thalamus and thence to prefrontal cortex. The nucleus accumbens also projects to various regions in the brainstem.

The nucleus accumbens is known to be associated with processing reward, reinforcement, pleasure, motivation, and goal-directed behavior.[236,237] The neurotransmitter dopamine, which is contained within axons that originate in a part of the midbrain called the ventral tegmental area, plays an important role in nucleus accumbens function, and also happens to be the target of most addictive drugs such as cocaine, amphetamine, and opiates. In Menon and Levitin's music study, parts of the midbrain, hypothalamus, and insula were also activated when listening to music versus "junk," all of these regions known from other research to form part of a "mesolimbic" network associated with the physiological manifestations of rewarding/emotional stimuli.[235] Finally, the orbitofrontal cortex was also active (Figure 4.3), a complex region that contains various subdivisions[238] and overall is involved in reward processing, learning, assessment of value, and decision making, and that we shall soon see is especially associated with our "positive" responses to music.

What about when listening to music that is perceived as being either "happy" or "sad?" Compared with the effects of "neutral" music, increased blood oxygen glucose levels (BOLD signal contrast) during the presentation of happy music were observed in anterior cingulate cortex (Figure 4.3), the left superior temporal gyrus (see Figure 2.7), an area of cortex adjacent to the hippocampus called the parahippocampal gyrus, and bilaterally in the ventral and dorsal striatum of the basal ganglia, including a structure called the caudate nucleus (Figure 4.2).[239] These regions are associated with various behaviors including reward, attention, and the planning, selection, and initiation of movements.

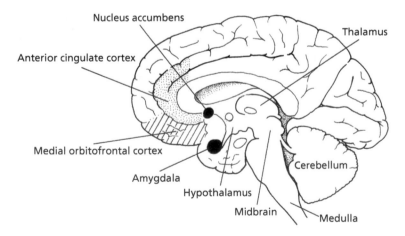

Figure 4.3 Medial view of half of the human brain, cut at the midline. Some of the regions are activated when listening positively to music (hippocampus not shown). Tasks that involve mutual cooperation activate similar areas (eg medial orbitofrontal cortex, anterior cingulate cortex, and nucleus accumbens). Other affective responses to music are associated with increased activity in the amygdala.
© Martin Thompson, 2016.

Similarly activated regions were seen in the chills intensity study described earlier. When music perceived as sad was presented, increased BOLD signal responses were noted in the right-sided hippocampus and amygdala, the latter of course being the same area that was activated in scans that were negatively correlated with chills. Auditory cortical areas in the superior temporal regions were, perhaps not surprisingly, activated under both listening conditions.

There even appear to be differences in the processing of minor and major harmonies—at least for subjects raised in the culture of western music. Different emotional meanings are attributed to different harmonic intervals,[240] and listening to minor chords rather than major chords increases activity in the amygdala as well as in parts of the cerebral cortex, brainstem, and cerebellum.[241] Another approach has been to use tests designed to analyze the neural responses to music that people find pleasant (consonant) or unpleasant (dissonant).[242,243] Dissonant music resulted in increased activation in the amygdala and also in the hippocampus and adjacent parahippocampal region,[242] areas we know to be involved in emotional processing (often negative valence) and memory function. Listening to pleasant music was associated with activation in auditory cortex, inferior frontal cortex, part of the insula, and the ventral striatum, incorporating the nucleus accumbens (see above). Activation of the ventral striatum/nucleus accumbens is especially obvious in the first few seconds after a presentation and is thought to play an essential role in the dynamics of the neural response to pleasant music.[243] There is also activation in premotor areas, but only when listening to pleasant music. Koelsch et al put forward the interesting idea that some of the observed activation was the result of a subliminal coding for vocal motor response—namely, mentally singing (or humming) along to the pleasant music. Subvocalization, as it is called, is hypothesized to be a mimetic act, which begins in infancy, covertly comparing other sounds with sounds we have learned and sounds that we make ourselves, imitating the motor activity (vocal or instrumental) of performers.[244] Indeed, when imagined singing is compared with overt singing there is enhanced neural activity in regions such as prefrontal and cingulate cortex, regions associated with the limbic system.[245]

Based on an earlier study,[220] Trost and colleagues defined nine "emotion factors": joy, sadness, tension, wonder, peacefulness, power, tenderness, nostalgia, and transcendence. They also examined various blends of these factors. These nine emotions fit into three "emotion clusters": vitality, unease, and sublimity. Positive, highly arousing emotions (joy, wonder) were correlated with increased activity in the left striatum (especially ventrally) and insula, while positive emotions that were "low-arousing" (tenderness, nostalgia) activated the right striatum and orbitofrontal cortex. High-arousal responses also activated auditory cortex, the caudate nucleus, motor cortex, and cerebellum; low-arousal responses "engaged a different network centered on hippocampal regions and ventromedial prefrontal cortex…"[246] I find it interesting that some emotions are rarely, if ever, aroused by music; these include guilt, shame, jealousy, disgust, contempt, and embarrassment.[220]

Unraveling the interaction between liking (enjoying) or disliking a piece of music, and whether that music is perceived as being happy or sad, was the aim of an interesting fMRI study undertaken on groups of musicians and non-musicians.[247] Expert musicians listening to music that they enjoyed showed enhanced neural activity in parts of the limbic system typically associated with processing salience; they also showed increased activity in brain regions involved in sensorimotor processing. However, in both groups, listening to music that was most liked activated (perhaps not surprisingly) areas and circuits associated with the complex processing of emotion and reward. The amygdala was active when listening to both liked and disliked music, though activation patterns differed, being greater in the right amygdala. Happy versus sad music resulted in relatively enhanced activity in auditory sensory cortex.

Changes in neural activity in the hippocampus are a common feature of "music-evoked emotions."[65] This is consistent with the observation that subjective, positive responses to music have a memory-enhancing effect,[248] and the commonly reported music-induced feeling of nostalgia may help remind us of a valued/significant past event.[220] It is also of interest that other imaging studies show that the hippocampus is involved not only in memory function but also in stress regulation and "the formation and maintenance of social attachments."[65] These links and associations have profound implications, which are considered further in Chapters 7 and 8 when discussing the roles of music in education and neurotherapy. Stefan Koelsch[66,221,249] and Kenneth Blum and colleagues[250] believe that using music to positively drive and stimulate limbic and mesolimbic structures such as the hippocampus and dopaminergic pathways may be of great benefit in the treatment of various types of depressive and anxiety disorders, and perhaps also various motor disorders.

The special role of the amygdala in music-evoked emotions has recently been summarized by Stefan Koelsch.[65] He emphasizes a diverse sensitivity of this complex structure to the prosodic elements of music, with a primary focus on its importance in aspects of social communication, emotional valence, joy, fear, and (in association with reward centers) "approach-withdrawal behaviour in response to socio-affective cues." The amygdala and part of the cingulate cortex are especially active when emotional information from diverse sources is congruent, for example when both facial expression and vocal prosody signify happiness.[251] Consistent with this, associating emotion-laden music with concurrent visual stimuli ("real world content") seems to have an additive effect, heightening responses in the amygdala as well as in the hippocampus and ventrolateral prefrontal cortex.[252] Music can even change our perception of neutral faces, influencing whether the facial expressions are interpreted as being happy or sad,[253] and subjective emotional responses to music are greater when we see as well as hear a musical performance.[254] In fMRI studies, when the emotion signaled by music and faces is congruent (both happy or both sad) there is increased neural activity in the superior temporal gyrus.[255] As pointed out by Dennis Dutton: "audiences worldwide find it natural and fitting that movies have musical scores to underline or interpret the emotions implicit in the story; even the earliest silent films were given musical accompaniment"[256] and the congruity or incongruity of background music has an effect on how we remember filmed events.[257]

Controlled laboratory studies confirm that the co-presentation of sad or scary music together with pictures expressing similar emotions produce the greatest limbic responses and strong affective experiences.[258] Consistent with all of this, damage to, or isolation of, limbic structures such as the amygdala in the temporal lobe adversely affects emotional processing and responses to music,[259,260,261] effects that may be lateralized, depending on whether the emotion is one of sadness or happiness.[262] Given the combinatory effects of visual imagery and fearful music, it is intriguing to note that, when listening to this type of music, closing one's eyes seems to increase amygdala activity,[263] yet that is exactly what many of us do when watching a horror movie!! I always thought it would make things better, but perhaps it actually makes things worse; perhaps I should keep my eyes open and actually watch the screeching shower scene in Alfred Hitchcock's *Psycho* next time it is on television!

From a neurochemical perspective, music affects a number of modulators known to influence our affective responses and emotional mood states.[264] Dopamine—which, as you may recall, is an important transmitter in mesolimbic pathways that mediate motivational behaviors and responses to rewarding stimuli—is clearly one such modulator.[250] When listening to music for the first time, initial evaluation involves processing in auditory cortex, the amygdala, and ventromedial prefrontal cortex, but when we are familiar with a song or piece of music, and we know what is coming, this expectation often increases our emotional response to the music in question.[265] This temporal anticipation is hard to reproduce in the visual art domain. In fact, listening to pleasurable music increases the binding of a radioactive analogue of dopamine in the dorsal striatum and nucleus accumbens,[266] a clear indication of the fundamental link between music and limbic reward systems, long embedded in the human brain. Importantly, the dopamine release occurs in the caudate nucleus during the anticipation of a rewarding emotional peak in music, whereas release in the nucleus accumbens occurs when experiencing the peak emotional response itself.[266,267] Robert Zatorre and Valorie Salimpoor argue that this striatal activation is linked to cortical circuits that "work together to make predictions about potentially rewarding future events and assess the outcome of these predictions."[268] Activity in the nucleus accumbens (and also the ventromedial part of the prefrontal cortex) is important in so-called "reinforcement learning," which is "driven by dopaminergic reward prediction errors that signal the discrepancy between expected and experience action outcomes."[269] Others have found increased activity in premotor regions as well as in basal ganglia and cerebellum when silently anticipating a known musical sequence, a pattern similar to that seen when learning motor sequence tasks,[270] perhaps to be expected given the close association between music and dance?

Levels of the peptide oxytocin, synthesized in the hypothalamus, are increased during singing[270] and have been reported to be increased in the plasma of patients exposed to music after open-heart surgery.[272] This hormone has long been known to be important during and after childbirth, when it is released from the pituitary gland in large amounts to accelerate the birth process itself and then stimulate lactation. But oxytocin does much more, and as I shall discuss in more detail in the following chapter, it reduces anxiety, facilitates approach and attachment behaviors, and enhances trust, altruism, and empathy in humans.[273,274,275,276,277,278,279,280,281,282,283]

Opioids are substances (some natural, some synthetic) that act on the central nervous system and are used therapeutically to treat pain, and recreationally to induce euphoric states. They are highly addictive. The body makes its own opioids, including endorphins, enkephalins and dynorphins, and these peptides and their receptors are recruited when processing natural (and drug-induced) rewarding stimuli.[284] Opioids are known to influence the release and activity of a number of neurotransmitters, including dopamine, and there is indirect evidence suggesting that musical activities (including choral singing and dance) may stimulate the endogenous opioid system.[285,286,287,288] Yet studies that directly measure the impact of music on these peptides are few, and the data not easy to interpret. Thus, peripheral plasma levels of the endogenous opioid beta-endorphin were found to be *reduced* after music imaging, but not when listening to music,[289] although what was going on in the brain at that time is unknown. In another study, music was found not only to affect opioid processing in a complex way, but also to alter levels of circulating mediators of inflammation.[290] Clearly more work is needed to understand the influence of these important neuroactive peptides on human emotional responses when confronted with music-related tasks.[264]

It should be noted here that activity in the human striatum associated with prediction and reward is of relevance not just within the musical domain, as we shall see in the next chapter when discussing the importance of music in fostering mutually beneficial social interactions and altruistic behaviors. The rewarding aspects of music are also, of course, crucially important in the context of education (Chapter 7) and neurotherapy (Chapter 8). Personally, at least in the pop/rock idiom, I usually get the largest emotional "hit" or reward—and find it hard not to move with the music—when listening to songs/albums that I grew up with and embraced during my teens and early twenties, years of considerable emotional turbulence. Many of my friends say the same thing: the music (and lyrics) that accompanied our early, overwhelming loves and losses retains an intense emotional presence and has the capacity to reawaken deep-felt memories of past experiences. Nick Hornby, in his book *31 Songs*,[224] communicates this love and passion for certain songs with some eloquence. The hormone/neurotransmitter norepinephrine (noradrenaline in the UK) is made from dopamine and works in numerous ways when we are stressed or hypervigilant, acting both within the brain and peripherally, for example by increasing heart rate, glucose availability, and blood flow to muscles associated with the so-called fight-or-flight response. In states of emotional arousal, norepinephrine activity potentiates molecular mechanisms underlying synaptic plasticity,[291] thereby enhancing learning and memory. We remember special things that happened to us, but on the downside we also remember stressful, perhaps harrowing, events that we would rather forget.

Recall that emotions associated with music affect neural activity in the hippocampus and amygdala. Perhaps this, together with the passionate rewards of music—intertwined as they are with profound emotional experiences—are so strong during our formative years that they continue to be a most effective driver of our memory and striatal dopamine reward systems later in life? In some instances I can clearly remember when and where I first heard a particular song or album, and perhaps even the person or significant other I was with at the time. Can you? These types of autobiographical, highly significant associative memories that are linked to a specific time and place also involve dopamine-based systems, but in this case the dopamine signal appears to act on specific circuits in the learning and memory center, the hippocampus, providing "a time stamp that labels particular events for storage as memories."[292]

Norman Mailer described jazz as orgasm (quoted in Shapiro,[72] p 299), which is perhaps just his own perception of how much he liked jazz, although it is intriguing to note that oxytocin levels increase when we are sexually aroused[293] and, as I alluded to earlier in this book, most of us would agree that music can evoke strong emotions and can have a profound impact on us in terms of sexual awareness/arousal. Interestingly then, some of the brain areas that are activated by music that produces chills and is perceived as being pleasurable and rewarding (eg medial prefrontal cortex, amygdala, and nucleus accumbens) are also activated in the brain of subjects viewing images of erotic and romantic couples, as revealed by imaging studies.[294,295] Is not music the "food of love?" The increased neural activity reported by Sabatinelli and colleagues was a reaction to the "pleasantness" of the visual stimuli, not an arousal (salience) induced by the pictures per se, because unpleasant images did not elicit this consistent pattern of neural responses. Some psychiatric disorders are associated with loss of feeling of pleasure, whether it be to food, intimacy, music, or some other stimulant. This is called "anhedonia," a condition in which the experience of reward is essentially absent. Interestingly then, there are rare cases of healthy individuals with apparently intact music perception but where the rewards of listening to music are selectively absent, while other types of reward (eg money) remain,[296] consistent with the idea that there are subtly different neural reward networks driven by different types of activity/stimulation.[295]

The neurotransmitter dopamine and the hormone prolactin are both involved in modulating sexual behavior, and their expression is altered by the sexual orgasm.[297] Is this similar to the dopamine surge when a person predicts and then experiences the peak emotional response to a piece of music[266,268]—the musical climax, if you will? Charles Darwin thought that music (and perhaps dance and therefore selection of fitness attributes) evolved primarily as a means for "charming the opposite sex" and attracting mates. We do know that definable structural and neurochemical differences (including dopaminergic systems) exist between male and female human brains.[298,299,300] Men, for example, have larger volumes of frontomedial cortex and amygdala,[298] whereas women have a larger caudate nucleus and an increased volume of the left superior temporal gyrus and parts of the frontal gyrus.[300] Luders and colleagues point out that because the superior temporal gyrus is more involved in language processing, "one could speculate that the observed larger grey matter volumes in females are associated with women's superior language skills." Comments on music perception and processing are generally lacking in such reports, but more imaging studies are clearly needed that individually analyze male versus female responses to pleasant versus unpleasant music-related activities.

In summary, numerous brain imaging studies have revealed defined areas of the brain that are activated by music and by emotional responses to music, along with measurable changes in brain chemistry and autonomic function. In his review on the neural processing of "music-evoked emotions," Stefan Koelsch[65] statistically analyzed results from many functional neuroimaging studies—including many of those mentioned above—and came up with a clear picture of the core regions that are active in the human brain. Most of the music-responsive networks that involve the amygdala, hippocampus, nucleus accumbens, parts of the basal ganglia, auditory and supplementary motor cortex, and cingulate and orbitofrontal cortex overlap with core areas involved in pleasure, reward, motivation, and executing goal-directed behaviors, including social attachment (Figure 4.3). I agree with Professor Koelsch that these relationships seem to confirm that music is an essential ingredient of what makes us human. Music does not transmit information or meaning in the same way as language, but it is a multisensory social experience, important in integrating neural activity and attention. In my view, music is just as important to humanity as language and speech, affecting our mood and sense of well-being and, as we will soon see, necessary for our development as children and our mental health as adults.

Why music? The evolutionary theories

The ancients understood the power of music in terms of bringing pleasure to people, and the role that music could play in lightening our mood and brightening our days. To quote some text that I first came across in a chapter by R.A. Henson[301]: "Many men are melancholy by hearing music, but it is a pleasing melancholy that it causeth; and therefore to such as are discontent, in woe, fear, sorrow, or dejected, it is a most present remedy; it expels cares, alters their grieved minds, and easeth in an instant"—from Robert Burton, when writing about "Music a Remedy" in *The Anatomy of Melancholy*. Nearly 400 years later, researchers have rediscovered these truths, finding that musicians seem especially sensitive to the emotion of sadness,[247,302] and music-evoked sadness can be aesthetically rewarding, can evoke feelings of nostalgia, peacefulness, and consolation, especially in people with a heightened sense of empathy.[303,304,305] Most importantly for the arguments marshalled in this book, the recognition of pleasant and unpleasant music, and an individual's emotional response to music (whether it is perceived as happy, sad, or scared/fearful), is universal and only partly modified by cultural experience.[306] Similarly, groups of westerners (Canadians) or Congolese Pygmies, each with no exposure to each other's musical cultures, both showed similar physiological arousal responses to music, suggesting that: "while the subjective dimension of emotional valence might be mediated by cultural learning, changes in arousal might involve more basic, universal response to low-level acoustical characteristics of music."[307]

Armed with all the new imaging information about how the modern human brain processes and responds to music, let us return to the fundamental question posed at the beginning of this chapter. If our immediate ancestors possessed a sophisticated protolanguage or musilanguage, why did we evolve, and now continue to possess, two separate types of universal communication, essentially running in parallel? Can we link the recent neuroscientific findings about music and emotions back to our pre-history, to perhaps 80,000–90,000 years ago when the spark was lit that enabled us to begin the journey to where we are now, with our novel cognitive architecture, our emerging sense of identity, and also perhaps with a disorienting awareness of our own finite lifespan?

As discussed in the previous chapter, language and speech allowed us to communicate across generations and essentially "short circuit" genetics because we were able to transmit information in a new way, each generation's knowledge and skills building on the discoveries and experiences of the previous generations. Modern language, and the necessary memory systems and circuitries that went with it, co-evolved with greater intelligence and new cognitive capacities, traits that have been the subject of positive selection. So why retain music and why does it remain a universal? Is this accident or design, spandrel or positive selection? Is it merely a cursory, idiosyncratic human pleasure, or is there some deeper evolutionary subtext? As Tecumseh Fitch has pointed out, music is energetically expensive, thus: "if music had no value whatsoever, one might expect strong selection against musical behavior. Recent evidence from subjects with congenital amusia indicates that the necessary genetic variance is present in human populations, albeit at a very low frequency. So why have not quiet, better-rested non-musical humans out-reproduced and replaced their musical conspecifics?"[7]

In truth we can never definitively answer these questions. Bah humbug, I hear you say—we've been conned … but many plausible reasons for the evolution and continued survival of music as a second communication system alongside language have been put forward. These proposals may not necessarily be mutually exclusive—in other words, there may have been multiple advantages for the founder "*Homo sapientior*" population to have music as part of their makeup. These various hypotheses "can peacefully co-exist. The only one that does not admit of alternatives is the cream pie theory, stating that music is completely useless—simply a form of self-stimulation that we practice with relish, without any obvious gain or any evolutionary advantage."[63]

Turn-taking is important when people are gainfully talking to each other; as soon as you get more than about four people nattering away at the same time, it becomes difficult if not impossible to sustain an intelligible conversation—unless of course you are declaiming something, and all are (willingly or unwillingly) hushed into silence to listen to your pearls of wisdom. But then the communication is *not* mutual. Music, however, allows large-group participation in which you can contribute as an individual but also allows the individual to be physiologically linked into the larger group network; the arousal patterns become yoked together—there is a sense of oneness, a sense of social community, where everyone is moving together with shared intentions and mutual goals.[40,308,309] Imagine four people sitting around a dinner table talking animatedly all at once—bedlam; now they stop talking, and either begin singing a four-part chorus (soprano, alto, tenor, bass), or else each person picks up an instrument and they begin to play a Mozart or Schubert string quartet, or the Beatles' "Eleanor Rigby." Now the four separate voices make a cogent whole; they make sense and tell a communal story. As Sandra Trehub and colleagues wrote: "Although music lacks communicative specificity in comparison with language, its power sometimes exceeds that of language in social, emotional and spiritual domains. In live contexts, moreover, music can communicate to greater numbers of individuals and over greater distances than language can."[310]

David Huron,[311] while leaving open questions about the evolutionary origins of music, nicely summarized many of the possible adaptive benefits of music in human life. There is, for example, mate attraction and mate selection (a favorite of Charles Darwin); being a good singer and dancer are attributes that could well reflect fitness and power, and may therefore help to attract a mate. In addition, because music and rhythmic beat help to structure time, music/drumming was likely used for distant communication—to signal to others far away. Signaling via sound can also be done at night or when visibility is poor. Other, not necessarily mutually exclusive, possibilities include social cohesion, group effort, perceptual and cognitive development, motor skill development, conflict reduction, and what Huron refers to as "safe time passing"; if it is dark and cold outside, with wild beasts roaming about, it is safer to sit in a cave around the fire and have a sing-song. Perhaps that is what the TV set or the PC/Mac does for us these days, rather than being out on the streets at midnight. In addition, from the perspective of physical health, there is good evidence that music has positive effects on the immune system and can influence the expression of various hormones, thus affecting the way we respond to events and stresses in our lives.[312]

I should also add to this list trans-generational communication (where music and song can be a useful combined mnemonic device for passing cultural information from one individual to another, and in particular, from one generation to the next). Music provides a framework that helps in memory formation and the organization of knowledge, and its emotional impact seems to enhance memory formation,[188] perhaps as described earlier through the specific activation of dopaminergic and related neural pathways. I can remember almost no poetry but I still remember the lyrics of a whole bunch of folk songs that I learned when I was a student at university. Music helps in the formation of a cultural archive of history, of context and place—a store house for oral tradition and knowledge. It is important for maintaining social traditions and engendering group-assimilated identity. There is evidence in aboriginal communities in Australia, for example, that music acts to help develop a repository of the oral tradition that contains the history of the group— the boundaries and important spiritual landmarks, the geography of the land they own, places for water and food, a history and knowledge that is passed on from one generation to the next. As in indigenous African cultures,[75] music is used throughout an aboriginal person's daily life; it is omnipresent, and "maturation can be measured in the esoteric knowledge he has acquired through song, and as an old man he knows that his honour is based partly on his mastery of the secret sacred songs of the band."[313]

In such cultures, it seems that any given individual may not necessarily know the whole song of a particular group, or if they do they may not have the authority to communicate all of it. In her studies on the songs and music of the Yolngu people of northeast Arnhem Land, who incidentally have no words for "music" or "performance" but do have words for "song" and "dancing," Fiona Magowan comments that: "senior men and women pass on selected segments of ancestral knowledge belonging to their own related networks of clans ... In turn listeners steadily accumulate patterns of ancestral knowledge through which connections between ancestral journeys can be made."[314] The upshot is that there may be various contributors to enable the group as a whole to know and recount the entire narrative. This is what I call the Coca-Cola idea. I have been told that no one person knows the complete Coca-Cola recipe or the Kentucky Fried Chicken recipe—several individuals know parts of it, but it only works when they get together and combine their parcels of information. It is possible to imagine groups where the cultural history—who they are, who their neighbors are, their land and boundaries, and their social traditions— are stored within a musical, ritualistic context; however, only when the group as a whole combines everything together can the complete story be told.

Steven Brown,[103] Ian Cross,[315] and others have long emphasized the importance of music at the level of the group. Music in an evolutionary context is associated with increased cooperative survival strategies; it promotes prosocial behaviors and helps to define kinships and delimit tribal boundaries. Music promotes collective thinking, group catharsis, and a shared sense of passing time. It helps to maintain social and cultural identity, bonds that underlie the concept of shared physiological arousal that links people together in a way that is not possible with any other form of communication—music embraces and enwraps all participants in its cohesive shell. Here it is pertinent to comment on some revealing and remarkable links between the genetic backgrounds of populations and their respective musical cultures. Analysis of DNA sequences (haplotypes) from paternal (Y chromosome) or maternal (mtDNA) lineages revealed that close musical cultures were significantly correlated with close genetic distances.[316] A similar correlation was found when comparing musical genres with the genetics of indigenous populations in Taiwan,[317] and a phylogenetic study of 58 distinct musical features shared by different populations in the West African country of Gabon again revealed the influence of ancestral inheritance on musical diversity.[174] These are important new findings that I consider as yet another indication of the social and cultural power of music and its influence on modern human evolution.

Ian Cross has argued that music, as an expression of emotion, is an "honest signal" that allows humans to interact and share experiences, even though at the individual level each person may have many different outlooks and ambitions: "Music allows participants to explore the prospective consequences of their actions and attitudes towards others within a temporal framework that promotes the alignment of participants' sense of goals."[318] In music, the coupling of action and perception allows coordination between individuals and allows us to infer the goal of other individuals and/or cooperatively interact with them.[319] Music can thus have a critical role in the management of real and imagined social relationships, "particularly in situations of social uncertainty."[320] Two-and-a-half thousand years ago, Confucius wrote: "When music and courtesy are better understood and appreciated, there will be no war" (quoted in Shapiro[72] p 222). And as language and the emerging sense of individuality in "*Homo sapientior*" inevitably led to even greater levels of social complexity and uncertainty, the links between music, dance, empathy, and group-related cooperation and bonding became especially important as an evolutionarily necessary counterweight, an idea fleshed out in considerably more detail in the next chapter.

Motherese

Over a century ago the German biologist Ernst Haeckel proposed that "ontogeny recapitulates phylogeny"—that is, an individual's biological development parallels or reflects in some way the evolutionary development of the species. This idea has less currency these days, but in the context of the proposal that our immediate ancestors possessed a musilanguage or protolanguage, what do developmental studies in young children tell us about how immature brains process language and music? A number of scholars have proposed that a major reason for the existence of music is its role in pre-linguistic, prosodic-like communication, necessary for parent–infant bonding, especially given that human infants are born so immature and helpless, and unable to feed themselves.[321,322,323,324] Daniel Levitin, in his important book "*This Is Your Brain On Music*," also writes a great deal about this pre-verbal, infant-directed communication, sometimes termed "motherese" or "baby talk." This early nonverbal communication, which includes sensorimotor exchanges with carers,[325] is usually slower in delivery and higher in pitch, and involves exaggerated pitch changes that often slide from one to another. But is it a type of speech, or is its basis in the structures that form the foundations of music? Or is the question irrelevant—why not just leave it as a nonverbal, multimodal communication system that is necessary early in life, which eventually separates (just as in evolution) into two distinct but interlinked strands as we mature—one we call music, the other we call language?

Ellen Dissanayake[323,326] argues, in a similar way to Trevarthan,[325] that music forms part of a multimedia presentation, including dance, mime, and so on, that emerges from this need for a pre-linguistic two-way interaction between mother and baby—a sensorimotor communication that is required before the neural architecture and circuitry of the brain mature, before the capacity to assimilate, generate, and express language comes on line. Motherese gets an infant's attention and is (or at least should be) calming and reassuring. These pre-verbal interactions are important for "survival-enhancing affiliative interactions between mothers and infants,"[322] as well as being important in driving the perceptual, behavioral, cognitive, and emotional development of a child. In an extension to these ideas, the anthropologist Dean Falk has suggested that motherese evolved when mothers needed to use both hands for foraging and so forth. Because they could no longer carry their infants and therefore became physically separated from them, it was essential for our ancestral mothers to orally communicate in a way that reassured infants and controlled their behavior,[324] that stopped them from crying and drawing attention to themselves and their caregivers. Indeed, happy sounds are what the baby wants to hear, whether in speech or in song.[327]

Pre-verbal, infant-directed communication has a high emotional content,[328,329,330] leading some to suggest that the prosodic-like nature of music is: "intimately connected with
emotional systems because care-givers use music to communicate emotionally with their
infants before they are able to understand language."[331] Newborn infants prefer the sound
of their own mother's voice,[332] but interestingly seem unable to discriminate between different male voices![333] In addition, however, when mothers interact with their babies in the
first few months after birth, as well as the use of so-called lalling sounds and vocalization
(crooning; oohing and aahing), critical elements of communication also include facial
expression (smiling), eye contact, and hand gestures. There is evidence that these nonverbal communications and the intentions contained therein are universal and constitute
an essential interactive link between mother and pre-verbal child (see also[326,334] for more
about these ideas). I have already discussed the importance of expression and gesture in
adult face-to-face interactions. In fact, humans have evolved very characteristic eyes; we
can see the sclera (the whites of our eyes) surrounding the iris and pupil, which means we
detect eye movements and direction of gaze very well. Interestingly, dysfunctional gaze
behavior with reduced eye contact is typical of autism-like disorders.[335]

Dopamine-driven reward circuits in the brain are active when mothers see images
of their own infants as opposed to unknown babies, especially when viewing happy
faces.[276,336,337] Mirror neuron areas and limbic regions related to emotion and/or empathy processing, such as parts of the prefrontal cortex, anterior cingulate cortex, insula,
and amygdala, are also activated, intriguingly more so in the right hemisphere. It is
worth noting here that many of these regions are also implicated in distributed networks involved in processing gaze and social attention cues,[338] and that these regions
are activated in humans when mimicking different types of facial expression.[339]

What we as adults call music (although it may not be distinguished as "music" by a
young infant!) probably has advantages over the medium of language early in life because
it can better facilitate perceptual motor skill development and encourage the collective
expression and experience of emotion. In the young of our species this is potentially of
profound importance, given that our offspring take many years to become self-supporting.
For a group to remain viable, there is a need for social networks, cooperative structures
to support mothers whose primary task is to rear the child—feed, nurture, and protect.
In his essay "Music, cognition, culture and evolution,"[315] Ian Cross emphasizes that music
is not directly functional and it can be "about" many things at the same time ("transpos-
able aboutness"); it has what he calls "floating intentionality," bridging across different
domains or modules of behavior. As a consequence he argues that, in early childhood,
music "can be … a free means of exploring social interaction and a 'play space' for rehearsing processes that may be necessary to achieve cognitive flexibility." Or, as he wrote in an
earlier essay: "music, or protomusical behaviours in the form of interactions and play, may
help to instantiate processes that integrate and redescribe information across domains."[340]
Musical interaction may help in the development of emotional (self) regulation—the
ability to express feelings but also control or modify one's emotions and level of arousal
depending on circumstance and interactive social context.

There is much to be said for the infant bonding idea and also the role of "protomusic" in assisting sensorimotor, cognitive, and social development,[340] and it is certainly true that many of us carry indelible memories of the songs we heard when we were very small. In the uterus, "sounds arising from maternal gastro-intestinal, cardiac, and vocal activity are ubiquitous," and words spoken by the mother are much louder than speech generated by others.[341] Furthermore, the fetal cortex can already discriminate sounds by 28 weeks, and late-term fetuses can process and discriminate various aspects of speech.[342,343] By measuring heart rate and body movement in utero, altered responses to music (eg "Brahms' Lullaby") between gestational ages 28–35 weeks have been noted[344] and it appears that late-term fetuses can attend to, discriminate, and remember—at least to some extent—different voices and different languages, with enhanced responses to the mother's voice and native language.[345] The auditory experience of the fetus influences the way in which the newborn infant responds to and analyzes speech and other auditory input,[343,346] and perhaps explains a preference for the mother's voice.[332,347]

After birth there are obvious difficulties in identifying and quantifying how uncooperative, pre-attentive infants respond to and process music.[348] Nonetheless, newborns do appear to be able to detect and respond to a regular beat in music-like sounds, and can process information about frequency, pitch relationships, melodic contour, consonant versus dissonant intervals, and so on.[206,321,349,350,351] Such observations support the comment by Sandra Trehub that "the rudiments of music listening are gifts of nature rather than products of culture,"[329] even though the cortical representation of pitch appears not to be properly established until about three to four months after birth.[352]

But—and this is an important "but" to my mind—as discussed before, features such as pitch, timbre, and rhythm are not exclusive to the musical domain but are characteristics of auditory processing and prosodic communication in general, including vocalized speech and song. As others have pointed out: "Sensing higher-order periodicities of sound sequences is similarly needed for adapting to different speech rhythms."[351] Importantly, various studies have shown that the brains of human infants already possess the functional circuitry needed for processing the emotional content in vocalizations,[353,354] some of which is right hemisphere biased.[353] Because infants can recognize and respond to prosodic features of both language and music, Ian Cross has suggested that "for human neonates, linguistic and musical channels are likely to be equally accessible and not discrete."[320] Similarly, others have found evidence for a shared "emotional code" in both speech and music.[355] The common involvement of the adult amygdala and other regions during the perceptual processing of both linguistic and musical prosody is clearly consistent with this. Based on their extensive pediatric studies in older children, Koelsch and Siebel have suggested that "the human brain, at least at an early age, does not treat language and music as strictly separate domains, but rather treats language as a special case of music."[356] Indeed, from a perceptual point of view, both Stefan Koelsch himself[357] and others[179,217] no longer regard music and language as entirely separate entities—what Koelsch has called the "music-language continuum."

The suggestion of core structures that can be activated in infant brains by prosodic information, whether contained within speech or song, is not inconsistent with the musilanguage precursor idea, because such fundamental structures form part of the interactive emotional bedrock upon which the more highly specialized, newly evolved linguistic frameworks were built. Of course, we must presume that Neanderthals, who would also have given birth to immature infants, would also have required some form of maternal–infant communication to promote bonding prior to more sophisticated interactions in adulthood—perhaps something akin to "musilanguage" was sufficient for this purpose. There is perhaps one fly in the ointment; as described in Chapter 2, congenital amusics who seemingly cannot perceive melodic content also have difficulty in interpreting the emotional content of speech.[105] So how, then, do such children interpret their mother's vocalizations in infancy—if they do not seem to have any other dysfunctional behavioral attributes, cognitively or socially?

Language or music, or a meld of both—is there anything in the neuroimaging or physiological literature that helps us decide whether a particular mode of acoustic communication is more dominant when parents and their infant offspring interact? Maybe, but it is complicated, with some of the difficulties relating to the small size of the infant brain and to the difficulty in defining landmarks when imaging neonatal cortex. The left cochlea nerve, which primarily but not exclusively drives the right (musical?) side of the auditory brain, is more anatomically and physiologically mature in fetuses and newborns, but lateralization of responses in the auditory cortex is less clear-cut.[341] In fact, an fMRI study that analyzed the resting-state networks in preterm infants, in the absence of any overt task, detected no clear lateralization of neural activity, unlike the strong lateralization of resting-state networks reported in adults.[358] As mentioned earlier, fetuses do seem to show "attention to and rudimentary memory of voices and language"[345] and seem to discriminate certain aspects of speech, important for later language acquisition after birth.[343,347] And we also know from MRI studies that newborn infants respond to music and that these responses already seem to be right hemisphere biased.[359] But also, as mentioned earlier, infants are sensitive to the prosodic elements of speech at a very early age,[320,360] a responsiveness that is associated with activation of regions involved in affective processing such as the frontal cortex and insula.[354,361] Furthermore, two- to five-day-old infants display distinct patterns of neural activity when presented with common versus ill-formed syllables,[362] similar to differences seen when imaging regional activation in adult brains.[363] Others have reported a left-sided predisposition to processing "linguistic"-type stimuli from birth.[364,365]

Then again, another study found that processing was less lateralized in two-day-old infants than in adults, and that speech (and even hummed speech, which contains only prosodic information) activated the right auditory cortex to a greater extent, the authors suggesting that: "very early in life, speech processing and music processing rely partially on the same neural substrates."[366] This observation fits with developmental data and with very recent MEG recordings (magnetoencephalography—see Chapter 2) from adults who lack, or have a highly reduced, corpus callosum—the major fiber bundle linking the two cerebral hemispheres.[367] Unlike normal subjects in which language-related activity was mostly confined to the left hemisphere, in subjects with agenesis of the corpus callosum language resulted in bilateral activation, activity that was sometimes even more marked on the right than on the left, leading the authors to propose that the corpus callosum is needed for experience driven language lateralization. Developmentally, myelination of fibers in the human corpus callosum, and hence onset of more rapid and effective transmission of signals between the two cerebral cortices, is detected about one to two months after birth and continues to mature throughout the first postnatal year.[368]

Sounds reinforce suckling behavior in newborns. In an interesting study, DeCasper and Prescott[341] found that unfamiliar speech reinforced suckling only when presented to the right ear, whereas heartbeat and familiar voiced speech reinforced suckling when presented through the left ear. Based on these data and their review of the literature, they propose that the newborn auditory system is similar to an adult's in that the "right cochlea/left auditory cortex differentially resolve rapid temporal variation, especially amplitude variation" while the "left cochlea/right cortex differentially resolve spectral information occurring over longer intervals, greater than 100ms." By two to three months of age, the presentation of speech results in a spatiotemporal pattern of activation of cortical regions remarkably similar to that seen in adults.[369,370] Regions first activated by a stimulus were in the superior temporal regions, then extended over time to more posterior regions of this gyrus towards Wernicke's area, especially in the left hemisphere, and eventually to the left inferior frontal gyrus in the vicinity of Broca's area. Interestingly, music resulted in bilateral activation in temporal cortex. The authors concluded that "there is a left hemisphere advantage for speech relative to music at the level of the planum temporale" and that Broca's area is active in young infants before the babbling stage, acting as an integrating region during the acquisition of language and the development of programs required for speech production.[370]

Consistent with earlier work,[332] Dehaene-Lambertz et al found a different pattern of infant brain responses when the sound of the mother's voice was presented, leading them to suggest that "the mother's voice plays a special role in the early shaping of posterior language areas."[370] Other work from this group has revealed clear left–right asymmetries in maturation of the superior temporal cortex in one- to four-month-old infants and early correlative maturation of pathways between inferior frontal and temporal cortex, the nascent arcuate fasciculus.[371] The maturation of the corpus callosum at about this time (see above) may also be important in the development of this cerebral asymmetry.[367] All this is consistent with a functional bias for language in the left hemisphere early in development that "becomes more focussed over time as children's language skills become increasingly complex."[372] Earlier, I cited a study describing the integrated processing of lyrics and tunes in the left hemisphere of adult brains,[192] and it therefore comes as no surprise that six- to eight-month-old infants have been found to learn lyrics and melodies more easily when they are paired with each other[373]—very much the substance of simple lullabies. As we shall see in Chapter 8, therapists can take advantage of this associative enhancement when working with memory-impaired patients. Development of linguistic skills in early childhood correlates with the myelination—and hence speed of signal conduction—of nerve fiber tracts associated with language-related brain areas,[374,375] changes that are especially evident before the age of four.[376] But language acquisition also requires memory and cognitive involvement, and imaging studies also reveal activity of frontal cortex, occipital cortex, and cerebellum in one- to two-year-olds listening passively to speech.[377]

In terms of what young babies can vocalize, for the first few weeks of life human infants (similar to monkeys and apes) cannot move their tongue when they vocalize (cry!), and the larynx "sits high in the throat."[85] Babbling sounds begin at about three to four months when the tongue and larynx have descended further down the throat, and by five to six months such nascent speech sounds appear to be driven by the left hemisphere. This early phase in vocalization likely involves activity in the ventral, and part of the dorsal, fiber pathways that are present at birth and connect the temporal lobes with the inferior frontal gyrus, including Broca's area,[378] perhaps suggesting that early infant—maternal vocal communication, at least, is not strictly musical in nature. Very young infants can apparently distinguish and discriminate between pairs of vowels or consonants typical of speech sounds, and Holowka and Petitto[379] found a right mouth asymmetry in babies during babbling and a left mouth asymmetry while smiling. Because each hemisphere essentially controls the opposite side of the body, the data were interpreted as indicating that there was a left hemisphere specialization for babbling in human infants, leading the authors to state that "babbling reflects babies' sensitivity to and production of patterns in linguistic input. We thus conclude that babbling represents the onset of the productive language capacity in humans, rather than an exclusively oral-motor development."

Given that mothers would generally have spent the most time with their babies, but noting that both infant girls and boys would have interacted with their care-givers to a similar degree, is there any evidence for sexual dimorphism in the way humans interact with babies, and subsequently create or perform music and dance later in life? An interesting fMRI study carried out at the RIKEN Brain Science Institute in Japan compared brain activity in parents and non-parents listening to infant-directed speech.[380] Mothers with pre-verbal infants uniquely exhibited greater brain activity in *language processing areas* (Broca's and Wernicke's) associated with the left auditory dorsal pathway, "regardless of whether they listened to the prosodic or lexical component of infant-directed speech." Increased activity in speech-related motor circuits was not obviously associated with music-processing regions, and was not seen in fathers, or in nonparents, or in mothers with older, now verbal, children. Given the evidence that mothers use language areas when they are listening to infant-directed speech, which cortical areas are activated when a mother is herself communicating with her pre-verbal infant child? If there is enhanced right hemisphere activity, that might help clarify whether music is indeed a carryover to facilitate the development of early interactions and the building of relationships between mothers and their infants.

As mentioned earlier, architecturally there are gray matter differences between males and females, differences that include auditory processing areas and parts of frontal and cingulate cortex.[137] Functionally, there are subtle differences in the way males and females process pitch: men lateralize more to the left hemisphere, although as the authors point out they found "no difference in behavioral performance between genders."[381] When comparing brain activity in subjects exposed to noise or music, the primary auditory cortex is relatively more activated by music in males than in females, and there are sex-related differences in deactivation of prefrontal cortex activity.[382] Taken together with studies showing increased suppression of repeated auditory stimuli in men,[383] the authors attributed these differences to gender-related differences in selective auditory attention, even speculating that "the present sexual dichotomy would be consistent with the concept of evolutionary advantages in a hunter-gatherer society where the inhibition of constant irrelevant stimuli in men may facilitate them to focus their attention to a single task, eg hunting"(!). But as my colleague Nick Bannon pointed out to me, there is of course another factor that needs to be taken into account: "male adults have to re-calibrate their vocal self-recognition both acoustically and timbrally during voice-change, which represents a 'bottleneck' in biographic continuity—much less evident, though not absent, in girls." Of course, there is a great deal of sexual dimorphism in the mature human voice, regarded as important in mate choice and mate competition.[92]

When listening to songs with or without lyrics, differences in perceived arousal state are greater in females than males, the vocal (language?) content influencing women to a greater extent.[384] Differences in the way adult female and male brains process various components of language have been described, although these differences may, to some extent, reflect social influences on gender behavior rather than intrinsic biology.[385,386] This must occur early in childhood because differences in the way language is processed in the brains of females and males are already evident in 9- to 15-year-old children, with greater activation in linguistic areas in girls.[387] The influence of upbringing may be important here because in some cultures, compared with the perceived dichotomy in western society, music and language are more fluid in their relationships, with subtle changes in the emphasis placed on text versus melody depending on social context.[217,388]

Finally, listening to music reduces testosterone levels in males but not females,[389] while exposure to the hormone oxytocin, which is increased during singing[271] and is regarded as important in prosocial behaviors, apparently has different effects on men and women, enhancing recognition of kinship interactions in women, and somewhat paradoxically, competitive traits in men.[390] Similar dimorphic effects have been observed in social approach behavior. Oxytocin, when give intranasally to women, "selectively promotes approach behavior in positive social contexts"—in other words, treated women get closer to attractive and friendly males.[281] Finally, oxytocin levels rise when mothers interact with their children and reward centers in the ventral striatum are activated,[276] an intriguing observation in the context of the maternal–infant bonding idea that is under discussion here.

In summary, there is no doubt that rhythmic, nonverbal, prosodic-like communication and associated motor responses are important in early maternal–infant interaction and attachment, but to me at least the available scientific evidence does not unequivocally establish whether this communication is "protomusical" or "protolinguistic."

Lateralization of brain function is rudimentary at birth, and as I suggested earlier in this chapter, perhaps such a distinction does not need to be made until the brain matures, when these two communication streams become more evident. Harmonically structured elements in infant-directed speech are almost certainly of critical importance, both in helping the auditory system to mature appropriately during early language (and music?) acquisition, and in facilitating the more general development of social interactions with other humans.[391] Infants respond most to the prosodic "happy voice quality" of a vocalization, irrespective of whether the mode of communication is speech or song.[327] Could it be that "motherese" is in fact an ontogenetic echo of our evolutionary history—an echo of our ancestors' musilanguage? When we interact with an infant, could we be interacting with a reflection of our immediate ancestor? Is this a window into our musilanguage past?!

Conclusion

Evidence from clinical neurology and from research into the perception and production of language and music in modern humans has undoubtedly revealed differences in the processing networks used by the two communication streams: more left biased for speech, and more right biased for music, in addition to separate processing areas within secondary auditory regions in the superior temporal gyrus. But it is also clear that certain aspects of language and music are processed in common, or at least that similar regions are activated in the brain.[209] As pointed out by Isabelle Peretz et al,[392] co-activation of brain regions in fMRI does not necessarily mean "evidence of the sharing of the underlying neural circuitry"; nonetheless, the weight of evidence is persuasive, and certainly such an overlap would be expected if both types of communication evolved from a common prototype/precursor. This sophisticated precursor would have comprised complex vocalizations accompanied by visuomotor cues including gesture and facial expression. It presumably required empathy, the ability to regulate one's own emotions, and the capacity to attend to, understand, and respond to the actions and emotions of others. It was clearly sufficient to enable communication of skills and cooperative work between individuals within groups.

Modern language and articulate speech capability was probably superimposed on circuitries that were mostly involved in the processing of the more prosodic aspects of interpersonal communication, such as arousal, emotion, reward, and social attachment. In our new communication system, in addition to some common early auditory machinery and modular/discrete templates relating to, for example, pitch analysis and processing the harmonic spectrum of a sound,[154,391,393,394] understanding and interpreting a multitude of more complex vocalized sounds that were linguistically relevant to an individual presumably now required considerable additional learning as well as the involvement of higher-level cortical processing to modulate earlier parts of the auditory pathway—a form of top-down processing.[395] Even today, the prosodic elements of language remain vital to understanding the meaning and intent of a phrase or sentence. Nonverbal elements such as gesture, eye contact, and facial expression all add to the mix; no wonder that emails and texting are subject to all sorts of interpretative misunderstandings—80–90% of the communication content is missing!

Music, side by side with language, has a profound impact on us throughout childhood and adult life, and it seems unlikely to me that the unique and specific responsiveness to music exhibited by adult humans is merely a hang-over from a requirement for a pre-verbal communication system in infants. Music continues to exert its power well beyond infancy, and we still need to explain why adults continue to respond in such rewarding and basic emotional ways to music, in ways that are so very different from other sensations and experiences. Music is fundamental to our biology: it continues to aid in the collective expression and experience of emotions, it facilitates cognitive and social development, and children who learn music seem to have increased capacity for various other perceptual motor skills (see Chapter 7). Returning to David Huron's suggestions about the possible adaptive benefits of music in adult human life,[311] as well as enhancement of perceptual, cognitive, and motor skills there is sexual fitness and mate selection, and perhaps also mate retention, protection and maintenance, long-distance communication, conflict reduction, and music-driven group effort. Music aids in the natural rhythmic alleviation of toil—people singing in a collaborative, synchronized way when they working, whether it be digging, marching, or when they're pulling on ropes and so on. And strenuous exercise feels less tiring if associated with the generation of musical sounds.[216]

Music coordinates activity, and many would argue that music is one of the only activities that can harmonize affective states and synchronize physiological arousal within a group. As discussed earlier in Chapter 2, our perception and response to rhythm are culturally dependent, thus music "may support cultural identity because it can facilitate interpersonal synchrony, consistent with theories that the function (i.e., adaptive value) of music and musical rhythm is to facilitate social cohesion."[396] The social, emotional mode of musical communication also seems critical to our psychological well-being. The anthropologist and evolutionary biologist Robin Dunbar[397] has developed some interesting ideas about gossip, suggesting that it acts as a linguistic instrument of social order and cohesion, akin to grooming behaviors in non-human primates. But as Dunbar himself implies,[286] the universality of music and the evidence for the power of shared musical experiences suggest that music may be just as, perhaps even more, potent an agent for linking individuals and bonding larger groups together, even acting to short-circuit the normal paths taken to establish a social relationship.[309] Music is the only phenomenon (apart, that is, from modern-day team sports) that can bring together a group of disparate humans, all of them isolated in the sense that they are all conscious of their own individual existence and their own mortality, yet all working in synchrony towards a "greater good." We sing together, and we move and dance together. Nothing else can do that—language cannot, unless the speaker is a great orator, oratory in some ways being a cross-over between speech and music. The great Australian author David Malouf said this about the power of music in his short story "The Domestic Cantata":[398] "The last notes died away. Miss Stanton sat a moment, as if she were alone out there, somewhere in the dark, and they, like shy animals, had been drawn in out of the distance to listen; drawn in, each one out of their own distance and surprised, when they looked about, that music had made a company of them, sharers of a stilled enchantment." This quote leads nicely on to the next chapter, which focuses exclusively on music and cooperative prosocial behavior: how music seems to tap into regions and networks of the brain that also process empathy, altruism, and social cooperation. A true good news story.

Chapter 5

Music, Altruism, and Social Cooperation

The man that hath no music in himself,
Nor is not moved with concord of sweet sounds,
Is fit for treasons, strategems, and spoils;
The motions of his spirit are dull as night,
And his affections dark as Erebus.
Let no such man be trusted. Mark the music.

—William Shakespeare, *The Merchant of Venice*

We often think of natural selection as a fight for survival, with reproductive advantage favoring the best adapted to a particular situation, competing for example for limited resources. But as the late Len Freedman, one of the dedicatees of this book, wrote in his summation of his evolutionary human biology teaching experience: "The competitive nature of evolution by natural selection remains the predominant, underlying emphasis in much present-day evolutionary thinking and writing ... (but) ... there is another important evolutionary mechanism, cooperation, the role of which is insufficiently appreciated and emphasised." This is an important insight, although the concept is not new. The great western philosophers Hobbes and Rousseau disagreed as to whether humans were naturally selfish or naturally cooperative. Post-Darwin, this idea of the evolutionary advantages of cooperation and mutually beneficial behavior has gradually received support in various quarters, for example by the Russian Prince Peter Kropotkin, in his book *Mutual Aid: A Factor of Evolution* (1902), "a prophetic work, though now largely forgotten."[1]

Altruism in the animal kingdom is a form of social behavior where there are consequences for both the giver (actor) and the receiver. Classically, altruistic acts result in an increase in "fitness" for the receiver and may (but by no means always) have some degree of negative consequences for the actor. While selfish behaviors that enhance individual fitness are relatively easy to comprehend, altruistic acts that negatively affect the actor may ultimately reduce his/her fitness—how then to evolve and continue to select for such a proximate behavior? "The evolution of cooperation remains a central paradox in biology."[2] The answer almost certainly lies in the beneficial impact of altruism and cooperative behavior on the viability and welfare not only of the individual but especially of the group as a whole. Initially hypothesized to involve genetic changes that conferred direct fitness benefits to the individual but that also indirectly maximized inclusive fitness by enhancing cooperation between family members,[3,4] group selection ideas have gradually been modified to include multiple levels of selection. "For example, cooperation could be favored if the benefits at the group level (between-group benefits) outweighed the cost at the individual level (within-group costs). It is sometimes suggested that in situations where kin selection or inclusive fitness could not account for cooperation or altruism, this new group selection approach provided an alternative explanation."[5]

The additional and important concept of "reciprocal altruism,"[6] where there is clear, mutual cooperative advantage, also extended the kin selection idea to non-related group members who, at some time in the future, could be relied upon to return a favor. Cultural group selection extends these ideas even further, with increasing emphasis on the profound impact of culture on gene–environment and/or gene–culture interactions (see also Chapter 3). Indeed, culture can be the sole driver of maintaining group identity and ensuring a competitive advantage at the evolutionary level. In *"Homo sapientior,"* while altruistic acts remain of benefit to genetically related individuals, in us—and this is a crucial distinction—altruism spreads a far wider net in both space and time, involving large-scale cooperation with much bigger groups of unrelated, but culturally compatible, individuals.

As alluded to earlier in Chapter 3 when discussing mirror neurons, cooperation and prosocial behaviors can be observed in primate species, but the nature of these behaviors and their relevance to our own evolutionary trajectory remain the subject of lively debate among experts in the field. Forms of empathy and associated altruistic behaviors can be recognized in non-human primates,[7,8,9] behaviors that often appear to be "biased in favour of genetic relatives and reciprocating partners."[10] The nature of these prosocial/cooperative activities varies substantially between primate species,[10] but can include assisting others in a fight, territorial defense, hunting, grooming, food sharing, and what may be interpreted as acts of consolation.

There are important differences in the quality and type of altruistic behaviors in humans versus other primates such as chimpanzees.[11] According to Warneken and Tomasello, altruism encompasses a number of activity domains—helping, sharing, and informing—and chimpanzees are poor at sharing resources and do not "inform others of things helpfully."[11] Children as young as three years old, when engaged in a collaborative enterprise, will share resources with others in an equitable fashion.[12] Even when vocalizing, chimpanzees are essentially competing, getting others to do as they require. According to Joan Silk and Bailey House, "chimpanzees (and other great apes) cooperate in a number of contexts, but do not have robust preferences for outcomes that benefit others."[10] And to quote from the work of my colleague Cyril Grueter: "Humans are the only multilevel species in which mere tolerance between interbreeding groups evolved into multigroup cooperative networks and the coordination of whole social groups, giving rise to many derived features of human sociality such as intense cooperation, prosociality, and cultural transmission."[13]

The better and more sophisticated the reciprocal communication system between individuals, the more likely it will be that collaborative efforts are appreciated and the fruits of these collaborations shared equally.[12,14] In fact, human altruism seems to extend beyond reciprocal altruism and involves what has been termed "strong reciprocity."[15] In this condition altruism is rewarded, usually at some time in the future, but individuals in a group who do not conform and cooperate to some degree, and who act in a selfish way, may be punished. Cooperative and altruistic behaviors can ultimately garner a selective advantage within an evolving species,[16,17] but an ostracized individual may have trouble surviving and finding a mate! Presumably, early in our history the best and most creative communicators would likely have been positively selected for—culturally and/or sexually (see discussion in Chapter 3, "Genes, language, and intellect"), and the ability to empathize and read the intentions of others would ultimately have favored prosocial attitudes in a population.[18] Note that the extent and importance of reciprocity can vary depending on whether it involves close or distant partners. We rarely (and perhaps should not?) keep a running cost/benefit analysis when socializing with close friends and partners, but we do tend to keep "tabs" of costs and benefits in interactions with more distant acquaintances.

My colleague Jim Chisholm has proposed that adult human cooperative activity "is the common developmental outcome of an innate capacity for attachment" between infants and their parents early in life.[19] The necessary long-term care of human infants meant that infants with the best multi-sensory "mind-reading" skills would receive the most secure, trustworthy attachments with kin and others ("alloparenting") and thus, presumably, the best early care.[9,20] Certainly, at an early age, children show a "biological predisposition to help others achieve their goals, to share resources with others" and "humans seem to have evolved a system of communication premised on cooperation."[11] The development of moral norms of behavior in children is strongly influenced by personal experience and prosocial interactions with others, including preferential interaction with other children who know, for example, similar songs![21] Receiving positive feedback in a social context is important in establishing how we perceive ourselves, our "self-concept."[22] "A human child is born eager to connect with others"[9] and our first instinct seems to be to cooperate, with more selfish behaviors developing later.[23] As Pascal Boyer has written: "Humans are unique among animals in maintaining large, stable coalitions of unrelated individuals, strongly bonded by mutual trust."[24] Fehr and Rockenbach went so far as to state that, in their view: "Human cooperation represents a spectacular outlier in the animal world."[25]

I have already mentioned the cultural group selection idea, where there is ongoing positive interaction between "like-minded" individuals. There may also be cultural flow between different groups, ultimately leading to the "spread of cooperative institutions within ethnic groups, which might then create a context favouring the genetic evolution of prosocial cognitive mechanisms through individual-level selection."[26] And when humans lived and thrived in interdependent, socially cohesive groups, a reputation for consistency and fairness must have been of value in the general population, and the "sense of reciprocal obligation must have been palpable."[1] The transfer of social, cultural, and intellectual skills and inventions requires tolerant behaviors and an interactive environment where new ideas are proffered and considered by the potentially affected group as a whole. A type of trade is established where there is division of labor; the exchange (and barter) of food, goods, and services; and the sharing of novel information. Such behaviors also require patience, foresight, risk, and delayed reward paradigms, very much the domain of an advanced prefrontal cortex. Even today, economic organization and market forces remain important drivers of prosocial attitudes, explaining some of the cross-cultural variation in exactly how we behave towards others.[27]

But social decision-making also requires that an individual considers the flux in any process, and must be "tailored and updated to the particular mental state of another."[28] Sharing is not always equitable, and as Sarah Brosnan writes in the journal Frontiers in Neuroscience (2011): "In joint situations, individuals cease cooperating with partners who consistently dominate better rewards, giving a selective advantage to those individuals who solicit other, potentially more equitable partners. Nonetheless, short-term inequity does not appear to disrupt cooperative relationships. Given that many interactions do not typically result in complete equality, this flexibility may clear the way for cooperation to persist despite modest inequality, while long-term inequity can be used as a cue that a particular cooperative relationship is no longer beneficial." There is a constant interplay between forces bringing us closer together or driving us apart, involving reputation and social reward-related circuits on the one hand[29] and "more primitive survival-enhancing" circuits on the other.[30] Indeed, not all human groups show the same prosocial/altruistic behaviors,[31] and even amongst people in WEIRD (western, educated, industrialized, rich, democratic) societies, there is individual variation, with so-called "extraordinary altruists" at one end of the scale[32] and psychopaths at the other.[33] Reappraisal of our social interactions with others is associated with altered neural activity in numerous brain regions, especially those known to be associated with emotional responses (insula, striatum, and posterior cingulate cortex) and with what is termed "mentalizing" (eg inferior and medial prefrontal cortex, temporo-parietal junction).[34] I should here clarify the term "mentalizing"; it is a term used by psychologists to describe our ability to imagine our own as well as others' mental states and to infer their intentions.

In an interesting and challenging series of papers, it has been argued that prosocial or altruistic behavior, even if costly to individuals, was needed to improve the likelihood of survival of a particular human group in times of conflict, when challenging environments and inter-group competition made extinction a distinct possibility.[35,36] Essentially, Professor Bowles suggests that warfare and lethal competition between disparate groups of early humans were commonplace, limiting population growth and driving the selection of cooperative "group-beneficial behaviors."[36] He argues that "culturally transmitted practices presuppose advanced cognitive and linguistic capacities, possibly accounting for the distinctive forms of altruism found in our species" and suggests that a predisposition favoring altruism in humans "may be the result of a gene-culture coevolutionary process in which, as Darwin wrote, group conflict played a key role."[35] In this context it is worth noting that, throughout recorded history, communal vocalization (war cries) and music-making have been used in the period leading up to, and during, battle: "Fighting morale and solidarity have always been fortified by musicality."[37] This association, what Johnson and Cloonan call "the dark side of the tune," nonetheless can be viewed as reinforcing the evolutionary links between music and cooperative behaviors that lead to collective action. Even at the genetic level, "from conflict can come forth harmony; the very selfishness of genes can give rise to cooperation ... if it pays to cooperate, natural selection will favour genes that do so. Thus selfish genes can come to be accomplished cooperators—selfish cooperators, pragmatic cooperators, but accomplished cooperators nonetheless."[38]

Our individual perception of risk and uncertainty in the face of adverse circumstances, and our behavioral flexibility and capacity to cope with such risks, may also have contributed to the evolution of greater intelligence[39] as well as the selection of altruistic behaviors favoring strong reciprocity in the great majority of a population.[40] The importance of "shared reciprocal access to resources in harsh environments with high resource uncertainty" and social behaviors that facilitate such interactions can be observed even today in hunter-gatherer societies around the world.[39] This idea is also beautifully captured by Robert Shorto in his book on the history of Amsterdam.[41] He argues that the constant life-threatening struggle against water in the massive northern European delta that became the Netherlands had a huge impact on the psyche of the people that eventually populated this region: "Individualism, as a theory and as an idea, is related to extreme conditions and, seemingly paradoxically, to the need to band together." Leadership is needed in such times of crisis, perhaps based on prestige rather than dominance, leadership of a kind that most usefully encourages cooperation and prosocial activities.[42]

Which areas of the human brain are active when actively performing mutually or socially cooperative tasks? Can we visualize the "neurobiology of social decision-making?"[28] Subjects have been scanned when performing tasks involving games such as the "Prisoner's Dilemma" or other trust games (see Matt Ridley's book *The Origins of Virtue* for an excellent description of these games and their historical development). Rilling et al used the Prisoner's Dilemma game to investigate which brain areas are active when performing acts of reciprocal altruism.[43] As discussed earlier, this form of cooperation seems to be of great importance to our species, involving some kind of gift—not necessarily material in nature—and the expectation that at some time in the future the recipient will eventually return the favor. Subjects (36 women) placed in an MRI scanner had to make decisions on whether to cooperate with another individual; each was then awarded a sum of money that was dependent on the level of cooperation or non-cooperation. Mutual cooperation, where the welfare of the other player was taken into consideration, was consistently associated with activation in areas observed to be linked to reward processing and assessment of motivation-value information, including the nucleus accumbens, caudate nucleus, medial orbitofrontal cortex, and anterior cingulate cortex (see Figure 4.2). Inferring generous, as opposed to selfish, play has also been shown to affect activity in ventromedial prefrontal cortex, there being some right-sided bias to temporo-parietal and also parahippocampal regions.[44] It is worth noting here that some of these regions, with the additional inclusion of the right superior temporal sulcus, are also active when we experience face-to-face social interactions with others.[45] Even *believing* that we are interacting "live" with someone else in an experimental setting (when in fact we are not) is sufficient to alter the neural processing of incoming speech.[46]

In discussing their data, Rilling and colleagues proposed that "activation of this neural network positively reinforces reciprocal altruism, thereby motivating subjects to resist the temptation to selfishly accept but not reciprocate favors." Further studies of various types of cooperative game-playing that require the subjects to appreciate the social context, infer/anticipate the behavior and intentions of others, and predict the potential consequences of a decision have confirmed increased activity in certain regions of prefrontal cortex as well as in regions such as the anterior cingulate cortex, temporo-parietal junction, and amygdala. These regions encode important aspects of insight, reasoning, and mentalizing, and help initiate and sustain complex social interactions.[47,48,49,50,51,52] The amygdala in particular is larger in volume in people termed "extraordinary altruists"—in those, for example, who volunteer to donate a kidney to a stranger.[32] The amygdala is also known to be reduced in size in aggressive individuals with psychopathic traits who are deficient in prosocial emotions such as empathy and remorse.[53]

Altruistic acts are rarely performed without expectation of external praise or advantage; some form of reciprocity is important. Interestingly then, imaging data support the idea that altruism is psychologically rewarding; it makes you feel good. Individuals usually desire positive social feedback about themselves, and will tend to bias their interpretation of any such feedback, helping them to develop and preserve a "positive self-concept."[22] The rewarding feeling that results from such social feedback is accompanied by increased activity in the ventral striatum, anterior cingulate cortex, and medial prefrontal cortex. Changes in how a subject's own concept of self are altered when feedback is received from others was found to be associated with activation of cortical areas more associated with mentalizing.[22]

The punishment of "defectors"—those that do not obviously comply with "social norms"—can sometimes come at a cost to the punisher,[54] but it can also be a rewarding experience. Punitive actions result in increased activity, again in the nucleus accumbens; thus we may gain a degree of satisfaction through the "punishment of norm violations."[55] The authors of these findings also obtained evidence for some genetic variation in the dopamine systems that mediate much of the neural interactions in this reward network. Others have reported that about 2–3% of the population in English-speaking countries exhibit some type of antisocial personality disorder, and it has been argued that the persistence of such people who cheat and take advantage of others may in fact be of long-term benefit to the social group as a whole, owing to "the necessity for society to fight against antisocial behavior, [and] play positive roles for society and/or human groups, especially in the ancestral environment."[56]

Interestingly, there is an emotional consequence to breaking a promise, a response that seems inbuilt because in fMRI studies involving healthy "*Homo sapientior*" subjects such dishonesty correlates consistently with activity in regions known to be involved in social interaction—the dorsolateral prefrontal cortex, anterior cingulate cortex, and amygdala.[57] Peer group pressure impacts on our decision-making: Do we conform? Are we in or out of the group? Imaging of subjects as they made decisions influenced by the judgments of "in-group" or "out-group" members has revealed increased conformity-related activity in part of the basal ganglia (dopamine/reward?), anterior cingulate cortex (affective behavior/social acceptance?), and posterior superior temporal sulcus and posterior insula (trust/perceive the perspective of others within the "in-group?").[58]

Overall, the lateral part of the cortex situated above the eye orbit (the so-called orbitofrontal cortex) seems to be associated with "norm-abiding behavior," or doing the right thing in case of punishment, while activity in the caudate nucleus and ventral striatum in the basal ganglia appears to be associated with reciprocal cooperation and the performance of charitable acts. Rilling et al suggested that activity in the anterior insular cortex may "mark negative social interactions as risky or averse," interactions to be avoided in the future.[28] Matthew Rushworth and colleagues have suggested that there are four frontal lobe regions in the cerebral cortex that make distinct contributions to those predictive and decision-making behaviors that are perceived as rewarding: these are the ventromedial and medial orbitofrontal cortex, the lateral orbitofrontal cortex, the anterior cingulate cortex, and the anterior prefrontal cortex (Figure 5.1).[59] Finally, Rilling et al reported that suppression of activity in the amygdala promotes trust by reducing the fear of being "let down." Interestingly, people with damage to this structure have significantly reduced eye contact with others during conversations,[60] a change in behavior that most of us would likely view as "shifty."

In Chapter 3, I introduced the concepts of "Theory of Mind," which describes an individual's ability to attribute mental states to others, and "empathy," which broadly

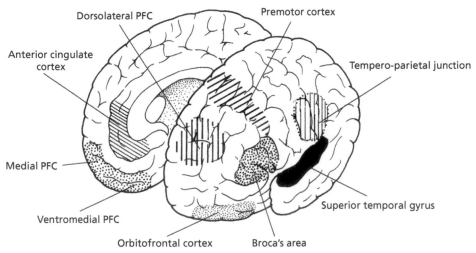

Figure 5.1 A summary drawing showing many of the common regions of the human cerebral cortex (orbitofrontal, ventromedial, and dorsolateral prefrontal cortex; anterior cingulate cortex; temporo-parietal junction; and superior temporal gyrus) that are activated either when listening to pleasurable music or when performing acts of engagement, social cooperation, and altruism. For specific information about right or left hemisphere laterality, please refer to text. Also shown for reference are Broca's area and premotor cortex. Regions not shown include nucleus accumbens and the caudate nucleus. PFC, prefrontal cortex.
© Martin Thompson, 2016.

describes the ability to infer intentions, desires, and emotional experiences in others. Each necessarily requires a concept of self, and both are regarded as essential components of social cognition and social interaction. In animals, including of course non-human primates, empathy has been suggested to be the "main proximate mechanism for directed altruism," an interactive, prosocial behavior leading eventually to advantageous evolutionary outcomes.[7] Neuroimaging studies in humans have revealed that Theory of Mind and empathy stimuli activate overlapping, but also separate, neural pathways.[61] Common regions include the medial prefrontal cortex and anterior parts of the temporal lobes. Theory of Mind stimuli preferentially activated orbitofrontal cortex and parts of the frontal, occipital, and temporal lobes, while empathy stimuli resulted in greater activity in the cingulate cortex, anterior insula, and amygdala, regions more associated with processing emotion.

In humans, empathy can be divided into two separate, but sometimes interactive, neural systems, one concerned with directly sensing and feeling another's emotions (emotional or affective empathy) and the other with more evolutionarily recent behavior—cognitive, self-reflecting, and autobiographical, and intuiting and understanding another's intellectual/psychological viewpoint (cognitive empathy), which is "unique to primates and humans."[62] According to Simone Shamay-Tsoory, emotion recognition and emotional contagion involve a network that includes the inferior frontal gyrus, inferior parietal cortex, anterior cingulate, and anterior insula, while so-called cognitive empathy involves parts of the prefrontal cortex, temporo-parietal junction, and medial temporal lobe (including the hippocampus), these regions also being key players in Theory of Mind, "self-other distinction," and declarative (autobiographical) memory processing. However: "Depending on the situational context and information available in the environment, empathic responses may involve a co-recruitment of so-called mirror networks and regions involved in Theory of Mind or mentalizing."[63]

The cortical regions described above are important in empathic responsiveness, in the ability to feel (and make cognitive predictions about) what others are feeling, for example empathy for pain.[63,64,65] This is not the same as sympathy for another's plight! In addition, some of the cortical regions that process somatosensation, but that also receive visual and auditory information, can be "vicariously recruited by the sight of other people being touched, performing actions or experiencing somatic pain."[66] Humans can guess the level of pain by looking at another's face[67]—we see someone else in what we perceive as emotional discomfort/pain and hope that we do not experience it ourselves. If we are asked to imagine pain in our own body when looking at images of pain or fear, the latter predictably activates the amygdala, but a cortical area driven by both thought processes is, once again, the anterior cingulate cortex.[68]

All of us know people who seem to be less empathic than others; we are not all the same in how we interact within a social context. Cooperating and empathizing with someone else requires that an individual can predict how another person will react to a particular situation, an ability that we have noted is associated with activity in anterior cingulate cortex. However, the extent to which this region is activated varies between individuals and is linked to the ability to feel emotional empathy. Activity is high in this cortical region in individuals who show high emotion contagion and who are interested in the rewards of others, but low in subjects low in emotional contagion, or interested (selfishly) in their own rewards.[69] It is therefore interesting that inter-individual differences in gray matter density and volume in various regions of the cortex have been found that seem to correlate with the level of either affective or cognitive empathy.[70,71] Another report found that individuals who perceive themselves as being lonely have a smaller left superior temporal cortex![72] However, as discussed in Chapter 2, from a nature versus nurture point of view, it is not yet clear whether these associations are due to intrinsic inter-individual variability (see also the discussion on oxytocin later in this section), or are a consequence of different "empathy-experiences" gained during childhood and/or adolescence, or—most likely—are some combination of the two, experience interacting with susceptibility.

Prolonged maternal–infant relationships, and later on cooperative social group behavior between adults, were presumably already supported to some extent by the pre-linguistic, primarily prosodic, mimetic-based communication systems used by our ancestors (see Chapter 4, also[9,73]). Modern human communication is highly complex and involves an inferred or predicted understanding between the sender and the intended receiver. This ability to communicate and share intention seemingly has its own processing system that is "distinct both from sensorimotor processes … and language abilities (with their largely left-hemisphere localization)."[74] Language-driven evolution of sustainable mutual cooperative behaviors more than ever would have involved shared goals and shared intentionality,[75] trustworthiness, prediction, value judgment, and in "*Homo sapientior*" the development of complex social networks and interactions beyond the immediate family.[76] Using various theoretical models, Nowak and Karakauer proposed that language could only have evolved if "information transfer is beneficial to both speaker and listener … the evolution of communication requires cooperation between individuals."[77] It is difficult to imagine the evolution of modern, syntactic language if speech was used only to deceive another!

One of Merlin Donald's conclusions in *Origins of the Modern Mind*—that "the Darwinian universe is too small to contain humanity"—is entirely consistent with my earlier comments that, because of language and culture, there is transmission of knowledge within and across generations, each generation accumulating knowledge and information from their ancestors. With language—this new and unique communication system built on the foundations of gesture, facial expression, and imitation—there is a concomitant increase in intelligence, associated with the evolution of the modern mind and, at some point, what we now recognize in ourselves and others as consciousness. As Philip Lieberman eloquently describes it in his book *Uniquely Human: The Evolution of Speech, Thought, and Selfless Behavior*, "the 'key' to the evolution of the modern brain is rapid vocal communication. That consequently is the key to human progress; the enhanced linguistic and cognitive ability that the human brain confers allows us to transcend the constraints of biological evolution."[78] BUT, trust, cooperativity, and mutually altruistic behaviors are necessary components of this cultural process, and "even before humans began actually speaking to one another in a behaviourally modern way, their immediate hominin ancestors already differed from other apes in their eagerness to share one another's mental states and feelings."[9] To again quote Matt Ridley from his book *The Origins of Virtue*: "Society works not because we have consciously invented it, but because it is an ancient product of our evolved predispositions. It is literally in our nature."[1]

Music and prosocial behavior

So how does the foregoing discussion relate to music, and how does it help convince you that music also had an essential place in the evolutionary trajectory of "*Homo sapientior*?" What is critically important here is that a great many of the brain regions implicated in Theory of Mind and empathic processing overlap, or at least are very closely associated with, those areas activated when listening to rewarding and happy music, music you are most likely familiar with and that gives you "chills." If we also compare such regions with areas of the brain that are active when performing acts of engagement, social cooperation, and altruism;[28] when you feel guilty about telling a lie;[57] and/or when processing reward-related behaviors,[59,79] then the extent of the overlap becomes remarkable (Figure 5.1).[80] Areas where there seems to be a close relationship include the frontal cortex (eg orbitofrontal, ventromedial, and dorsolateral prefrontal cortex), anterior cingulate cortex, temporo-parietal junction, superior temporal gyrus and sulcus, ventral striatum, nucleus accumbens, and caudate nucleus. Importantly, reminiscent of certain aspects of music processing, at least some imaging studies indicate that there is a right hemisphere bias when subjects are involved in social interactions of one kind or another.[45,81] However, when subjects make judgments about social concepts such as honor and bravery, imaging reveals activation of the left superior anterior temporal cortex,[82] in the vicinity and on the same side as one of the regions activated when comparing responses to happy versus sad music.[83]

There is evidence that membership of a group influences how individuals experience both affective and cognitive aspects of empathy.[84] It is therefore fascinating that emotional responsiveness to, and participation in, musical activities is rewarding and activates brain areas that share common features with affective empathic processing circuitries.[85,86] When playing music together, recording of brain wave activity points to activity patterns in the right ventrolateral frontal cortex that reflect "empathic processes in musicians observing their own musical performance in ensemble."[86] Musical training enhances these links, presumably by also strengthening cognitive empathy (and perhaps mirror neuron) circuitries. Overall, the take-home message is that music and associated synchronized behaviors reinforce empathy and "affective engagement,"[87] and enhance the recognition and sharing of emotional states, all indicators of the importance of music as a social glue in "*Homo sapientior*." Music, and with it dance, brings individuals together, providing a special social context that unifies us in body *and* in mind.[88]

Evidence for close links between music, empathy, altruism, and cooperative behavior is also to be found in studies that focus on brain neurochemistry. The impact of music on dopamine release and signaling in the brain was discussed in the previous chapter, noting that mesolimbic dopaminergic systems are also involved in goal-directed behaviors and reward-related activities, including decisions about reciprocity. Another neuromodulator, serotonin, also appears to be important in enhancing cooperative behavior between individuals, diminishing the likelihood of retaliatory responses and punishment behaviors.[89] Interestingly then, mutations in one of its receptors has been reported to affect artistic creativity.[90] The hormone vasopressin has long been known to be important in the control of blood pressure and in promoting the reabsorption of water from the kidney (vasopressin is also known as antidiuretic hormone). More recently it has become clear that this hormone has neuromodulatory functions. Variations in the gene encoding the vasopressin receptor AVPR1a are correlated with how subjects perform in the "dictator game," a laboratory trial that measures altruistic decision-making,[91] but as discussed again later in the section on musical heritability, mutations in this receptor are also linked to creativity and musicality.

In addition to vasopressin, there is a considerable body of evidence showing that the hormone oxytocin enhances social awareness and prosocial behavioral traits.[91,92,93,94,95,96] Oxytocin "enhances socially reinforced learning and emotional empathy in humans,"[97] but not cognitive empathy (which may be associated more with dopamine signaling). It has an antidepressive, positive impact on emotional behavior,[94] and may also increase sensitivity to reward[98] and induce prosocial altruistic behaviors.[99] Intranasally administered oxytocin increases trust in subjects, associated with decreased activity in regions such as the amygdala and striatum, consistent with a reduction in fear about "social betrayal."[100,101] Not surprisingly then, genetic variants of the oxytocin receptor have been discovered that are also associated with differences in the way humans empathize, engage in prosocial and affiliative behaviors, and respond to stress.[102,103] At the extreme end of the spectrum, children and adolescents displaying so-called "callous-emotional" traits—perhaps a precursor of diminished prosocial behavior and sociopathy/psychopathy in adulthood—also showed polymorphisms in the oxytocin receptor gene.[104]

In her book *Why Music Moves Us*,[105] Jeanette Bicknell discerningly focused on this hormone, suggesting that oxytocin may act as a link between emotional responses, music, and social bonding—including the neurobiology of parent–child attachment. In one therapeutic study, oxytocin levels were reported to increase in postcardiac surgery patients who had been exposed to music,[106] but whether this type of proximate neural response to music is also influenced by genetic polymorphisms in oxytocin sensitivity is, to my knowledge, unknown. A more recent and fascinating study on four members of a vocal jazz group revealed that plasma oxytocin levels rose in the singers, but only when they were improvising together, perhaps indicating enhanced social interactions during that particular activity.[107]

Music can act as a delineator of social groups and is also a powerful unifier in times of conflict; just think of the bagpipe players striding out of the allied trenches during the First World War, the ubiquitous military marching bands, and the drummers and buglers playing for all they were worth as battlegroups marched towards each other ... Drumming, dancing, and synchronous singing can bring on ritualistic trance-like states, entrain neural activity, and elicit a unified, collective state of consciousness[108,109,110]—a "battle trance" in which there is reduced fear, reduced perception of risk, and a willingness to sacrifice for the whole, for the common good. So in addition to all the prosocial- and cognitively/ psychologically enhancing aspects of music and dance pertaining to each individual, this communication stream forges coalitions and alliances within and between culturally like-minded groups, deters enemies, advertises group strength, and delineates territory.[109] And yet, given that the males would have been the hunters and fighters, it is odd that in males, but not females, music has been reported to *decrease* testosterone levels, which would be likely to reduce aggressive tendencies![111]

Group music-making and dance, in which individuals have positive expectations and enjoy their own activity/ability, while at the same time receiving the approbation of other group members, are likely to act as a major driver of the positive reward circuits intrinsic to the brain of "*Homo sapientior*." This urge for social contact and the need to share "physical, affective, and ideational experience" may even have been important in helping to shape the emerging sense of self and helping to create our own meaningful identity within an evolving social network.[88,112] In human pre-history, the stirring and rewarding feelings elicited by music and dance (sound and action) may well have acted to "synchronize and harmonize the emotional mood of a group of individuals at a time when they are called upon to act in the interests of the group, the better to further their own interests."[1] Indeed, as discussed previously, in the present day it is clear that mutual music-making can accelerate the formation of social bonds between like-minded humans.[113] And in promoting group interactions, social networks, and collective arousal, music and movement have almost always been an essential element of ceremony and ritual, helping to facilitate the faithful transmission of culture from one generation to the next—maintaining ritual traditions.[114]

Is there evidence of inheritability of musicality?

The universal that we call music has been preserved since the very beginning of "*Homo sapientior*" and has presumably continued to evolve since then. I have argued that music was, and continues to be, of profound importance to the human species. So, from a Darwinian perspective, any genes that contribute to the complex behavior that we call musicality, including creation, performance, and response, might be expected to be at worst neutral and at best positively selected for in some way, presumably involving both sexual and social selection.[115,116] It is also likely, given the phenotypic complexity of human communication, that many of these genes or clusters of genes would be linked to genetic machinery involved in other cognitive, prosocial, and/or emotional behaviors that were evolutionarily advantageous to our species.[117,118]

There is of course a general sense that musical families often have musical children—many of the married couples (the Kays, Blues, Barnes, Firkins) with whom I have played in various bands over the years have very talented musical children who have formed their own bands, and several of these children have made recordings. My own children had lessons and enjoy music but did not continue to play, and while my wife likes to play the flute I am not a great one for rehearsing and we rarely play at home, whereas the friends' households mentioned above were filled with music all the time. Sending the kids off to another room to practice their piano pieces is not the smartest idea—I had a Homer Simpson "d'oh!" moment when I later realized this; after all, music is a social not a solitary experience!

The seven generations of musicians in the Bach family are perhaps an exemplar of musical heritability, but as ever the nature versus nurture issue is difficult to disentangle. An early study by Scheinfeld and Schweitzer found that, in a sample of 122 outstanding instrumentalists, principal opera singers, or music students, when both parents were musically talented about 70% of their offspring were regarded as also being talented.[119] A much more recent twin study in which subjects were asked to rank their own abilities found evidence for the heritability of aptitude and "exceptional talent" across a number of cognitive, creative, and sporting domains, including music.[120] The effect was similar for both men and women.

Availability of, and perhaps parental insistence on, early musical training in a supportive home environment is obviously an important and rewarding parameter in many instances,[121] although in music at least, truly exceptional creative talent often exhibits itself very early in life. And of course, there is a difference between aptitude (eg absolute or at least a well-developed sense of pitch, sense of rhythm, and so on) and talent: "Aptitude is the basis for technique, but while technique is highly essential, by itself it cannot produce talent."[119] But talent also requires training and hard work to achieve greatness, sometimes to the exclusion of all else. As discussed by Scott and Moffett, persons of genius with exceptional creative and/or interpretative gifts often have no direct descendents (that are known about).[122] The same authors also tell the remarkable story of the Hon Daines Barrington, who in 1781 gave a lecture to the Royal Society about five exceptionally gifted child prodigies, one of whom was Mozart. One of the others, W. H. Crotch, became Professor of Music at Oxford at the age of 21 years. At two-and-a-half years of age he picked out the National Anthem on his father's organ. Imagine if it had been he and not Mozart destined for musical immortality? Would his abilities have been handed down, from Crotch to Crotch—or should that be from Crotch to crotchets?

Although "musical talent is in all probability inherited through a number of genes acting together …,"[119] there is now at least some emerging evidence for a hereditary basis for certain aspects of music and dance ability in humans. For example, absolute pitch capability seems to be present in some children even before any musical training,[123] and evidence of a hereditary component for absolute pitch has also been obtained.[124] As is often the case in studies weighing genetic influence against upbringing/environment, twin pair studies can be very revealing. Using data from a large twin study in Sweden, Mosing et al found that about 50% of the observed variation in the ability to detect and discriminate differences in sequential presentations of either pitch, rhythmic stimuli, or melodic stimuli was "due to genetic influences."[117] Furthermore, a clear link was found between musical discrimination ability and IQ, indicating some shared genetic factors. As the authors suggest, this covariation may be related to the need to use working memory and other executive functions in both the musical discrimination and non-musical cognitive tasks. Others have shown that the size and functionality of auditory cortex in children is related not only to potential musical ability but also to literacy and attentional skills.[125]

In an earlier study it was found that identical twins were more likely to be able to detect "wrong" notes in a popular tune than fraternal twins.[126] This was a very specific task, and I stress here that we must be very, very careful to distinguish between basic or core sensorimotor and emotional responsiveness to music and rhythm, which almost all humans possess (except perhaps for the very few with true congenital amusia), and exceptional creative, interpretative, and/or performance aptitude in music and dance. As described in Chapter 2, the core musical elements seem to be primarily right hemisphere driven, but musical training and higher levels of perceptual processing entail interactions that also involve the left hemisphere. In recent human history it is clear that there is indeed considerable variation in musical ability, but perhaps this is only to be expected 4,000 generations or so on from our founder population in Africa? Similar variability exists in languages and dialects, and in our ability to paint oils or watercolors, play golf, solve algebraic equations, answer IQ tests, and so forth.

A large-scale hunt for links between musical aptitude (discrimination of pitch, sound patterns, etc) and variation in the human genome has revealed several SNPs in genes that encode proteins that are important in auditory pathway development, including genes implicated in the development of receptive components in the cochlea as well as parts of the auditory brainstem.[127] As mentioned earlier, the hormone vasopressin has been implicated in cognitive function and seems likely to modulate certain social and affective behaviors. It is thus intriguing that sequence variability in a gene that encodes a receptor for this neuroactive peptide (AVPR1a) has been linked to the quality of creativity in dancers[90] and musical memory.[128] As Granot et al point out: "Given the role of vasopressin in social behavior, the association found in our study between musical memory and vasopressin could serve to support evolutionary accounts postulating a social adaptive role in music."[128] Consistent with these views, in another study involving 15 families, various musical processing tests revealed evidence for a genetic contribution to musical aptitude,[129] which was later followed up by examining polymorphisms in 19 Finnish musical families; the study confirmed the importance of the AVPR1a haplotype and musical ability.[130] The most recent work from this study group has identified several other genes that appear to be positively selected in association with musical aptitude and creativity.[131,132] In addition to genes associated with inner ear development, the authors identified genes broadly linked to reward, cognition, learning, and memory—although it should be noted that the (474) subjects were all musically experienced, and presumably from WEIRD backgrounds. In these studies there was over-representation of genes encoding the AMPA glutamate receptor and some cell adhesion molecules—all important in synaptic plasticity, particularly in the cerebellum.

Finally, polymorphism in a receptor for the neurotransmitter serotonin has also been associated with episodic memory performance[133] and creativity,[90] while altered function of the dopamine system (eg by mutation in the gene encoding the enzyme that makes dopamine, COMT) is correlated with altered connections with prefrontal cortex[134] and measurable changes in certain aspects of working memory performance, cognitive ability, and lexical decision-making, as well as with reward and addictive behaviors.[135,136,137] Polymorphisms in COMT influence creative potential,[138] consistent with the hypothesis that the influence of mesolimbic dopamine systems on reward behaviors is modified by genetic changes that may also influence how individuals respond to music.[139]

I mentioned in the previous chapter that research has identified a significant correlation between genetic variance and specific melody styles. In an analysis of 31 Eurasian populations, the data suggested that "maternal lineages have a more important role in folk music traditions than paternal lineages."[140] These observations indicate that women can have a significant influence on the transmission of musical culture in a particular population. A similar correlation between folk music genres and genetic lineage as assessed by mtDNA sequencing was found among indigenous populations in Taiwan, a correlation that was not observed with language, leading the authors to state that analysis of music types "might be capturing different aspects of population history than language"[141]—it may in fact be a more reliable indicator than others when studying human lineage and migration.[142] Finally, the most recent phylogenetic study on musical diversity in farmers and hunter-gatherers in Gabon confirmed that vertical transmission (ancestor to descendent) is far more important in delineating musical styles (especially metrics and rhythmic/melodic content) than horizontal transmission (between living populations).[143] In these "non-WEIRD" populations, the authors obtained evidence for both matrilineal and patrilineal descent, dependent on particular social and cultural contexts/practices. Based on comparisons of musical structure and style, a similar claim—"Echoes of our forgotten ancestors"—was also made several years ago by Victor Grauer,[144] although direct genetic correlations were not available to him.

I will go further, stimulated by an article by Mark Moffett[145] on his thoughts as to how human society forms distinct and coherent groups, and the need for stable "societal labels" to identify not only individuals but at the same time help to sustain cooperative group identity when there is a sizable increase in population numbers. Language (including dialects), symbolic ornamentation, and body art would act to individualize and perhaps also mark members of a particular group. In addition, although Moffett does not raise the possibility, the correlation between genetic identity and musical content described above—perhaps along with specific ceremonial and/or dance-like traditions—would seem to me to be a perfect label, defining and demarcating increasingly bigger groups in early modern human hunter-gatherer societies: "Societal labels...provide the solidarity upon which complex systems of altruism can be created, making possible anonymous societies large enough to build civilizations."[145] What you wear and what you listen to still makes a difference today. I well remember the raging battles in southern England in the 1960s between the mods in their tailor-made suits and the rockers in their black leather jackets—scooters versus motor bikes, and (of course) a clear differentiation in musical tastes: rhythm & blues, soul, and ska for the mods; Eddie Cochran, Gene Vincent, and rock 'n' roll for the rockers!

In sum then, it is surely no coincidence that the diverse brain areas that are associated with social cooperation and interactions, altruism, empathy, and reward overlap with areas that are activated when listening to pleasant or uplifting music (Figure 5.1). This is entirely consistent with a critical role for music in fostering social cooperativity, honesty, trust, and beneficial collective behaviors within groups of "*Homo sapientior*" (see also Chapter 4), and perhaps a major reason why music "is a permanent part of our mental furniture."[146] In close association with the evolution of language and the modern mind, music and dance were of critical and fundamental importance to our early ancestors. Increased fitness and reproductive advantage of a group was gained not only by an individual's success and sense of identity, but also if cooperative social behaviors enhanced one's self-esteem and at the same time benefited other members of the group. Importantly for our ancestors, these benefits extended to others who were not necessarily of the same family. There would have been inter-breeding between different kin within groups, and presumably also liaisons with members of other groups, sharing genetic material over time. Nonetheless, it seems clear that vertical inheritance is a dominant influence, with recognizable links between the genetic backgrounds of populations and their respective musical cultures.

Steven Brown has argued that "the straightforward evolutionary implication is that human musical capacity evolved because groups of musical hominids out-survived groups of non-musical hominids due to a host of factors related to group-level cooperation and coordination."[147] Music is uniquely suited for this purpose because, as Ian Cross[148,149] has proposed, music has what he terms "floating intentionality": it is usually consequence (and risk) free, and has indeterminate meaning that differs between individuals and between contexts. Thus, in a group, a given piece of music can embody "various simultaneously co-existing referential frameworks for each participant, and it becomes possible for multiple individuals to share a common musical act" that permits "engagement in co-ordinated interaction in time while minimising possible inter-individual conflict."[148] Trust in others is associated with a decreased fear of social betrayal. In his important book

Brain and Music, Stefan Koelsch uses the term co-pathy rather than empathy because "co-pathy refers to the social function of empathy."[150] It is when an individual responds in a congruent emotional fashion to what he/she perceives others are feeling at that moment—perhaps what communal music and dance do best? And as I will argue in the next chapter, music may have assumed critical importance during the evolution of "us," as we became blindingly self-aware, and as we developed language-driven individualities and identities, and confronted our own mortality.

Chapter 6

The Consequences of Owning a Modern Mind

Still thou art blest, compar'd wi' me!
The present only toucheth thee:
But Och! I backward cast my e'e,
On prospects drear!
An' forward tho' I canna see,
I guess an' fear!

—Robbie Burns, *To a Mouse*

In discussing the role of music in human existence, Anthony Storr[1] asks whether music is a refuge, a temporary escape from reality, from the day-to-day exigencies and tribulations of life, or whether it is—and here he quotes Nietsche—life-affirming, reconciling us to its vagaries, confronting tragedy, the "artistic conquest of the horrible." But perhaps these are not necessarily mutually exclusive positions if, by doing the latter, we identify with other members of our species and thus come to accept our individual lot as a mere transient on the planet's surface. To acknowledge life as it actually is, whether ecstatic, painful, joyful, and so forth, can be a source of wonder and reconciliation.

As described in Chapter 4, our brains process music that is perceived as happy or sad, pleasant or dissonant, in different ways. Music-evoked emotions can drive activity in reward centers such as the nucleus accumbens, or limbic structures such as the amygdala. There is evidence that some elements of this diverse responsiveness to music are present very early in life, but our subtle, individualistic responses are influenced by our autobiographical and cultural experiences and fueled by our expectations, resulting in a full range of emotional triggers, most having social, interpersonal relevance within and across space and time. Positive responses to music tap into emotional and reward circuits as well as circuits associated with cooperative, prosocial behaviors. "Wherever humans live, and however they have organized their societies, they exhibit a behavioural peculiarity of gathering from time to time to sing and dance together in a group. By featuring both human song and entrainment (in the dancing movements and perhaps clapping performed in synchrony with the singing/music), such behaviour qualifies as human music. Indeed, the fact that it occurs in every human culture, and indeed subculture, without exception, unless deliberately suppressed by severe sanctions against it, marks this phenomenon as the most universal human behaviour of a musical kind on record."[2] Can this universality tell us anything about the evolutionary history of our species—why we may have survived, and why we have retained two communication systems, interrelated yet distinct from each other?

In a fascinating article about "the ties that bind us,"[3] Harvey Whitehouse and Jonathan Lanman argue that: "While humans could rely on kin altruism and reciprocity to reap the benefits of cooperation in small, face-to-face social groups, new psychological adaptations were required to benefit from cooperation and accumulated cultural knowledge in larger communities defined by symbolic identity markers." The need for stable societal labels in large groups[4] was briefly discussed in the previous chapter. With our advanced autobiographical memory capacity (ie a memory of our own, unique personal experiences throughout life, as well as accumulated general knowledge about the world around us), and of course with the evolution of language and articulate speech, we could now share experiences and information with others in a more personal way: "The perception that one shares with others' important, self-defining experiences encoded in episodic memory, we argue, produces a powerful sense of psychological kinship."[3] And to effectively enhance cooperation and overall social/group identities, what better vehicle for encouraging large-scale social and cultural cohesion than cooperative music-making and dance?

Mortality and positive thinking

With the evolution of modern articulate speech and an advanced cognitive architecture, through our mutual comprehension of the past, present, and future, at some point we came to realize the transience of things, to comprehend that we are mortal: "We are alone among animals in foreseeing our end."[5] This was also beautifully described by Peter Medawar some years ago: "Only human beings guide their behaviour by a knowledge of what happened before they were born and a preconception of what may happen after they are dead; thus only humans find their way by a light that illuminates more than the patch of ground they stand on."[6] In the barest and bleakest of terms, and in the absence of religious faith, life could be regarded as a sentence of sentience trapped in a vehicle shrinking into nothingness. Language and the still ill-understood phenomenon of consciousness may well have co-evolved, but did it come at a potential price? "There is a tragic dimension to consciousness … there is madness, depression, guilt, and dread. There is the fear of death—and strangest of all, the fear of life … For some people, in some circumstances, consciousness becomes so unbearable that they commit suicide to bring it to an end. 'To be or not to be?' is a peculiarly human question."[7]

In a letter to the journal *Nature*, Professor Ajit Varka discussed comments made to him by a colleague, Danny Brower, about human awareness (and denial) of mortality.[8] In his view, it is the evolution of neural mechanisms for denying mortality that allowed our species to survive. In Varka's words: "If this logic is correct, many warm-blooded species may have previously achieved self-awareness and inter-subjectivity, but then failed to survive because of extremely negative immediate consequences."[8] I was fascinated to read this because I have long had similar thoughts in relation to hominin species that may

have evolved language and a modern mind similar to ours, but did not maintain something akin to music as a parallel integrating and socializing communication stream. These
were hypothetical species that did not survive as a consequence—did not make it through
potential bottlenecks that confronted our own small founder population.

The biologist Tali Sharot suggests something that is perhaps complementary to my
music idea: that to counteract intimations of mortality humans had to evolve neural
substrates that allowed us to think positively, to increase the odds of survival. Indeed,
via neuroimaging studies he found that positive, optimistic thoughts activate specific
regions such as the anterior cingulate cortex, amygdala, and parts of the prefrontal
cortex.[9,10] The concordance with areas associated with emotional responses to music
(see Chapter 4) is revealing, and while I appreciate the need for care in causally relating
imaged neural activity to complex behaviors, it surely further supports the idea that
the music universal is of fundamental importance to our cognitive makeup. In fact,
I have yet to meet anyone whose mood was not lightened by singing and then whistling
Monty Python's "Always Look on the Bright Side of Life." Optimism is not the same
thing as hope, although I imagine without optimism there is little chance of hoping that
something good is going to happen soon. Hope is perhaps more context-specific and
goal-directed, related to desire for a particular outcome; it has an affective component.[11]
In Greek mythology, when Pandora opened her box, evil was released into the world
but the spirit of hope remained inside—hope, or perhaps it was optimism? With "*Homo
sapientior*," the arrival of self-awareness involved very great risk, and a vulnerability that
was perhaps offset by an intrinsic cognitive substrate for optimism and an emotional
need for hope....

In the earlier quote from David Lodge's novel *Thinks*,[7] the word "guilt" was used. The
concept of guilt is associated with moral values and moral emotions, something that may
also be uniquely human. Morality in this case is as defined by Jorge Moll et al in a review
on the neural basis of cognition: "considered as the sets of customs and values that are
embraced by a cultural group to guide social conduct, a view that does not assume the
existence of absolute moral values ... Morality is a product of evolutionary pressures that
have shaped social cognitive and motivational mechanisms, which had already developed
in human ancestors, into uniquely human forms of experience and behaviour."[12] It seems
to me that there are obvious links here to proximate norm-abiding behaviors, reciprocal
altruism, and so forth, as discussed in the previous chapter. Being fair and kind to another
individual eventually leads to "an agent-neutral morality in which individuals follow and
enforce group-wide social norms."[13] Regions of the human brain most clearly associated
with moral cognition[12] include those we have encountered before when discussing music
and cooperative social behavior—prefrontal cortex, medial and lateral orbitofrontal
cortex, insula, the superior temporal sulcus region, and—subcortically—the amygdala,
parts of the hypothalamus, and the ventral striatum. Again, we see these regions linked to
behaviors and positive emotions that are associated with the interests or welfare of self as
well as of others in an empathic, social, and cultural context, and yet again the links with
music are clear.

Burials and grave goods

Is there any evidence for a change in the perception of self in *"Homo sapientior"*—can we look back and detect a change in social structure and whether our evolution was linked to any new sense of identity, a new concept of self, and our interrelations with others? What about an emergent sense of mortality, a sense of the spiritual, a need to conjure up notions of an after-life? Obvious clues come from the emergence of more sophisticated tools and technologies, the innovative use of decoration, paintings, the creation of artifacts for symbolic representation, and so on. But anthropologists believe you can also acquire information about our "state of mind" by examining how the dead were buried.[14,15] Evidence of ceremony and ritual in or around skeletal remains is generally taken as an indication of mourning for the dead, which in turn suggests sentience and a sense of loss, of mortality. There is the idea that, when you start to bury people in what may appear to be a purposeful and ritualized way, then that goes hand in hand with a certain level of consciousness and awareness, of modern thought processes. An element of ritual would invariably be associated with some form of group music-making and perhaps dance, and presumably also accompanied by some type of formalized communication or incantation.

It has been claimed that occasional Neanderthal skeletons found in caves are evidence of deliberate burial practices, and perhaps signs of the emergence of ritual belief systems. In some cases the bodies seem to have been cut up, the flesh deliberately removed, and the bodies arranged in some way. There are a number of examples in Europe, the Middle East, and Asia: for example, skeletons in the Kebara Cave in Israel, which is about 60,000 years old, and the Shanidar Cave in Iraq, which is between 44,000 and 60,000 years old. In La Ferrassie in France, the fossil remains of eight Neanderthals (two adults, four children, and two fetuses) have been found close together lying head-to-foot, interpreted as being a deliberate burial site.[16] The age of these fossils is between 35,000 and 70,000 years. Flint tools were found nearby—perhaps so-called grave goods? And a cave in Drachenloch in Switzerland has been found to contain what seem to be systematic arrangements of bear skulls and bones, again interpreted by some as indicative of ritual and cult-like behavior.

In one cave, pollen was found near to the Neanderthal remains, leading some scholars to assume that the dead individual was buried with flowers. However, others now suggest that it is not possible to be certain that this is an indication of some sense of consciousness in Neanderthals, perhaps similar to ours. It is quite possible that the pollen just blew in there at some later date, or perhaps the flowers had been used prior to death for some medicinal/curative use? In another example, what seem to be Neanderthal remains that were deliberately covered over may only be the result of a subsequent rockfall. Problems with interpreting other so-called purposeful burial sites have been extensively discussed, and the evidence for such burials regarded as "equivocal."[14,17] True, or ritualistic, burials need to be separated from so-called funeral "caching," where multiple skeletal remains are found together in deep shafts or at the back of deep caves. Neanderthal remains have also been found in pits and seemingly left with general detritus. In summary, there are both advocates and sceptics in terms of the debate about Neanderthal burials, and we can only make guesses about their level of sentient and symbolic thought. An "abstract" rock engraving in Gibraltar is believed to be Neanderthal in origin, and has been dated to at least 39,000 years old,[18] but—at least until now—such intimations of culture in our cousins are rare.

Even if, in relatively much more recent paleolithic times, Neanderthals were more formally burying their dead, could it have been an idea that they learned from their far more sophisticated, intelligent, mortally self-aware, language-driven neighbors? Could they just have been copying their modern cousins, "Homo sapientior," with whom they had co-existed for thousands of years—at least in Europe and the Middle East? These now extinct hominins clearly possessed intelligence and excellent observational powers; they were reasonably smart people and very good mimics. Perhaps they knew that if they did not bury the dead the corpses would smell and decay, and attract insects, scavengers, and predators to the camps. So the living would perhaps place the dead in trees or take them to exposed higher ground, or occasionally put them in holes in the ground. And in those Ice Age days the ground was hard, so the living would likely make the smallest hole possible, meaning that it was necessary to break up a body prior to burial. Some species of animals are known to notice the death of others and may even stay with or manipulate the now lifeless body, but the critical question is whether the animals know that this too will be their fate, that it will happen to them. I doubt that they do. Similarly, Neanderthals may have perceived the death of another member of their group differently from the death of strangers or the death of other animal species. Perhaps they did sense and mourn the passing of others. But did each Neanderthal comprehend that death—or should I say permanent lack of movement and responsiveness—would at some time in the future happen to him or her as well?

My own view is that true burials, true fearful intimations of mortality, only arise with us because, with language and the evolution of the modern mind, we alone have the capacity for imagination, for mental time travel, and the ability to truly communicate with others across generations and comprehend the continued existence of the world, before, during, and after our own brief lifetime. We alone worry about what happens after death, when our perceptual window closes. Belief in a supernatural, other-dimensional existence after death to sustain lineage and ancestral rights to land and so on may also have had economic and political significance.[19] Yet we strive, we create—to give purpose and meaning to this transience—a biological imperative that underlies the individual narrative. To quote David Lodge again: "Homo sapiens was the first and only living being in evolutionary history to discover he was mortal ... so how does he respond? He makes up stories."[7] In his book on language, Rod Mengham goes so far as to suggest that "the secret purpose of language may not be to further communication between the living and the living, but between the living and the dead."[20]

In his book about religion and "conceiving God,"[19] David Lewis-Williams points out that religious belief is also, in a sense, a universal that persists worldwide, but he argues that Homo sapiens would also have seen and experienced death all the time and that invention of a spiritual realm and beliefs in an after-life "could not flow simply from an *awareness* of death." Perhaps what was different was an awareness of our *own* mortality? Certainly when examining modern *Homo sapiens* fossils and looking at their more frequently encountered burials, these sites seem to differ quite markedly from Neanderthal sites. In Qafzeh in the Middle East, for example, there is evidence of a burial of a young woman and (presumably) her infant, and at this site there appear to be artifacts associated with burials dated to about 90,000–100,000 years old.[21] According to Vanhaeren et al, the discovery of perforated shells associated with a 76,000-year-old burial is the "first known instance of an ornament used as a grave good."[22] With human burials the bodies are more obviously laid out, and the presence of various types of precious grave goods—objects and ornaments, which would have taken time to make—placed in the burial site may indicate spiritual significance, perhaps related to concepts of (desperate desire for?) an after-life.

Together, these anthropological findings indicate respect for the dead and clearly reveal an emergent knowledge about the difference between being alive and being dead, and in particular an awareness of one's own mortality. "Unlike other social animals, humans are very good at establishing and maintaining relations with agents beyond their physical presence ... It is a small step from having this capacity to bond with non-physical agents to conceptualizing spirits, dead ancestors and gods, who are neither visible nor tangible, yet are socially involved."[23] In a similar vein, when writing about the emergence of belief systems and spiritual awareness in *Homo sapiens*, Ian Tattersall wrote: "The Neanderthals had occasionally practiced burial of the dead, but among the Cro-Magnons [au: oldest known modern humans in Europe] we see for the first time evidence of regular and elaborate burial, with hints of ritual and belief in an afterlife."[24] The anthropologist Maurice Bloch suggests that what distinguishes us from other primates is our imagination, a key neurological adaptation required for our unique sociability; religion, including belief in an after-life, is just one aspect of our new, imaginary world.[25] And it is almost certainly specific to *"Homo sapientior."*

Maurice Bloch proposed that we have two types of social interactions: one he terms "transactional social," found also in baboons and chimps for example, which he regards as Machiavellian, "the product of a process of continual manipulation, assertions and defeats,"[25] and the other "transcendental social," regarded as unique to humans because it requires a new kind of imagination and encompasses what he terms essentialized roles and groups. These roles and groups exist separately from the individual; we exist in "imagined communities," like supporters of a particular football team, with imagined obligations and duties. It is, he argues, because of this transcendental mentalizing that the distinction between natural and supernatural, now and tomorrow, becomes blurred. And the transcendent nature of music, its "floating intentionality,"[26] is of course an ideal vehicle to support this new cognitive and cultural capacity.

In Chapter 4 I briefly described Steven Mithen's proposal—neatly encapsulated in the title of his book *"The Singing Neanderthals"*[27]—that our cousins, and perhaps also our ancestors, used a gestural, prosodic, protolanguage communication system in which, according to Mithen, "music" was an essential part. Did they chant, or something like it? If so, could such communal "proto"-chanting have been one of the drivers for the evolution of imagination and awareness, perhaps by eliciting altered perceptual states (ecstasy, rapture, trance) and imaginary worlds that were important in further developing hominin proto-consciousness?[28,29] Lewis-Williams suggests that human consciousness comprises a spectrum of shifting and adaptive states that incorporate alert consciousness and problem-oriented thought, dreaming during sleep, and day-dreaming (introspection, reverie), through to visions and hallucinations.[19] To "deal with the weird, non-real experiences that their brains sometimes generated, humans developed a parallel realm of existence—the supernatural, a realm that evolved alongside the emerging sense of self." Trance-like group behaviors integrate thoughts and emotions, and can mediate transcendental experiences. As Alondre Oubré writes in her book, chanting perhaps provided "a somatic and cognitive vehicle for psychological and social catharsis" and "mitigated the pathos of emotional despair which undoubtedly increased as early hominins gradually developed greater self-awareness."[28]

Our new brain architecture, superimposed on our "modern" skeleton, takes us from the *Homo sapiens* dated at about 195,000 years old, to what I have presumptuously presumed to call "*Homo sapientior*," a new type of hominin perhaps only about 75,000–85,000 years old. As mentioned earlier, this is roughly equivalent to about 4,000–4,500 generations of our unique species. Was the "brutal high beam of consciousness"[30] that transfixes us something that required a counterweight? Was music and dance a critical element in generating social cohesiveness and social interaction as we became self-aware, as we developed language-driven individualities and identities—a way of satisfying our desperate need for connectedness? With music we are no longer, because of the evolution of the conscious mind, a "society of selves."[31]

Even today, "rituals with synchronous body movements [are] more likely to enhance prosocial attitudes," and increase "perceptions of oneness," especially rituals judged to be sacred.[32] The indivisible association between music and religious/spiritual ceremonies and rituals supports the importance of music production and participation in creating, for example at funerals, "a sense of public order out of the inner turmoil of emotions,"[33] building bridges between the living and the living, between the living and the dead, and providing a buffer between fact, superstition, and fear. In the words of the famous conductor Sir Thomas Beecham, quoted in *Beecham Stories*,[34] compiled by H. Atkins and A. Neuman: "The function of music is to release us from the tyranny of conscious thought," or as Sir Colin Davis was reported to have said in a BBC interview in 2007: "[Music] doesn't put off death unfortunately, but it gives you a very good time while you're still alive." Amen to that, maestro!

When we are singing in choirs or playing in a band or an orchestra, all participants contribute as individuals, but there is a collective or group outcome where the individual is subsumed within a greater, physiologically aligned, whole. Although accents and dialects in language can be used to define social/geographical group identities,[35] speech is in many ways an isolator, an individualizer. We can talk to only several people at any one time, usually taking turns, and of course it helps enormously if the listeners speak and understand the same language as us. Language, along with the modern human cognitive mind, is associated with an increased sense of self. Was music—this emotionally rewarding, rhythmic, and melodic communication system that was almost certainly derived from the pre-"*Homo sapientior*" musilanguage, protolanguage, or 'Hmmmm'[27]—embellished and universally retained as a necessary counterbalance to this heightened sense of individuality, to the unfathomable and growing realization of our mortality that came with the evolution of the modern mind and a new level of trans-generational communication? Was harmonization needed to balance individualization?

I suggested in Chapter 3 that our species has attained an almost Lamarckian type of evolution where the genetic code has, to some extent, been short-circuited. We can pass on newly acquired information to the next generation of human beings, who do not have to be genetically related to us to receive this knowledge, and they then pass on what they learn and what they have been told, and so on, and so forth. With the development of external databases (books, tapes, and now the world-wide web) there is an exponential learning curve of information and knowledge (although not necessarily wisdom). This, as far as the archaeological evidence shows, is like nothing else that has ever happened on the planet. We are a new type of animal. Yet at the same time there is still the need for connectedness, to be noticed, to link "me, myself, I" to others, increasingly so through social media channels such as Facebook, Twitter, YouTube, and so on. In this context it should be remembered, as eloquently pointed out by Anthony Storr in *Music and the Mind*,[1] that the human being as a solitary *listener* is a modern phenomenon; it depends almost entirely on modern technology. Even sitting still and quiet in a concert hall listening to trained musicians with one or two thousand others in the audience is a recent development in the history of music. As Storr says: "Music began as a way of enhancing and coordinating group feelings. Today, it is often a means of recovering personal feelings from which we have become alienated."[1]

The listening habits of the young all over the world are changing rapidly;[36] and people are presumably obtaining a positive, perhaps even addictive, reward from listening to hours and hours of music on their mobile phones and MP3 players, even when asleep. Paradoxically, the use of headphones and personalized music equipment has made the isolationist element of music even more significant; instead of acting as a type of glue, music sometimes seems to be used as a barrier to shut out the real world! Or perhaps these solitary listeners, to use Anthony Storr's expression, are actually vicariously connected to others in an imaginary auditory space ... with music acting as a salve to a modern mind craving for stimulation of any kind. The consequences of this transformation as our youngsters grow up are yet to be played out. And speaking of modern technology, we know from scientific studies that group-singing in unison "makes the hearts of the singers accelerate and decelerate simultaneously."[37] I wonder if this same phenomenon also occurs if physically isolated individuals are linked together in a coordinated musical activity via modern-day computer technology, via the internet? Interestingly, synchronizing movements with a virtual partner makes the partner more "likeable."[38]

Thousands of years ago the Greek philosopher Aristotle wrote: "It is not easy to determine the nature of music or why anyone should have a knowledge of it. Why do rhythms and melodies which are mere sounds resemble dispositions while tastes do not, nor yet do smells." It is not possible to put into words this musical, multi-individual, corporate entity that may be a unique invention of our species. Nobody has ever satisfactorily described it. In an interview with Susan Chenery published in the *Weekend Australian* newspaper (Jan 11–12, 2014), Donald Fagen of Steely Dan fame said: "When everything's working right, you become transfixed by the notes and chords. In the centre of it, with drums, bass and guitar all around you, the earth falls away and it's just you and your crew creating this magical stuff that can move 10,000 people to snap free of life's miseries and get up and dance and scream." But the same question remains—why is it that, when we listen and/or participate in musical events, just about all of us one way or another experience emotional reactions and responses to them? There is a broader sense of well-being, immune responses, emotional responses, and so on. It surely is no accident. Music has always been a communicative social medium, important for our well-being from the moment that we began, a core component of the brain of our founders some tens of thousands of years ago. The inner, knowing self seems to be linked to other inner selves, in a mesh of physiological, emotional, and cognitive empathy. As Marcel Proust put it (quoted in Storr's *Music and the Mind*): "I wondered whether music might not be the unique example of what might have been—if the invention of language, the formation of words, the analysis of ideas had not intervened—the means of communication between souls."[1]

Chapter 7

Music, Development, and Education

...and if I had to live my life again, I would have made a rule to read some poetry and listen to some music at least once every week; for perhaps the parts of my brain now atrophied would thus have been kept active through use. The loss of these tastes is a loss of happiness, and may possibly be injurious to the intellect, and more probably to the moral character, by enfeebling the emotional part of our nature.

—Charles Darwin, from his autobiography

When I watched young Venda developing their bodies, their friendships, and their sensitivity to communal dancing, I could not help regretting the hundreds of afternoons I had wasted on the rugby field and in boxing rings. But then I was brought up not to cooperate, but to compete. Even music was offered more as a competition than as a shared experience.

—John Blacking, *How Musical is Man*

In my dictionary the word "educate" is defined as "to bring up and instruct: to teach: to train," and the word "education": "bringing up or training, as of a child: instruction: strengthening of the powers of body or mind: culture." The online encyclopedia "Wikipedia" defines it, I think, very well: "Education in the largest sense is any act or experience that has a formative effect on the mind, character or physical ability of an individual. In its technical sense education is the process by which society deliberately transmits its accumulated knowledge, skills and values from one generation to another." In general, the best training-induced learning paradigms are those that lead to "performance improvements that generalize beyond the training context and persist over time."[1] According to these authors, only a few such paradigms exist—in their view these include playing action video games, taking part in athletics, and engaging in music.

In this chapter, which focuses on the importance of music in child development and education, I will describe some of the evidence showing that musical training not only improves auditory perceptual skills, but also enhances a range of other sensorimotor abilities. Because listening to, and participating in, musical activities "involves a tantalizing mix of practically every human cognitive function,"[2] we shall see that including music in school curricula has benefits well beyond the musical sphere, aiding in an individual's general cognitive and perceptual capabilities, emotional development, and social interactivity. Individual music-making has its own benefits, but working in groups may be even more useful. To quote Stefan Koelsch in his recent review about the neural basis of music perception: "Making music in a group is a tremendously demanding task for the human brain that elicits a large array of cognitive (and affective) processes, including perception, multimodal integration, learning, memory, action, social cognition, syntactic processing, and processing of meaning information."[3]

For those in the know, at least since the time of the ancient Greeks, an education that included music in its curriculum has been thought to be of great benefit to the human mind and the human body. In addition to instruction in grammar, logic, and rhetoric, the harmonic (mathematical) structure of music was previously taught along with arithmetic, geometry, and astronomy. This latter quartet later came to be known as the "quadrivium" and was an essential teaching practice right through the Middle Ages. In 1588, the great English composer and musician William Byrd gave this advice in his *"Psalmes, Sonets & Songs,"*[4] some of which is quoted below:

> Reasons briefly set down by th'auctor, to perswade every one to learne to sing.
>
> *First* it is a knowledge easily taught, and quickly learned where there is a good Master, and an apt Scoller.
>
> 2. The exercise of singing is delightfull to Nature & good to preserve the health of Man.
>
> 3. It doth strengthen all the parts of the breast, & doth open the pipes.
>
> 4. It is a singular good remedie for a stutting & stammering in the speech.
>
> 5. It is the best meanes to procure a perfect pronunciation & to make a good Orator …
>
> … Since singing is so good a thing, I wish all men would learne to sing.

In modern western society, the majority have experienced at least some kind of musical training,[5] although access to music programs at school may be less likely in poorer socio-economic areas/countries. In my view, music in schools is for everyone. There are even some who advocate that individuals with congenital amusia (see Chapter 2) can be taught to sing, given the appropriate environment and encouragement, although if that ambition fails there may still be advantages to participating because group activities that emphasize rhythm appear to have their own cognitive benefits.[6,7]

Normal subjects

In early childhood, for a notably prolonged period of time compared with other primates, the human brain is especially adaptable, sensitive as it is to environmental input and experience-dependent events. As discussed in Chapter 3, considerable growth and maturation of the human cerebral cortex occurs in the first two to three postnatal years. Importantly, the most recently evolved and expanded regions of the human cortex—those associated with higher cognitive functions—are the most immature and capable of modification by postnatal experience.[8] The critical connections between frontal cortex and temporal and parietal cortex also take several years to mature. Note also that, while the majority of neurons in the brain are already present at birth, neurons continue to be born postnatally in the cerebellum, the region so important in ensuring the coordination and synchronization of voluntary movements. Accelerated evolution of multiple ways to subtly regulate and control gene expression, together with sophisticated mechanisms for altering synaptic strength, underpin the postnatal flexibility of the developing human cortex. Overall, the quality and nature of an individual's experience early in life influence the selection, and then maintenance and plasticity, of neurons and their connections—influences that persist into adulthood.

We have seen that very young human infants respond to prosodic communication (motherese) and music-like sounds, sounds that are perhaps an echo of our ancient musi-language, and we also know that regions of the cortex known to be involved in language/music processing are already selectively active just several months after birth. From the neuroscience perspective at least, our developing brains are ready and waiting for appropriate linguistic and musical input. In fact, a great many studies have reported that music training in normal subjects, especially when started in childhood, has a significant impact on brain plasticity and cognitive development. Of course not all will necessarily benefit to the same extent because, as reviewed by Merrett et al,[9] there is a need to take into consideration factors such as genetic predisposition, intrauterine learning, postnatal age when training began, whether or not training is ongoing, the type of instrument that is used, and an individual's personality/motivation.

So what is the evidence that musical training in children, even if only for a relatively short period of time, can continue to enhance auditory function even years down the track, into adulthood and old age? Overall, for auditory processing at least, the accumulated evidence consistently shows that musical training is correlated with changes in brain morphology and altered, usually enhanced, acoustic discrimination and processing at almost all levels. Affected regions include the brainstem[10,11,12] and primary as well as secondary areas of auditory cortex.[12,13,14,15,16,17,18,19,20,21,22,23] Remarkably, early intensive musical training for as little as 15 months results in observable structural changes in the developing brain,[24,25] including an increase in volume in the right primary auditory cortex.

One longitudinal fMRI and MEG study in seven- to nine-year-old children reported considerable individual variation in the size of Heschl's gyrus, but for a given individual the cortical regions that process music are morphologically stable by primary school age. Nonetheless, during this period there is ongoing functional plasticity that is associated with musical training.[26] Presumably these functional changes reflect complex molecular, cellular, and connectional changes that are not reflected in gross changes in gray matter volume. According to Seither-Preisler et al: "a large right Heschl's gyrus signifies high musical potential, which increases a child's intrinsic motivation to learn and practice a musical instrument regardless of social influences." But as discussed by them, and by myself earlier in this book, inter-individual variation in the size of different cortical regions may have a genetic (nature) or early-learning (nurture) basis, or of course a combination of both. Twin studies do in fact show that the size of the auditory cortex is influenced by heritability[27] but that this influence is not absolute, leaving some room for experience-dependent influences.[16,24,25]

The beneficial changes that result from sensory experience may also include more subtle types of plasticity that involve certain specific aspects of auditory processing. For example, in the developing auditory cortex, animal studies have revealed considerable use-dependent plasticity in terms of tonotopic frequency maps, responses to sound intensity, and spectral tuning of acoustically responsive neurons.[28,29,30] The neurotrophin BDNF, which was discussed in some detail in Chapter 3, plays a role in at least some of these experience-dependent developmental changes.[31] In human trials it has now been shown that interactive auditory experiences that require the attention of an infant significantly alter physiological responses in the auditory cortex, enhancing sensory processing and fine-tuning auditory maps.[32] Importantly, there is also evidence in animal studies for continued plasticity of auditory cortex into adulthood, potentially allowing for compensatory changes in older individuals,[33] including those with impaired hearing—a topic considered further in Chapter 8.

Learning and playing a musical instrument is a multisensory experience that involves neural processing within, and interconnections between, a number of sensory, motor, and higher order integrative areas. These areas include the superior temporal sulcus, the lateral part of the parietal lobes, the intraparietal sulcus, and the prefrontal cortex (Figure 5.1). So it is perhaps to be expected that early musical training, in addition to the development of enhanced auditory perceptual skills, also leads to changes in parts of the brain not directly involved in processing auditory information, changes associated with enhanced motor and visuomotor performance.[34] Improved sensorimotor capability is associated with increased neural activity in diverse brain areas, and numerous changes in gray and white matter architecture have been documented, especially in the brains of highly trained individuals who began learning early in life and who continue to practice.[19,35,36,37,38] Connections between auditory, motor, and premotor cortex are strengthened,[21] and in string players there is expansion of areas in the motor and sensory cortex that process information to and from the hand,[39,40,41] and altered processing in regions associated with the lips in trumpet players.[42] An increase in the size of the massive bundle of fibers that interconnects the two cerebral hemispheres—the corpus callosum— has been reported,[20,24,43] perhaps related to increased coordinated activity between the hands.[44] Training before the age of seven years produces the greatest changes in the structure and connectivity of the corpus callosum, changes "that may promote plasticity in motor and auditory connectivity that serves as a scaffold upon which ongoing training can build."[45]

Early musical training and ongoing musical performance also result in significant changes in the size of the cerebellum in the brainstem, although the changes are complex and show both regional and gender-specific variation.[46,47] Musicians also possess larger cerebellar peduncles—huge white matter structures that connect the cerebellum to the rest of the brain—but changes seem limited to the right-hand side for some reason.[48] Interestingly, lesions or degeneration of the cerebellum itself—the structure that houses learned patterns of fine motor control—are associated with deficits in certain aspects of musical ability.[49]

Recent neuroimaging research has also found evidence of positive effects of musical training on gray matter volume and plasticity in a declarative memory processing region, the hippocampus; these changes presumably relate to the learning and memory required during the training program.[16,50] Finally, a longitudinal imaging and psychological testing study on subjects aged between 6 and 25 years (testing was repeated two or three times, each two years apart) found a significant effect of music practice on gray matter volume in the temporo-occipital and insular cortex.[51] These authors also found that music practice gradually improved reasoning and working memory capacity, the latter positively correlated with the number of hours spent practicing! Overall, and as considered more fully in the following chapter, such findings may explain why learning a musical instrument can even protect against dementia and cognitive impairment much later in life. Furthermore, there may be an additional "cognitive reserve" as a consequence of music training, perhaps similar to the protection afforded to older humans who are bilingual, especially those continuing to speak more than one language.[52]

A word of caution here: about 1% of professional musicians who play and practice *too much* develop a debilitating loss of function and control of skilled movements in the fingers and hands. These so-called dystonias probably arise from abnormal processing in the cortex and other parts of the brain such as the basal ganglia, which code sensorimotor information from the hands and fingers.[53,54,55] Expansion of mapped representations of the digits seems to cause interference in sensorimotor integration, a deficiency that can be improved by proprioceptive training after enhancing brain plasticity using a "non-invasive" technique called transcranial magnetic stimulation (TMS), which uses pulsed magnetic fields to generate weak electric currents in the underlying brain tissue.[56] Interestingly, TMS in normal, highly trained pianists can be detrimental, but in musically untrained individuals it improves fine control of finger movements.[57]

Musicians and individuals who are "good" at music often have improved memory and discrimination for pitch, but such people have also been reported to have improved language and literacy skills, including reading and verbal memory.[58,59,60,61] A large-scale statistical analysis of 13 previously published studies that examined the effect of music training on reading skills confirmed that training significantly improved language awareness and some literacy skills, but not fluency in reading.[62] Training for as little as four years in childhood has measurable effects on the perception and responses to speech in older adults.[63] As described in Chapter 2, while there are differences in the way our brains process the spectral characteristics of music and speech, certain aspects of speech such as vowel sounds are more music-like. There are also elements of prosody and temporal structure (rhythm) that are common to both music and speech. Indeed, there are now many studies showing that musical experience and training improve our ability to process and encode many of the basic and emotional elements of speech, enhance the overall accuracy with which we detect speech, and may aid in verbal fluency and vocal communication abilities.[64,65,66,67,68,69]

The social importance of childhood participation in group music-related activities is discussed later in this chapter, but it is worth noting here that high-school music classes have been found to improve speech processing.[70] Similarly, a recent US study examining the effects of a two-year community music program on otherwise normal children from "underserved backgrounds" at high risk of learning and social problems found that these children possessed improved perception of some aspects of speech.[71] Relevant here are studies showing that early musical training improves a child's ability to encode and process speech in the presence of background noise.[72,73,74] As discussed by Kraus and Chandrasekaran: "Classrooms, for a variety of reasons, are inherently noisy … an effective music training program in schools could reduce the negative influences of external noise and better prepare the child for everyday listening challenges beyond the challenges that directly relate to music."[18]

Learning to move in time to a rhythmic beat—even just tapping a finger or a foot—may be sufficient to enhance synchronized activity in the brain, potentially enhancing cognitive and linguistic skills.[6,7] In fact, musicians are better at accurately detecting and discriminating between syllables that require "resolution of temporal cues."[75] Recording electrical signals from the human brainstem using evoked responses has revealed that music training enhances the early sensory processing of both music and speech, in both the auditory and audiovisual domains.[76] Perhaps because of this, general aspects of attention and concentration often seem to be better in musicians than in non-musically trained individuals. In the cortex, the left planum temporale, a region important in sensory language processing (Wernicke's area), is larger in musicians and is associated with better and faster processing of speech sounds.[14]

In healthy individuals, listening to and performing music enhance "cross-modal" performance and skill sets that are not limited to the aural and linguistic domain. For example, it was reported that children given music lessons possessed a slightly higher IQ,[77] and children with at least three years of instrumental music training showed enhanced nonverbal reasoning skills.[65] The beneficial effects of keyboard training versus other training tasks on children's spatio-temporal reasoning have also been reported.[78] Listening for as little as ten minutes to a Mozart sonata was reported to increase the coherence of brain activity of some cortical regions and enhance spatio-temporal performance,[79,80] although subsequent work has not always been able to replicate this "Mozart effect"[81] and any positive effects seem only to be short-lasting and may be more related to arousal levels.[82] But could certain types of music have more impact on social and cognitive development than others? We have already seen that happy and sad music, music we like or dislike, activates different parts of our brain, but is there more to it? Maynard Solomon, in discussing the concept of beauty in his great biography of Mozart,[83] writes about beauty's transience and strangeness, how it remains an image of instability, of impermanence, of mortality. Solomon suggests that music "through its juxtaposition of formal materials rather than solely through its rhetoric is capable of representing mortal contests, in particular symbolizing clashes between generative and disintegrative forces." Music: "balances the tension between form and disorder, the familiar from the alien." Beneficial physiological and behavioral effects in boys with "special educational needs" have been reported when Mozart was played as background music in class.[84] Could it be that Mozart's music is somehow on the cusp between formal academic constructivism and emotional uncertainty and fragility, and thus is uniquely able to stimulate diverse regions of our brains because of that?

Trained musicians exhibit enhanced performance in visuospatial tasks such as mental three-dimensional rotation of objects, tasks in which the subject must use mental imagery to rotate drawings to see whether they fit with the three-dimensional shape of a real object.[85] fMRI analysis revealed a statistically significant increase in brain activity in Broca's area, but only in trained musicians who were performing these virtual rotation tasks. This led the authors to state there was a: "transferable benefit of music training to alter brain function and enhance cognitive performance in a non-musical visuospatial task."[85] Gray matter volume in part of this region—the pars opercularis—is statistically larger in orchestral musicians,[13,86] and the effects of maintained musical activity in improving performance in visuospatial and various cognitive control tasks are still measurable in the aged.[87] The involvement of Broca's area in the performance of complex auditory-related and visuospatial tasks again shows that this region is not just a motor speech area, although it is intriguing to note that individuals with congenital amusia perform less well on these types of spatial processing tasks.[88]

Since the time of ancient Greece there has been an implicit relationship between music and mathematics, as well as with astronomy. In other words, there is a link not only to the emotional core of human well-being but also to non-musical cognitive domains, to the rational intellect. These links are explored in Thomas Levenson's book *Measure for Measure*,[89] in which he details the way music and science have influenced each other across the history of western culture. In Jamie James' book *The Music of the Spheres*[90] he also discusses these links at length, tracing through history the overlap between music and science, the great dreams of celestial harmony, the harmony of numbers, the "sublime cosmic order." Pythagoras showed that altering the length of a string resulted in a calculable change in the frequency of the note, and that when the ratio of notes was simple (2:1, 3:2) they sounded pleasant but complex ratios produced discord. In seeking the mathematical rules governing the movements of the sun, moon, and planets, Pythagoras argued that their orbits must generate particular harmonic notes, creating a heavenly music. James' comment on the great Pythagoras is that he defies categorization: a primary thinker in philosophy, mathematics, music, and cosmology. In our era, music still has the capacity to educate, and Pythagoras might be gratified to know that we now know that the cognitive skills and strategies established during musical training are useful in other "spheres."

As reviewed by Wan and Schlaug,[21] the capacity for music to impact other, non-aural and/or vocal modalities may be because music-making can affect higher level "polymodal integration regions...which may alter task performance in other domains." In recent times, for example, tantalizing fMRI evidence relating to an impact of music training on mathematical ability has been reported.[91] They reported that the pattern of brain activity in adults, while mentally adding or subtracting fractions, was—compared with that of controls—consistently different in individuals who had had musical instrument or voice training/lessons since early childhood, with increased activation especially in the left frontal cortex and inferior part of the temporal lobe. In musicians, improved mathematical ability may be related to improved proficiency in symbolizing and abstracting visual numerical representations, and also to enhanced working memory and the ability to discriminate between correct and incorrect calculations. Such an interpretation is entirely consistent with the conclusions of Jeanne Bamberger almost two decades ago: "the goal of musical development is to have access to multiple dimensions of musical structure, to be able to coordinate these dimensions, and most important, to be able to choose selectively among them, to change focus at will."[92]

Most studies on the influence of music training on the structure and function of the developing human brain have examined individuals who have worked hard at learning an instrument—the piano, violin, and so on.[17,18] But most children are not going to spend hours a week on their own practicing an instrument, owing to either boredom, loss of social interaction, or intrinsic lack of sensorimotor ability. As I stated in an earlier chapter, I realized too late as a parent that sending my own boys off to another room, alone, to practice the piano or other musical instrument was a dumb thing to do ... I should have known better. When teaching music using the famous Suzuki method, the parents play a crucial and cooperative role in helping their children learn to sing or play an instrument—making music should be fun!

What we need to know is whether inclusive and enjoyable involvement in musical classes, *at whatever level*, has a beneficial effect on the participants. Lack of skill or perseverance at learning an instrument does not necessarily mean that a child does not respond to, or benefit from, exposure to music. Most children, even the very young,[93,94] spontaneously enjoy and respond to music and dance, especially in a group/social context. In fact, there is good evidence that joint music-making, including singing and group drumming, enhances cooperative behavior and positive social interactions between young children, just as it does in adults.[95,96] Children prefer to socialize with other children who know (and presumably enjoy) similar songs and thus have some shared cultural knowledge.[97] Moving in time with others acts in a similar way;[98] dance training has been reported to enhance sensorimotor skills in ways that differ from music training.[99]

Participation in music-related activities is crucial because, compared with passive musical exposure, active involvement is especially conducive to the development of social as well as linguistic skills.[100] Unfortunately, singing, playing instruments, and dancing "become significantly de-emphasized in the learning environment when formal schooling starts and 'the arts' become relegated from the cognitive learning core,"[101] yet ongoing engagement with the "arts" enhances our sense of mental well-being.[102] Michael Thaut even argues that "the artistic pursuits of young children (may be) an ontogenetic repeat of a critical evolutionary cognitive development of the human mind." As briefly discussed in Chapter 4, we learn how to speak and sing by watching and listening to others, and later on we covertly vocalize (subvocalization) when listening to music. This is a type of mimesis, a type of motor imagery, and it has been argued that sounds need to be produced—for example singing aloud—in order for us to recognize and understand the musical (and speech?) sounds emanating from others.[103]

But we must be careful not to make exposure to, and participation in, music (and dance) too competitive or too dependent on sensorimotor competence. As quoted at the beginning of this chapter, John Blacking lamented the competitive, isolating aspects of his own western musical education. His experience with the Venda in the Northern Transvaal taught him that music and dance are social/cultural activities and that "technological development brings about a degree of social exclusion" and "the technical level of what is defined as musicality is therefore raised, and some people must be branded as unmusical... these assumptions are diametrically opposed to the Venda idea that all human beings are capable of musical performance."[104] When the Venda dance, drum, and play music associated with ritual occasions, known as "Tshikona," this is a group activity in which each individual (traditionally male) has a pipe that can only play one note, women play drums, and the whole is critically dependent on the sum of the parts. Synchronous movement (dance?) also forms an essential element of such occasions, and both dance and ritual synchrony help to bind individuals together and promote social interaction.[105,106] Music, through the integration of perception and action, allows us to make predictions about our own and others' actions, facilitating adaptive cooperative behavior between individuals.[107]

Given the mounting evidence that exposure to music and some degree of musical training improve prosocial skills and offer more general cognitive and sensorimotor benefits to children, it therefore seems reasonable to question whether exposure to music in one form or another not only improves development in normal children, but may also have an important therapeutic impact in children where development is delayed or abnormal in some way. Can music help in situations where children have learning difficulties? Can it be an important educational tool? Paula Tallal and Nadine Gaab[61] believe that strategies that involve, among other things, musical training may offer important benefits to children with language-learning impairments. The dynamic temporal processing that is such a feature of music, coupled with improved attention and processing skills, may all act to improve language, reading, and perhaps other cognitive skills in these children.

Music training in children with developmental disorders

In the following chapter I review the use of music therapy in treating individuals who have some form of acquired neurological and/or physical dysfunction, usually in adults, but of course such problems can also arise in infants, children, and adolescents. The use of music to help treat children with developmental disorders is also a type of therapy, but in the next few pages I will briefly consider exposure to music therapy in such children as an extension of the educational process. For example, music lessons are a useful way of enhancing auditory perception, cognitive performance, and speech-language development in profoundly deaf children with hearing aids and/or cochlear implants.[108,109,110] Music can also improve listening and reading skills in dyslexic children.[111,112]

Autism and Asperger's syndromes are developmental genetic disorders of the nervous system characterized by complex behavioral deficits, particularly with regard to emotional responsiveness, social interactions, and developing nonverbal empathic understanding with others. Williams syndrome is a rare genetic disorder characterized by various physical defects as well as altered morphology of a number of brain regions. Individuals with Williams syndrome generally have lower intelligence than the rest of the population, and behaviorally they can exhibit substantial social disabilities and high anxiety levels, and have reduced visuospatial and motor capabilities. Perhaps paradoxically, individuals with this syndrome are notable for their high (often uninhibited) sociability, their loquacity, and their love of music: "a tribute to the extraordinary affective power of music."[113] In his book *Musicophilia*,[114] Oliver Sacks devoted an entire chapter to describing case histories of people with Williams syndrome, referring to them as "A Hypermusical Species!" Music permits young people with autism and similar disorders to experience what might be called a virtual sense of social and emotional interaction, entirely consistent with what we have already discussed in earlier chapters. Again quoting from Heaton and Allen,[113] they cite the autistic poet Craig Romkema, who wrote: "Music is the regulator of my nervous system, the shelter for my frazzled mind."

Autistic pre-school children have been found to discriminate between musical instrument sounds more quickly than between instrument names,[115] and it may therefore be of significance that the left temporal cortex shows abnormally reduced activity in very young children who develop autism, with correspondingly high activity on the right-hand side.[116] The authors hypothesize that a failure of left hemisphere specialization during language comprehension in early life "may not only delay basic language acquisition in infants and toddlers with autism, but may also impair the development of social language behaviours."[116] Might some compensatory right hemisphere processing therefore take place in these circumstances? This is reminiscent of what happens in people born with no, or only a very small, corpus callosum[117] (Chapter 4). Such people have language, and sometimes also cognitive, deficits—would music training help these individuals as well?

Autism is also associated with reduced eye contact and reduced recognition of emotion in faces,[118] and is thought to be associated with deficits in the mirror neuron system. Remember that this system encodes both viewed and self-directed actions and appears to be important in the empathic way we perceive and interact with others (described in more detail in Chapters 3 and 5). Again referring back to an earlier chapter (Chapter 4), music can affect the subjective way we look at faces—that is, whether expressions are happy, neutral, or sad—and enhances our emotional identification with others.[119,120] Music also affects various neurochemicals and hormones known to influence our affective responses and emotional mood states.[121] Given these observations, together with the established relationships between networks that process musicality and social interactions (Chapter 6), it seems reasonable to mount the argument that "interventions incorporating methods of music making may offer a promising approach for facilitating expressive language in otherwise nonverbal children with autism."[122] There also appear to be deficits in the connections between cortical regions that encode the voice and areas associated with reward—including the orbitofrontal cortex, ventromedial prefrontal cortex, amygdala, and nucleus accumbens.[123] But these are also regions where a great deal of music processing goes on (Chapter 2), again suggesting a neural basis for the profound impact of music on autistic children. Singing may be especially helpful, given that there are strong interconnections between voice- and face-recognition areas in our brains.[124]

I have presented perhaps an overly exhaustive set of examples, but one that I hope convincingly demonstrates the ability of music to enhance both normal and "abnormal" developmental brain function. The more we study music and its place in the evolution of the modern mind, why we have retained this form of sophisticated communication in parallel with language—complementary but distinct—the more we will reveal clues and construct cogent arguments that will help put music (and dance) back into the center of the educational spotlight. And as we shall see in the next chapter, we will also identify more situations where neurologists and therapists will have no alternative but to accept the scientific rationale for the healing power of music. In a 1961 article by the musicologist Alexander Ringer, in a world—as he puts it—"beset by sputniks, race tensions, inflation, and crumbling political alliances" he laments the rise of the technologist and the demise of the liberal arts: "the bankruptcy of an educational philosophy which in its zeal to promote technical knowledge has sadly neglected the formation of creative men and women." He goes on: "in this scientific age, a more general understanding and appreciation of the arts imposes itself, possibly for the first time in history, as an educational imperative rather than a luxury."

Anthony Storr, in his wonderful book *Music and the Mind*,[125] also promulgates the importance of music in education, and here I will quote from the introduction to his book. It is worth quoting in full: "Many people assume that the arts are luxuries rather than necessities, and that words or pictures are only the means by which influence can be exerted on the human mind. Those who do not appreciate music think it has no significance other than providing ephemeral pleasure (and here I think of Steven Pinker in this regard and his well-known 'auditory cheesecake' quote). They consider it a gloss upon the surface of life; a harmless indulgence rather than a necessity, of no great importance to our species. This, no doubt, is why our present politicians seldom accord music a prominent place in their plans for education. Today, when education is becoming increasingly utilitarian, directed toward obtaining gainful employment rather than toward enriching personal experience, music is likely to be treated as an 'extra' in the school curriculum which only affluent parents can afford, and which need not be provided for pupils who are not obviously 'musical' by nature." Even group teaching of music at high school seems to improve neural processing capacity and encoding of speech, and thus the benefits of musical training are "not limited to expensive private instruction early in childhood but can be elicited by cost-effective group instruction during adolescence."[70]

So, no excuses, ministries of education, school boards, administrators, and bean counters—some degree of music training and group music-making should be an obligatory component of the educational curriculum, especially in pre-primary and primary schools. It is unfortunate that in recent times we have separated almost all forms of human activity into either scientific or artistic categories, something I will return to in the final chapter. I regret that music was ever labeled as "art." Music just "is"; it is a core component of what makes us human, an essential and core element of our cooperative makeup, however it is labeled. To treat music as an "art" is to suggest music is peripheral to our day-to-day existence, relegating it to merely a leisure-time activity, allowing administrators of all kinds to find excuses for disengaging it from mainstream education. But there are champions: in modern times, the Musikkindergarten Berlin, established by Daniel Barenboim, is "the first kindergarten in which music is not only used as an occasional add-on but as the central education medium for the child every day."[126] Perhaps the last word here can go to the great diarist Samuel Pepys, a champion of music in education: "Even in his grief Pepys worked on one of his great letters, a disquisition on the place of music in education, 'a science peculiarly productive of a pleasure that no state of life, publick or private, secular or sacred; no difference of age or season; no temper of mind or condition of health, exempt from present anguish, nor, lastly, distinction of quality, renders either improper, untimely, or unentertaining. Witness the universal gusto we see it followed with, wherever to be found.'"[127]

Chapter 8

Music, Therapy, and Old Age

In the end there is one dance you'll do alone

—Jackson Browne, "For a Dancer"

In ancient Greek tradition many of the gods had musical links, as of course did the Muses, the nine goddesses who provided the inspiration for literature, dance, music, and so on. Music (derived from the Greek: *mousike*) can be interpreted purely as we understand it as music, or in ancient writing the word can have a more all-encompassing meaning in relation to all the muses—including theatre, art, poetry, music, literature, and dance. Music itself was ascribed great healing and educational powers and was considered indispensable for the preservation of mental and bodily health. Music provided a link between the harmony of the cosmos and the harmony/health of the human body and soul. As paraphrased by Jamie James in his book *The Music of the Spheres: Music, Science, and the Natural Order of the Universe*,[1] in Iamblichus' biography of Pythagoras he describes a scene in which Pythagoras comes upon a potential violent scene of jilted passion: "He convinced the piper to change his tune from the Phrygian mode to a song in spondees, a tranquilizing meter. The young man's madness instantly cooled, and he was restored to reason." Plutarch, just after the death of Christ, wrote that "medicine, to produce health, must know disease; music, to produce harmony, must know discord" (Shapiro, p 37),[2] and not long before, the poet Horace in his Odes wrote: "Black care shall be lessened by sweet song"[2] (Shapiro, p 186).

Michael Thaut, a professor of both music and neuroscience, and a strong advocate for the therapeutic powers of music, has reviewed the cultural importance of music therapy in other early civilizations in Mesopotamia, Egypt, and Israel.[3] Music therapy also has a long history in Asia and in Muslim countries, specific modes of music being used to treat different diseases, often at specified times during the day. For further reading on the widespread use of music as a therapeutic and educational resource in the Ottoman Empire, readers may wish to access an informative article by Professor Nil Sari on the "Muslim Heritage" website http://www.muslimheritage.com/article/ottoman-music-therapy. To this day, indigenous healers in different parts of the world continue to employ singing or rhythmic vocalizations when giving advice or some form of curative therapy.

Familiar music can unlock multidimensional recollections, and revive past emotional experiences and feelings, subjective experiences that are of course very different for each listener. The composer Paul Hindemith wrote this in 1952: "There is no doubt that listeners, performers and composers alike can be profoundly moved by perceiving, performing or imagining music, and that, consequently, music must touch on something in their emotional life that brings them to this state of excitation. But if these mental reactions were feelings, they could not change as rapidly as they do … The reactions music evokes are not feelings; they are the images, the memories of feelings." And later: "If music did not instigate us to supply memories out of our mental storage rooms, it would remain meaningless; it would merely have a certain tickling effect on our ears. We cannot keep music from uncovering the memory of former feelings, and it is not in our power to avoid them."[4] The more familiar the music, the greater the activity of reward and emotion-related limbic and paralimbic structures, and the greater the positive emotional response.[5,6,7]

As we have seen in earlier chapters, we now know that different parts of the brain are activated when listening to happy versus sad music, and when listening to music that gives you emotional chills or scares you. But we also know that listening to music, whether we perceive it as "sad" or "happy," can elicit pleasurable feelings—positive affective responses that result in increased activation in areas also shown to be involved in reward behaviors, attachment, social interactions, and altruism. These regions are associated with what are presumed to be beneficial psychological changes and contribute to our sense of well-being, our sense that "all is right with the world." In their recent review about the pleasures of sad music, Matthew Sachs et al argue that music, especially sad music, can "promote homeostasis," correcting an imbalance in our emotional and/or physiological state caused by other real-life stresses.[8] In the same vein, a large-scale review of the music therapy literature found that patterns of neural activity linked to emotional regulation— the ability to maintain "a comfortable state of arousal by modulating one or more aspects of emotion"—are elicited by listening to "preferred and familiar music, when singing, and (in musicians) when improvising."[9] What Moore describes as "undesired activation patterns" occur when "introducing complexity, dissonance and unexpected musical events."

Altered mood states induced by music are associated with changes in neurochemical modulators such as catecholamines (eg norepinephrine), endogenous opiates, and various hormones.[10,11,12,13,14,15] Such neurochemical responses are particularly important to bear in mind when thinking about music in a therapeutic context. So, to remind the reader, there are changes (usually a reduction) in "stress" hormones such as adrenocorticotropic hormone and cortisol,[16,17,18,19,20,21,22] changes in testosterone,[21] oxytocin,[16,23] and endorphins,[24] and altered dopamine binding in the brain when listening to pleasurable/ relaxing music—especially music that an individual enjoys and LIKES to hear.[7,25] Finally, and of potential therapeutic relevance, pleasurable music mimics the effects of dopamine when subjects are learning and being tested on some reinforcement tasks.[26]

Playing music also affects our molecular makeup. In Finland, Kanduri et al took a blood sample from professional musicians after a two-hour concert performance and analyzed their blood transcriptome, comparing it with samples taken from matched subjects after a "music-free" control period. Although the RNAs were not obtained from the brain, and so do not necessarily only reflect central neural activity, a great many genes were found to be upregulated, especially those related to dopamine transmission, motor behavior, and neural plasticity.[27] Much more needs to be done, but this type of molecular approach may reveal insights into many facets of music, evolution, and cognition, and in the context of the current discussion these types of data may provide important information on "the neurobiological background of emotions, neurology and neuropsychiatric diseases, and attempts to understand the molecular mechanisms that mediate the effects of music therapy."[27]

Music as a potential therapy can be either active or receptive. The former involves playing—and often improvising—music, alone or socially with others, while the latter involves listening and perhaps also moving to music. Modern-day advocates of music therapy believe it can be used to enhance cognitive and sensorimotor function, as well as improve a patient's (or client's) psychological health and the quality of their social interactions with others. Music is motivating. It can aid in the expression of feelings that might otherwise be too hard to express, and music listening "may be helpful to bring up and make available therapeutically relevant issues (emotions, associations, memories, identity issues)."[28] Thus, music therapy can also help to increase attendance and group participation in treatment sessions involving patients with drug-related problems.[29] The motivational aspect of music is crucial because of the importance of motivation and attention when using therapies to enhance neuroplasticity in the brain after trauma or stroke, or in neurodegenerative conditions,[30] topics that will be considered in more detail later in this chapter.

Nonetheless, in talking to neurologists, psychiatrists, and neuropsychologists over the last 10–15 years, my impression is that most really appreciate music as an art-form but they do not necessarily think of music as a useful and/or proven therapeutic alternative, especially when considered in the context of conventional medical treatments. Many regard music therapy in the same sort of alternative therapy basket as acupuncture, reflexology, aromatherapy, iridology, and so on (see also Chapter 1). But acupuncture, for example, has now been shown to activate classical pain-suppressing systems in the body, and is more mainstream, and I believe we make a serious mistake if we ignore the genuine curative power of music in mental and physical health. Indeed, the major reason for compiling this book was to provide a comprehensive scientific rationale for moving the "art-form" of music and its associated physiological and behavioral effects out of the "alternative medicine" basket, turning it into a recognized medical discipline, part of the accepted armamentarium of neurologists, psychiatrists, and clinical psychologists. As Silvia Bencivelli wrote: "what happened some time ago to physical therapy may happen to music therapy in its turn: it may come to be increasingly accepted by official medicine, until it joins, with full status, the therapies already taught and practiced in medical schools and hospitals."[31]

This is not to say that music therapy does not already have its passionate adherents and practitioners.[32] In the United States, music therapy was used as early as World War I to help treat victims of shell shock and was widely used in a number of countries during World War II. The first music therapy program was apparently taught at Michigan State University in 1944,[33] and in 1950 the National Association of Music Therapy was established. Key post-war developments in the establishment of professional music therapy programs in Europe included the inaugural Society for Music Therapy and Remedial Music (later renamed the British Society for Music Therapy) and the Austrian Music Therapy Research Group. More recent developments in the UK are summarized by Darnley-Smith and Patey in their book, *Music Therapy*.[32] The following passage from their book (p 13) exemplifies the problems that music therapy has had in being recognized as an independent clinical discipline: "It was not until 1982 that music therapy became recognized as an effective form of treatment within the National Health Service in Britain and gaining recognition had not been a swift or easy process. Music therapists needed to demonstrate that they had a serious form of treatment to offer, more specialized than, for example, the use of music as a recreational activity which had been common in hospitals for many years. Crucial to official recognition was the need to show that the therapeutic treatment had some objective purpose which supported the treatment aims of mainstream medicine or psychiatry, and that there were recognizable skills and a body of knowledge which a music therapist could acquire through training.... Most importantly of all, music therapy needed to convince critical outsiders that it was a discipline that could survive scrutiny and detailed questioning of its methods and claims."

Many US colleges and universities now offer degrees in music therapy, and there are graduate and masters programs in the UK and elsewhere. Worldwide, a number of organizations (eg the American Music Therapy Association, the Institute for Music and Neurologic Function, and the British Society for Music Therapy) continue to flourish, with aims to promote research into music therapy and its clinical applications, including stroke rehabilitation, enhancement of motor function, and use of music in language and memory disorders. In 2009 the profession of music therapy in Austria became legally recognized and licensed. In Australia, music therapy was established as a profession in 1975 (the Australian Music Therapy Association) and clinical training programs have been offered in a number of Australian universities (eg University of Melbourne, University of Queensland, and Western Sydney University). A clinician's guide to music therapy and neurorehabilitation has been published[34] and the recent book *Communicative Musicality*, edited by Stephen Malloch and Colwyn Trevarthen,[35] has a section devoted to articles on "musicality and healing."

Obviously, music needs to have a clear clinical and evidence-based foundation, with rigorous observation and scientific analysis, even if, to quote Darnley-Smith and Patey again, early pioneers of modern music therapy possessed "an intuitive, and in some cases spiritual, belief in the power of music to affect the lives of their children and adult clients." As Mona Lisa Chanda and Dan Levitin argue in their comprehensive review on music and neurochemistry[12]: "If the notion of music as medicine is to be taken literally, it is crucial to employ as rigorous designs for its investigation as for testing traditional forms of medicine." Among their many suggestions for future research is the proposal for more controlled, multifactorial designs and larger experimental groups (to increase statistical power); they also maintain that studies should include music therapists as consultants or members of the research team "because their perspective on the application of music in clinical settings may be informative."

Decades ago, the teacher Clive Robbins and pianist/composer Paul Nordoff established music therapy programs designed to help children acquire linguistic and social skills, treating conditions as diverse as developmental autism, stroke, psychiatric illness, Alzheimer's disease, and miscellaneous learning disabilities. Their approach was predicated upon the belief that *all* humans respond to music and that music is a communication tool that enhances wellness and facilitates inter-individual interactions at many levels. Music is used in psychiatry and neurology, but sometimes also in oncology, pediatrics, gerontology, and palliative care.[33] There are some who believe that familiar music, through the activation of distributed neural cognitive and emotional networks, may even be of therapeutic value to patients in a coma or vegetative-like state, although the authors suggest that: "Proof-of-principle and open-label studies, followed by controlled trials on this topic" are needed "to improve the evidence-base of music as a therapeutic tool in neurological early rehabilitation patients with disorders of consciousness."[36] Thankfully, such work is starting to happen: patients with "disorders of consciousness" showed changes in their brain activity when listening to complex sound sequences[37] and when told their first name, but only after being played music that was of emotional and autobiographical relevance to the patient.[38] Variable autonomic changes in response to different types of music have also been reported in patients with severe disorder of consciousness.[39]

Music and "healthy" aging

Before I describe in a little more detail some new and fascinating evidence supporting the effective use of music therapy in a variety of clinical conditions, what about the importance of music in the otherwise healthy aged population? Aspects of this question have been considered in the previous chapter when discussing the benefits of music education on developing brain function and behavior. Here I focus on the long-term benefits of musical training, experienced either at an early age or later in life.

As we age we lose partners and friends, we suffer from chronic but not necessarily life-threatening illnesses such as arthritis and diabetes, we lose mobility and muscle strength, we often have poorer vision and increased hearing loss, and so on and so on. Anatomically, there is an age-related reduction in gray matter volume in Heschl's gyrus and the superior temporal gyrus as well as in anterior cingulate cortex, changes that are evident even when controlling for hearing loss.[40] Presumably as a result of deteriorating processing power both centrally and out in the peripheral auditory apparatus, the aged population generally has greater difficulty in understanding speech than younger adults, with poorer word recognition in background noise.[40] Remember that speech perception requires the analysis and processing of pitch as well as rapidly changing sounds, and the capacity to code and then decipher temporal information. Inability to segregate and then group temporal patterns of speech from background noise impedes a listener's ability to perceive speech.[41]

Trained musicians who have improved timing and temporal resolution early in the auditory pathways in the brainstem isolate and hear speech in noise better than non-musicians, and this capacity is retained throughout life.[42,43,44] Because rhythm forms such an important component of both music and speech, and is processed in neural networks essentially common to both communication streams,[45] musical experience and training may help protect against an age-related decline in auditory perceptual abilities and better communication in noisy environments. Enhanced pitch processing in the brainstem is also found in speakers of tonal languages.[46] The benefits that musical training bring to linguistic capacity are hypothesized to depend on overlapping networks that process acoustic features of both communication streams, as well as on the impact of additional precision, emotion, repetition, and attention (OPERA) that comes with musical training.[47,48] Recent evidence from fMRI studies suggests in fact that trained musicians are able to additionally recruit areas of the right hemisphere when discriminating speech sounds.[49] Thus music training can, in the longer term, be of use to older individuals who have developed problems hearing speech when there is background noise.

In Chapter 7, I discussed how, in healthy individuals, early training in—and exposure to—music improves not just auditory performance but also language and literary skills, and enhances capability in several non-musical cognitive domains. Regular music lessons or activities can improve affective mood states, reduce anxiety, enhance working memory and other essential cognitive and executive functions (planning, problem solving, reasoning, etc), and improve visuospatial abilities, and overall may mitigate cognitive decline.[50,51,52,53,54,55,56] In fact, a population-based twin found that a twin who played a musical instrument had a comparatively reduced risk of developing dementia compared with his/her non-playing sibling.[55] Musical activity, even music training that occurred much earlier in childhood, continues to enhance motor performance and cognitive function.[57] People of all ages, including older people, who sing in choirs report less depressive symptoms, have better lung function, are less stressed, and perceive themselves as healthier and more socially connected, with an overall higher quality of life.[58,59] At the physiological level, relaxing music in particular reduces stress-induced feelings of anxiety and prevents increases in systolic blood pressure and heart rate,[60] and in a recent randomized control trial it was reported that combining music intervention with lifestyle modification significantly reduced diastolic blood pressure in pre-hypertensive subjects.[61] Choral singing can also be used to increase motivation and help deliver key health messages to at-risk communities, for example as part of a program in Western Australia aimed at reducing the prevalence of diabetes and associated diseases in aboriginal people, contributing to "Pulkurlkpa—a deeply soul-felt sense of joy, hope, optimism, and resilience."[62]

Sustained stress has adverse effects on the immune system and it is therefore of interest that potentially beneficial changes in reducing stress and associated immunological changes have also been reported after participation in positive music-related activities such as dance, group drumming, and choral singing.[12,63,64,65] Of course, as reviewed by Fancourt,[11] the beneficial impact of music on the mind and the body's physiological and immunological systems (what the authors rather dauntingly call the "pyschoneuroimmunological" effects of music), while universal, is complex and likely to vary depending on the cognitive and mental state (and age) of an individual at the time of testing. It is worth noting here that chronic stress also affects fundamental components of our DNA, the so-called telomeres. These structures form protective caps on the end of DNA strands, reducing the likelihood of damage to the DNA as cells divide. Telomeres get shorter with age, and decreased length is unequivocally associated with an increase in disease incidence (eg cardiovascular disease, diabetes, and cancer) and overall mortality.[66] Interestingly, many factors can result in shorter telomere length, including inflammation, lack of exercise, and chronic stress. Telomere length can be readily measured in circulating white blood cells—but I am unaware of any study that has examined whether exposure to, or participation in, music has a measurable beneficial impact on telomere length. I suggest such a study would be most enlightening!

Music and dance are inseparable partners. The rhythmic dynamics of music and its links with movement and dance mean that music has sensorimotor attributes, important not only for physical rehabilitation after stroke, for example, but also with potential health and fitness benefits to the general population (eg calisthenics, "jazzercise"). During one of my musical hobby periods I played keyboards and rhythm acoustic guitar in a band called "Chain Reaction," with my friends Phil and Di Firkin, mainly doing covers of '50s, '60s, and '70s favorites. We played at many jive and rock 'n' roll nights, and I remember thinking—as I watched the 50-somethings, 60-somethings, and sometimes 70-somethings dance and gyrate and sweat for two to three hours—that we ought to apply for funding from the health department. Group dancing presumably results in an increased level of endorphins, the endogenous opiates, as is thought to occur in other synchronized activities such as rowing.[10,67] Endorphin activity in the brain has not been measured directly, but dancers have been found to have an increased pain threshold (a proxy for endorphin activity)[68], especially in a social context and when dancing in synchrony.[69] How many of us have danced through the evening only to realize on the way home, or next morning, that we had twisted an ankle or a knee, but didn't realize it until the music stopped?! Without doubt, the potent and heady mix of favored music, exercise, and convivial company must be about as good a psychological and physiological boost to the aging body as you can get, and encourages social harmony to boot!

Exercise is now well known to be an essential element in maintaining mental and physical health in the aged. The hippocampus, so important in learning and memory formation, is known to atrophy with age, but greater volume in this region is associated with a higher level of cardiorespiratory fitness.[70,71] The beneficial effects of exercise have some specificity because, when imaged over a three-year period, changes were not evident in the thalamus or parts of basal ganglia in the same individuals who showed enhanced hippocampal volume. In another, nine-year study, much longer-term exercise—involving walking about six to nine miles a week—was, however, found to be associated with greater gray matter volume in several regions, including prefrontal and temporal cortex, as well as the hippocampus. As described in Chapter 3, new neurons continue to be made in adult hippocampus, including human hippocampus, and in mice at least, the number of new neurons made is directly related to physical exercise. The longer the exercise duration, the greater the neurogenesis, which in turn is correlated with levels of the peptide BDNF and, as has recently been discovered, levels of a hormone called adiponectin, which is made by fat cells.[72] Another growth factor related to insulin may also play an important role in this exercise-related enhancement of memory,[73] as may other by-products of intense physical activity.[74] In humans, serum BDNF levels decline with age, but BDNF levels are positively correlated with the volume of the hippocampus in older adults,[70,71] and it is tempting to speculate that this relationship is due to altered levels of neurogenesis.

Remarkably, and of particular relevance to my earlier comment about dancing and communal rock 'n' roll nights, some have suggested that music itself may impact positively on the birth of neurons in the hippocampus.[14] Certainly, in experimental studies it has been shown that social interaction between animals increases hippocampal neurogenesis via a BDNF-dependent mechanism.[75] This animal work ties in with evidence that human hippocampal formation is active in studies that target the neural correlates of attachment, empathy, compassion, and tenderness,[76] and this important structure is actually smaller in individuals with a reduced tendency to experience tender positive emotions.[77] Hippocampal function is also related to the ability to reason quickly and develop abstract concepts (termed by psychologists "general fluid intelligence"). In musicians, but not non-musicians, there is a relationship between hippocampal volume and general fluid intelligence that appears to reduce an age-related decline in cognitive function.[78] Finally, I should add that there is an additional beneficial impact of exercise on the immune system,[79] but of course there is a need to tailor exercise regimes to each individual because extreme exercise may do more harm than good.

Happily, any form of physical exercise is perceived as less strenuous if the activity involves music.[80] Dance in particular has reported benefits on cognition/attention, posture, and sensorimotor performance in the elderly, although these may not necessarily be related to cardiovascular performance.[81] Perhaps there is enhanced cortical plasticity due to (i) increased visuomotor integration and the spatial navigation needed during dancing, (ii) the emotional rewards obtained from wheeling around to your favorite songs, and (iii) the fun of improvising new steps and interacting with partners such that "a large array of networks is thus being activated."[82] Rewarding aspects of music involve the nucleus accumbens, which is not only an essential component of the brain's reward circuitry but can also act as a dynamic interface with motor control centers.[83] By connecting with regions such as the amygdala and hippocampus, this nucleus may serve to integrate the motivational value of diverse goals that help select how we interact with others.[84,85] Taken together, these assorted observations reveal the potential power of communal music-making to significantly enhance the quality of life in the elderly. There should *not* be silence in retirement homes and residential care facilities for the elderly, and in the home environment carers of the aged might reap some benefits from singing, and even dancing, with their relatives or clients.

The positive effects of music on neurologically normal members of our species, whatever their age, surely suggest that music will also have profound benefits on those with some form of psychological or physiological dysfunction. In 1997, during a seminar on music and the brain, I carried out a test in which I played different types of music and asked people to indicate, via a checklist, how they responded emotionally to the music and how they characterized the music they heard. The possible ways they could describe their feelings to the music were: graceful, whimsical, tragic, spiritual, erotic, sad, cheerful, peaceful, angry, sensual, fearful, uplifting, or neutral/no feelings. When the Star Wars theme was played, just about everyone in the audience used the term "uplifting", so—as I said at the time—if someone is suffering from anhedonia or depression, why not play music and see how subjects or patients react and respond?

As pointed out by Stefan Koelsch,[86] the likely impact of music on the limbic system, and in this context especially the amygdala (see Chapters 4 and 5), has potential therapeutic power, given that the amygdala has been implicated in various anxiety and depressive disorders[87] and is smaller in volume in aggressive people with psychopathic tendencies[88] (see also Chapter 5). A large-scale review and statistical analysis of 15 studies that used music to help treat people with psychotic or non-psychotic mental disorders such as depression and bipolar disorder concluded that, when given in addition to standard care: "music therapy is an effective treatment which helps people with psychotic and non-psychotic severe mental health disorders to improve global state, symptoms and functioning."[28] Beneficial outcomes of music therapy did not depend on the type of mental disorder, but what was clear was that longer courses and/or more frequent sessions of music therapy were most ideal. In fact, there is evidence that music therapy helps to reduce depressive symptoms and associated anxiety in working-age subjects.[89]

Listening or moving in time to music is not the only way of using music therapeutically. Others have reported the benefits of encouraging individuals with a range of psychological or neuropathological conditions to write songs.[34,90] Therapeutic song-writing is reported to help individuals manage their responses to emotional, social, and physical adversity. According to Felicity Baker, (at the time of writing) President of the Australian Music Therapy Association, the process helps to clarify thoughts and emotions, helps re-establish a sense of identity and self-confidence, reduces anxiety and anger, and allows thoughts and experiences to be voiced and shared in a musical, and perhaps therefore less threatening, context.

Menon and Levitin proposed that music offers a "simple and elegant way to probe the neural basis of anhedonia (loss of pleasure in daily activities) in a number of psychiatric disorders, including depression, schizophrenia, and bipolar disorder."[91] This was essentially confirmed in an fMRI study of "healthy" controls versus depressed subjects briefly exposed to neutral versus their favorite music in a scanner.[92] In healthy controls, favorite music activated regions known to be associated with the rewarding aspects of music (medial orbitofrontal cortex and nucleus accumbens), but activity was significantly less in these regions in the depressed group. Interestingly, the nucleus accumbens is also important in mediating the placebo effect.[93] Because combined visual and auditory presentation of happy faces and happy music enhances neural activity in the cortex, the use of such congruent stimuli could be especially beneficial in patients with affective disorders.[94]

Nonetheless, and despite the advocacy of many in allied health fields, it seems to me that this potentially game-changing therapeutic approach remains, stubbornly, somewhat peripheral. In addition to music's rewarding role in facilitating cooperative social interactions, in Chapter 4 I described how music appears to be an especially effective activator of memory circuits, in part owing to the functional involvement of regions in the temporal and cingulate lobes, both known to be associated with the limbic system and memory processing.[95,96,97,98] We have also discussed how dopamine, clearly an important player in our affective responses to music, assists in labeling salient autobiographical memories for storage and subsequent recall. And because learning and recall capabilities are enhanced during moments of heightened emotion and arousal, music can have great mnemonic power.

Memory and dementia

The learning that occurs when singing or practicing a musical instrument has a number of components.[97,99,100] After rehearsal involving short-term memory, encoding and consolidation of memory "traces" take place, probably in the cerebral cortex. To remind the reader, working memory, which likely involves processing in prefrontal cortex, is an important cognitive capacity. It is the ability to sort through, and actively keep in mind, diverse but relevant pieces of information for short periods of time when undertaking complex computational tasks such as reasoning, decision-making, and problem-solving.[101] Although there may be subtle differences in the respective networks, there is considerable overlap in the neural structures (mainly the left lateralized Broca's area, premotor cortex, and inferior parietal cortex) that process both verbal and tonal working memory.[102] Importantly, in older people it seems that music training can enhance cognitive function as well as verbal working memory to a greater degree than other general lifestyle activities.[52]

Some of the molecular and cellular mechanisms thought to underpin plasticity and different types of memory were discussed in Chapter 3. To remind the reader, long-term memory is generally divided into procedural (implicit) and declarative (explicit) memories. The former mostly relates to the learning of perceptual and motor skills and habits, skills that can become automatic, and is processed primarily in cerebellum, basal ganglia, and probably parts of motor cortex. Declarative memories, however, can be consciously recalled and explicitly recalled and/or stated. Such memories are essentially the life experience of an individual; they are his or her autobiography. Importantly, both types of learning are believed to be enhanced by exposure to music.[97,103] Declarative memories contain both generalized/conceptual stores of knowledge (facts, ideas, concepts—called semantic memory) and more specific memories of particular events (time, place, person, associated emotions—called episodic memory). Declarative memories require the involvement of the hippocampal region and surrounding cortex—the limbic system and prefrontal cortex. Associative memories involve the retrieval and linking together of different aspects and modalities of autobiographical data, memories that are often evoked by listening to music. For example, when we listen to a particular song that is familiar to us, the music (and/or lyric) can trigger the nostalgic recall of autobiographical circumstances that forever remain associated with that particular piece of music.[104] This interaction between music and autobiographical memory requires the participation of circuits in, for example, the medial prefrontal cortex (see Figure 5.1).[105]

It is therefore not surprising that, in Alzheimer's disease (AD) and other dementias, especially familiar songs can unlock memories. AD is a neurodegenerative condition that is associated with death of neurons and widespread disruption of neural connections. Its pathology is associated with characteristic changes including cell loss, deposition of focal aggregations (plaques) of a protein called β-amyloid, the presence of filamentous tangles inside neurons, and widespread changes in glial morphology and reactivity. Pathological changes are normally first seen in the temporal lobe, especially the hippocampus and adjacent regions of cerebral cortex. Early-onset AD invariably has a major genetic and therefore heritable component, but the pathophysiological mechanisms that contribute to late-onset AD remain more problematic and are probably multifactorial in most cases. Neurological signs of AD include progressive memory loss (short- and medium-term memories mostly), problems with speech, depression, increased isolation, and a reduced level of social interactions. There are also other forms of dementia, some associated with vascular disease, and other syndromes that involve chronic neurodegenerative changes in the frontal cortical lobe and also sometimes the temporal lobe (frontotemporal lobar dementia). The latter in particular is also associated with problems in processing musical information, especially the recognition of emotion in music.[106] Such individuals also find it difficult to recognize happiness, sadness, anger, fear, and so on, in voices and faces, which is intriguing because the brain networks that encode musically evoked emotions appear to differ slightly from those that recognize emotion and facial expressions.[107,108]

A number of studies from many countries around the world have examined the usefulness of music in reducing agitation and withdrawal in people with AD, encouraging interaction with others and participation in social activities, and generally enhancing their mental state and sense of well-being. Music therapy also appears to have more general beneficial physiological effects on cardiovascular health in elderly patients with dementia.[13] In earlier studies, group choral singing was reported to enhance social interactions, reduce dependence on medication, and improve mood and memory recall in AD patients.[109] More recent research supports the generally beneficial impact of this type of group activity on the quality of life not only of AD patients, but also their carers at home and in more formal care facilities for the elderly.[110,111,112]

We have seen that music and memory are closely linked, but there is often remarkable and specific preservation of memory for tunes and lyrics in AD patients.[111,113] Memory for music is relatively spared, even when episodic and verbal memory is poor.[114] The preservation of musical memories in otherwise amnesic individuals supports the idea that: "learning and retention of musical information depends on brain networks distinct from those involved in other types of episodic and semantic memory"[114] and may be related to the comparatively widespread neural architecture involved in music processing and memory. One study reported that these networks include parts of the anterior temporal lobe and prefrontal cortex—on both sides of the brain;[115] more recently, parts of the cingulate cortex and supplementary motor area have also been implicated in encoding well-established musical memories.[116]

In people with mild or moderate dementia, exposure to music in one form or another clearly improves their capacity to recall autobiographical details about their lives[117] and improves general cognition, working memory, and overall quality of life.[118] New episodic memories are also better learned and retained in patients with mild AD when text is sung rather than spoken.[119] Music familiar to the individual therefore offers a doorway into the Alzheimer brain, a way through to find an old memory, a past adventure. Singing with carers may be even more efficacious, but because of likely differences in age and cultural background the challenge there is to find music that has meaning not only for the person with dementia but also for the person providing the support. In his book *Musicophilia*, Oliver Sacks describes the remarkable preservation of musical aptitude and its emotional relevance to Woody, a man with AD. I quote here from a transcript of an interview that Professor Sacks conducted with Robyn Williams, presenter of the Australian Broadcasting Corporation's *Science Show* in 2008: "He has no idea what he did for a living, where he is living now or what he did ten minutes ago. Almost every memory is gone except for the music." Sacks found it "really very, very remarkable to see that this man who was so confused and not there, disorientated, seemed completely there when he sang a song, and not only technically, but he would turn to his wife and his daughter and all the sensibility and intelligence and humour which had gone into the learning of the song originally still seemed to be there."

I described in the previous chapter how at least some form of musical training benefits cognitive development. Registration of new memories may be aided by using music as a mnemonic device, by organizing new non-musical information into a musical context with pitch sequences and rhythmic patterns.[120] The recall of words is better some time after a learning trial if the words are sung rather than spoken, not only for healthy subjects but also for participants with mild AD;[121] thus the therapeutic door may well remain open. While AD seems to impact on the ability of individuals to recognize emotions in people's faces (such as sadness, disgust, and fear) or prosody in their voices, the emotional, dynamic aspects of music appear to be retained,[122] with music able to generate intense emotional experiences in the listener.[123]

Music and allied social interactions may have direct neurogenic effects on the hippocampus, increasing the incorporation of new neurons, and thereby potentially improving memory performance in the elderly. But not all areas of the cortex are equally susceptible to AD, and degenerative pathological changes are known to develop at different rates in different regions as the disease progresses. Remarkably then, those areas of the cerebral cortex that exhibit less pathology in AD correspond to cortical areas involved in musical memory, which might "explain the surprising preservation of musical memory in this neurodegenerative disease."[116] At the very end of his book on music, Oliver Sacks wrote: "Music is part of being human, and there is no human culture in which it is not highly developed and esteemed. Its very ubiquity may cause it to be trivialized in daily life: we switch on a radio, switch it off, hum a tune, tap our feet, find the words of an old song going through our minds, and think nothing of it. But to those who are lost in dementia, the situation is different. Music is no luxury to them, but a necessity, and can have a power beyond anything else to restore them to themselves, and to others, at least for a while."[124] Amen to that.

Disorders of movement

Music can also be used for a wide variety of rehabilitation therapies aimed at improving gross and fine motor coordination and function. Music and dance obviously involve the activation and processing of many sensorimotor areas in the brain. As described in Chapter 2, listening and responding to the rhythmic aspects of music in particular are inherently associated with activity in interactive networks between auditory and motor cortex, the latter including motor and premotor cortex, and other subcortical structures involved in movement—the basal ganglia and cerebellum.[125,126,127] Specific circuits between the cerebral cortex and cerebellum are activated when tracking rhythmic patterns and when tapping to a beat,[128] and there are extensive interactions between auditory and supplementary motor areas in cerebral cortex.[129] Basal ganglia activity is also seen when tapping to certain types of visual, as well as auditory, triggers.[130] Indeed, neuronal activity can be synchronized and entrained by beat and meter.[131] fMRI studies have also revealed an interactive network in the brain—including regions in the superior temporal gyrus (processing of heard music), cerebellum (beat information), parts of the basal ganglia (selection and organization of movements), auditory thalamus, and various sensory and motor areas of cerebral cortex—that are activated when performing spatially patterned dance steps in time to music.[132]

Together, over various durations of time, these various brain regions process and integrate information relating to auditory perception and the timing, sequencing, synchronization, and spatial organization of movement.[133] These temporally precise interactions are most highly evolved in our species, the motor regions involved in the planning of movement hypothesized to provide a signal that "helps the auditory system predict the timing of upcoming beats."[127] Positive emotional responses to music usually involve unconscious movement—tapping, dancing, and so on—almost certainly enhancing the perception of the rhythm itself[134,135] and eliciting a pleasurable state, symbiotic events that are unlikely to be accidental and probably have deep evolutionary origins. We get special satisfaction when anticipating and then moving perfectly in time to a beat. Predicting the beat requires a mental model of time, movement usually being even more rewarding when you see others dancing around you, presumably processing and anticipating the beat in exactly the same way—a great way to bond socially and tune into the mental state of others (see earlier discussions in Chapters 3 and 5 on "Theory of Mind").

These aural–motor links are established early in life—thus, as I am sure any reader who has had children will acknowledge, one- to two-year-old infants move and respond rhythmically to musical and other metrically regular sounds, and really enjoy doing so![136] Happy sounds really grab their attention.[137] It is therefore not at all surprising that music-associated physical therapy in children and in adults improves gross and fine motor control, coordination, and rehabilitation. Music gets us moving and dancing, it patterns sensorimotor activity, it motivates, it is a pick-me-up that can boost a person's energy. This is especially important in older people; music has been shown to improve balance and gait in the aged, thereby reducing the risk of falls, which often lead to life-threatening complications.[138] The rhythmic element to music regulates motor function via arousal and motivation, and also acts to entrain motor activity in the brain, the choice of music being important, both in terms of enjoyment but also in terms of tempo.[139] In Parkinson's disease (PD) and other movement-related disorders, although perception of, and synchronization to, the beat can be impaired,[140] music and dance are consistently reported to be of great benefit. Benefits include improved mental concentration, better gait and balance, improved initiation of movement, and an enhanced range of motion.[141]

PD is a complex neurodegenerative disease that involves a number of areas in the brain and affects only particular types of nerve cell. Most clinical emphasis is focused on a pathway involved in motor control that runs from the ventral midbrain in the brainstem to the basal ganglia in the forebrain (the so-called nigrostriatal pathway). As the disease progresses there may also be significant cognitive decline, and it is therefore intriguing that some PD patients have problems in recognizing facial expression as well as aspects of emotional content when expressed in music.[142,143] In mostly older people with PD (although there are genetically linked cases and instances of drug abuse where parkinsonism begins much earlier in life), the vast majority of the midbrain neurons that contribute axons to the nigrostriatal pathway die, for reasons that remain not entirely clear, with a consequent loss of input to the basal ganglia. These neurons contain the neurotransmitter dopamine (importantly, the same chemical associated with reward circuits involving the nucleus accumbens) and their death deprives the basal ganglia of this important neuro-chemical mediator.

The control and timing of movement is complex and involves many regions that have multiple interconnections with each other, some excitatory and some inhibitory. Every skilled movement you make involves these complex circuits, involves planning and the selection and initiation of the appropriate learned program(s), with constant reference to sensory feedback from the moving part of the body to ensure that the planned movement is actually being executed properly. Loss of this midbrain-basal ganglia pathway, along with the loss of dopamine input, contributes to throwing the system out of balance, the end result being that there is increased inhibition in the system—it is like putting your foot on the accelerator with the handbrake still engaged. Most pharmacological therapies involve the administration of a precursor of dopamine called L-dopa, which can cross from the bloodstream into the brain and is there converted into dopamine. Other drugs can also be given with L-dopa.

I remember many years ago the English comedian Terry-Thomas, who had Parkinson's disease, talking on television about how he found it difficult to start moving and how he could move better by thinking about tap-dancing through doorways. This difficulty in initiating or continuing movements is a frequent symptom in parkinsonian patients and is called "freezing." It is a major cause of falls in PD and is very debilitating. L-dopa treatment works well, at least for a period of time, but has less impact on gait disorders and this freezing phenomenon. A number of clinical trials now support Terry Thomas's anecdotal comments. For example, training Parkinson's patients to walk while they are listening to rhythmically accentuated music of some kind or mentally singing to themselves has been shown to improve mobility, the quality of their gait, and their sense of body position.[144,145,146] Other studies have shown that rhythmic musical cues can help to reduce the effects of freezing,[147] especially when auditory stimuli are provided along with physical therapy such as treadmill training.[148] Improvements in the precision and coordination of arm and finger movements have been reported when patients listen to "stimulating music,"[149] and the ability to perform a skilled reaching task involving grasping and eating a small item of food is similarly improved if Parkinson's patients are also listening to a preferred choice of music.[150]

If drugs are used to temporarily deplete dopamine in otherwise normal subjects, these individuals became less accurate in their perception of time, which is associated with altered activity in the putamen and supplementary motor area in the cortex.[151] So the perception of time, and perhaps the ability to anticipate and then move in time to regular sensory inputs such as beat, requires dopaminergic activity; perhaps this is one of the reasons why successfully moving in time to music, whether by small body movements or full-on dancing, is such a rewarding experience for most of us, and why it is so beneficial in movement disorders such as PD.[152] As Oliver Sacks described in his interview with Robyn Williams for the Australian Broadcasting Corporation in 2008, even in patients "who were frozen, transfixed, often unable to initiate any movement or any speech, music would allow them to move, music would give them its flow, music would let them walk and dance and sing in the most astonishing way." And in *Musicophilia* he emphasizes the importance of combining music with dance in therapies aimed at unlocking movement in PD patients and in others similarly "frozen in a trancelike state" as a consequence of other neurological conditions such as encephalitis.

Stroke and trauma

Stroke is an increasingly prevalent neurological condition, primarily owing to the increased longevity of our population. Loss of brain function can result from an obstruction to blood flow and supply, hence depriving the brain of oxygen and energy, or—less commonly—trauma occurs because of an intracranial hemorrhage. The nature and type of functional loss vary depending on which blood vessels are affected, and thus which areas of the brain are compromised.

Early studies using rhythmic auditory stimulation in hemi-paretic (partially paralyzed) stroke victims revealed that, when used with physical therapy, there was measurably improved gait and length of stride.[120,153] More recent work combining a subject's preferred music with game technology and feedback during repetitive, activity-driven rehabilitation of arm function has also produced promising results.[154] Exciting new data clearly suggests that recovery in motor function is due to enhanced plasticity and functionality of spared brain circuits. For example, intensive training results in remodeling and expansion of white matter fiber tracts.[155] There are also reports that music-supported training programs that involve playing a keyboard or drum pads that emit piano tones enhance motor skills after stroke, again with evidence that some of this recovery is related to increased plasticity in cortical circuitry.[156,157] Consistent with these reports, in a selected group of stroke patients it was found that delivery of music therapy, involving intense music learning, altered the organization and excitability of parts of sensorimotor cortex, resulting in improved movement in partially paralyzed hands.[158]

"Music-supported therapy" (MST) is a training program designed to involve all sensorimotor, affective, and cognitive systems. In an important innovation in the rehabilitation field, fMRI was carried out on chronic stroke patients before and after MST, revealing a restoration of activity and connectivity in auditory and motor regions in the affected hemisphere, accompanied by improved hand function.[159] These changes were not seen in the healthy control group. In support of the importance of music in prosocial contexts, the rehabilitation of stroke patients using keyboard training was found to improve mood states as well as fine finger control, but beneficial effects were greatest in patients who played in pairs, one after the other, attributed by the authors to an additional benefit gained by observing the actions of others.[160]

Musically assisted speech is used to treat non-fluent aphasia (or Broca's aphasia), a disorder associated with an inability to vocalize meaningful words, phrases, and sentences, sometimes encountered following a stroke.[161] So-called melodic intonation/speech therapy can aid in partial recovery from aphasia resulting from left hemisphere damage, probably via recruitment of areas in the undamaged right hemisphere that show additional activation when singing the text of a song.[162] Familiarity with a song (melody and text) may be especially beneficial in such cases.[163] Even simple "singing" containing complex rhythmic patterns that drive left-hemisphere activity may be useful as a tool in language rehabilitation.[164] In fact, rhythmic speech may also be effective in stimulating right-hemisphere activity in aphasics,[165] although the added motivational and rewarding elements of music-related activities would likely enhance therapeutic outcomes.

Improvements in cognitive function and mood states in stroke patients who listen to music for at least one hour a day have also been described.[166] Some of the quotes from these patients are worth repeating: "When I put the music on I don't have to think about this stroke or other sad things all the time" and "With the help of music I can do dishes and other work in my household. Without music I would have just sat down feeling miserable." While admittedly dependent to some degree on cultural background, the playing of major, rather than minor, modes of music is more effective in reducing cortisol levels in conditions of perceived stress.[18] Stroke is a sign of cardiovascular problems and it is therefore of interest that, in a study of patients with coronary heart disease, "recreational music making" involving group activities reduced stress and altered the pattern of gene expression in circulating blood cells, especially genes associated with immune function.[167]

A Scandinavian study[168] published in the prestigious journal *Brain* extensively documented changes in cognitive recovery and mood after middle cerebral artery stroke in patients exposed to music versus language or a control group. The music (of any genre) was familiar to, and liked by, each of the subjects being studied. Not all tested cognitive parameters were found to have improved, but members in the music group showed better recovery of verbal memory, improved focused attention, less confusion, and less depression. Listening to "pleasant" music also increases awareness and positive emotional responses in patients with cortical lesions that result in so-called sensory or spatial neglect, where the subjects are unaware of information presented to one side of their body space.[169] Such carefully conducted studies properly reveal the potential efficacy of musical therapy in neurological disorders.

Loss of cognitive capacity also occurs in people affected by other types of acquired brain injury. Often these are closed head injuries resulting from a direct blow or sudden rotation of the head, causing the brain to crash against the inner surface of the skull. Less frequently the injury is due to a penetrating trauma caused by, for example, the entry of a bullet or bone fragments. After traumatic brain injury a procedure termed neurologic music therapy (NMT) has been found to improve executive functions such as decision-making, problem-solving, and switching attention from one cue to another. This therapy has also been shown to reduce anxiety and improve the overall sense of emotional well-being.[170] This was after only four 30-minute sessions! In a case that deservedly received widespread publicity, music therapy has been used, seemingly with great success, on Congresswoman Gabrielle Giffords, who suffered a terrible injury to the left hemisphere after being shot at close range in the head. Lyrics of favorite songs with melody and rhythm helped her to reacquire speech. Finally, music therapy has also been used in children with various types of severe neurological dysfunction.[171] When standard occupational and speech therapy was supplemented with a type of NMT, an "auditory attention plus communication protocol," behavioral and electrophysiological assessments indicated enhanced neural plasticity in prefrontal and cingulate cortex, and improved attention and communication in treated children.

Spinal cord injury

We have seen that music we enjoy activates parts of the limbic system and the nucleus accumbens, the latter acting not only as a "reward center" but also as a link between motor control centers and other structures involved in motivation and goal-directed behaviors. Presumably then, the nucleus accumbens forms part of the link between music and that elemental compunction to move and dance in time with the beat? Lack of motivation and depression are typical following a stroke or after a spinal cord injury, and it is of great interest that a recent study in primates found that the nucleus accumbens plays a "critical role in processing of motivation" during rehabilitation after experimental spinal cord injury.[172] Connections are apparently strengthened with motor cortex and with other regions such as orbitofrontal cortex and anterior cingulate cortex. By now we have encountered these regions many times—they are activated when listening to pleasurable music, and they are also activated when thinking positively, being optimistic in outlook. So the question is, when re-learning sensorimotor tasks after injury, why not routinely use music to help motivate patients and drive the recovery process? Singing has been reported to improve physical outcomes as well as "mood, energy, social participation and quality of life" in people with quadriplegia.[173] Makes eminent sense to me, yet having visited various spinal injury centers around the world, physical rehabilitation, including for example rhythmic walking on treadmills, is rarely if ever accompanied by music chosen by the injured patient. It should be.

Brain–machine or brain–computer interfaces are thought by many to be the future of restorative therapies for sensorimotor dysfunction, including of course the treatment of people paralyzed after spinal cord trauma.[174,175] Monitoring neural activity in appropriate parts of the cerebral cortex using a range of recording methods can be used, in association with complex algorithms, to stimulate muscle activity or drive external agents such as robotic arms. In a clever series of trials carried out in the UK at the University of Plymouth and the Royal Hospital for Neuro-disability, paralyzed musicians (the "Paramusical Ensemble") have been able to create music by looking at flashing images that correspond to short musical phrases. The visual input is recorded by an array of electrodes positioned over the visual cortex, which then transmits the selected musical phrase to a computer interface. The resulting music is played by partner musicians. Exciting as this is, the potential to use motor imagery to drive movement[175] leads me to dream of the day when paralyzed individuals think about playing a piece of music on an instrument and use that imagery to drive either synthesizers or robots to play for them!

Sleep

We know that—with luck—lullabies put babies to sleep, and I have sometimes seen more mature members of the audience fall asleep during a concert at our wonderful Perth Concert Hall. But for those who have chronic difficulties in falling or staying asleep, insomnia is a debilitating disorder that can affect day-to-day function, with potential psychological and physiological sequelae. Can music help adults with sleep problems? Sleep disorders are especially prevalent in the elderly, and may result from emotional stress, disease, acute events such as stroke, breathing issues (sleep apnea), chronic use of medications, and so on. A meta-analysis was recently carried out on ten studies that examined the impact of music therapy on various types of sleep disorder.[176] Although there was considerable heterogeneity in outcomes, taken together the authors found that music did indeed improve sleep quality in individuals with either acute or chronic sleep disorders. Music also improves the quality of sleep in those with fibromyalgia, a condition that is associated with—among other things—heightened sensitivity to pain.[177] Which is a convenient segue into the next section....

Pain and anxiety

It has long been believed that music can be used as a tool to alleviate pain, or at least influence the perception of, and reduce the stress induced by, pain. A review by Guenther Bernatzky et al[178] collated much of the data that points to the potential value of music therapy in nonpharmacological pain management. As quoted by Henson, in a manuscript from 1529, Caelius Aurelianus mentioned the reputed benefits of music in relation to treatment of insanity and sciatica: "A certain piper would play his instrument over the affected parts and these would begin to throb and palpitate, banishing the pain and bringing relief."[179] Modern-day reports confirm that listening to pleasant or cheerful music reduces the perception of pain.[180,181] Note here that subjects also experience less pain when viewing images of a "romantic partner," an effect that is associated with activation of reward circuits such as the caudate, nucleus accumbens, and parts of frontal and prefrontal cortex.[182] These circuits are of course active when listening to preferred music, so perhaps, along with activation of the endogenous opioid system,[10,68] this is an additional mechanism by which music assists in the relief of pain?

In the clinical context, an early study reported that music reduced the subjective experience of pain in the vast majority of dental patients,[183] and music appears to improve relaxation and perception of pain, and reduce anxiety in patients after cardiovascular or intestinal surgery.[184,185] In Sweden, Ulrica Nilsson has published numerous reports describing the "analgesic" impact of music.[186] For example, in a randomized controlled trial of patients undergoing hernia repair, intraoperative music reduced perception of pain soon after surgery, while postoperative exposure to music was associated with reduced cortisol levels (less stress?) and less anxiety—and these patients required less morphine for pain control.[187] Similar results were obtained when studying children's experiences after minor day surgery.[188] Music also reduces stress and anxiety levels in patients undergoing cerebral or coronary angiography[189,190] or colonoscopy.[19]

Music has also been used in the treatment of acute and chronic pain in palliative care situations.[191] In her review, O'Callaghan points out that music therapy diminishes the perception of pain, perhaps via a number of mechanisms—psychological and physiological—but that care needs to be taken in the type of music chosen and how the music is presented. For any given patient I would expect that pieces of music that have autobiographical significance and/or that are especially rewarding are likely to be of greatest benefit.[9] There may also be emotional benefits to carers and "significant others." But this field requires more prospective, carefully controlled clinical trials, coupled with studies that carefully analyze how music affects the neurochemistry of pain, and its subjective impact. Both are needed because the benefits may be great. Systematic reviews of randomized controlled trials, such as the one showing significant beneficial effects of music on reducing pain and anxiety in children undergoing medical and dental procedures,[192] should help to convince clinicians to use this approach more frequently, alone or in conjunction with so-called conventional palliative pain treatments. To quote Clare O'Callaghan's eloquent words at the conclusion of her short review: "Some of the most vulnerable members of our community, the severely disabled and dying, do not have access to the nourishment of aesthetic experiences. We have a humane mandate to offer palliative care options, such as music therapy, to deal with their pain experiences arising from degenerative conditions."[191]

Tinnitus

Tinnitus, or ringing in the ears, is the perception of sounds when no external sound is present, and is an incredibly common problem affecting about 10–20% of the population, with no truly effective cure as yet. It can have many causes, and many of us can adequately co-exist with this aural interloper by not paying it too much attention, but in some people tinnitus can become so intrusive and unbearable that it leads to sleep disturbances, attention deficits, severe depression, and worse. Management involves counselling, sometimes medication, and different types of sound therapy to mask a specific tinnitus frequency. There are different sound therapy options, recently evaluated for their clinical effectiveness,[193] which are often used as part of a broader management plan when dealing with tinnitus.

In this context, clinical research is now using specific types of musical training aimed at cancelling out tinnitus sounds and thus reducing the impost to sufferers. A study group based in Germany have developed what they call the "Heidelberg Model of Music Therapy," useful in those with chronic "tonal tinnitus," meaning tinnitus that consists of a continuous sound/noise of narrow bandwidth, usually with a characteristic frequency or pitch.[194] The therapy is complicated and involves first externalizing the sound, then active filtering and habituating to the tinnitus, as well undergoing some cortical retraining: "the patients shall be enabled to actively control the sounds in order to reorganize the underlying neuronal mechanisms maintaining the tinnitus." Therapy is tailored to each individual and his/her tinnitus sound. It would seem to be pretty intensive, involving nine consecutive stages, but the therapy does seem to be useful as an early intervention, reducing the likelihood of the tinnitus becoming a chronic condition.[195] Neuroimaging has revealed that these long-lasting therapy effects appear to be associated with changes in cortical organization, with increased gray matter in specific frontal and auditory cortical regions.[196]

Pregnancy and newborns

The congenitally deaf have a normal-looking auditory cortex,[197] learn to communicate with their hands as infants, and eventually use signing, lip-reading, and so on, to communicate via language networks in the brain, However, for most of us, auditory experience in the final third of gestation is important in beginning the maturation of patterned auditory processing, especially in the developing cortex. For preterm, low-birthweight babies the normal intrauterine sounds such as maternal heartbeat and "filtered but structured linguistic and musical input from the external environment" are absent in the intensive care ward.[198] These authors recommend that there is a need to design "neonatal intensive care units for preterm infants, who are deprived of a typical prenatal auditory environment." Careful use of appropriate, positive auditory input for preterm infants is especially important because neonatal intensive care units can be noisy, potentially affecting later hearing, language, and cognitive development—"preterm infants … often close their eyes in response to bright lights, but they cannot close their ears in response to loud sounds."[199]

In addition to such general potential benefits in the aural domain, there is increasing evidence for the specific usefulness of music therapy in enhancing the physiological wellbeing of preterm infants. In early studies in this field, in neonatal intensive care units sedative music was found to affect systolic blood pressure, heart rate, and respiratory rate in premature infants,[200] and the requirement of premature, low-birthweight infants for oxygen was less when they were played music (lullabies) as compared with recordings of their mother's voice.[201] Music also seems to relax preterm infants; it stabilizes their arousal state and reduces signs of stress.[202] Live music may be even more effective, if you have a caregiver who is available and capable! In a neonatal intensive care environment, live music as opposed to recorded music results in a reduced heart rate and deeper sleep in preterm infants,[203] an observation supported by a later meta-analysis of the effect of live music therapy in, for example, pacifying preterm infants and reinforcing sucking behaviors; these benefits appear to be greatest for infants weighing less than 1,000 g and at a gestational age of less than about 28 weeks.[204] Remarkably, music therapy may also benefit the caregivers: one recent study on the postpartum care of premature babies reported that listening to music increased the quantity and quality of breast milk expressed by the mothers![205]

Conclusion

The current (2016) director of the Music and Neuroimaging Laboratory at Harvard, Gottfried Schlaug, nicely summarized from a neuroscience perspective why music therapy might be expected to be useful in the clinical domain.[155] Music can modulate attention (distraction—relevant, for example, for pain and anxiety), emotion (relevant for affective disorders), cognition and memory (relevant for AD and other dementias), motor behavior (relevant for PD and other motor disorders), and communication/auditory perceptual processing (relevant for autism, language dysfunction, stroke, etc). Since that brief review was written there have been a number of important advances, many of them discussed in this chapter. In 2014, the effectiveness of music therapy was examined using a meta-analysis approach, incorporating randomized controlled trials, 21 in total, that had been published between 1995 and 2012.[206] The original studies involved testing the efficacy of music therapy in various disease paradigms associated with nervous, endocrine, cardiovascular, or respiratory systems, as well as examining the impact of music during pregnancy and childbirth. The conclusion was that music therapy treatment improved: "global and social functioning in schizophrenia and/or serious mental disorders, gait and related activities in Parkinson's disease, depressive symptoms, and sleep quality." Evidence for the treatment of other conditions was—at least at present—equivocal, but no adverse effects were noted.

Music has obvious effects on the central nervous system and on the endocrine system (hormones), autonomic nervous system (influencing, for example, blood pressure and heart rate), and immune system; moreover, it can help alleviate stress and alter perception of pain, and promote and enhance rehabilitation. Interestingly, while relaxing to music reduces both subjective and physiological measures of stress, stress-reducing effects are even further enhanced when listening to music in a social environment.[207] To quote Fancourt et al at the end of their detailed review on the "psychoneuroimmunological" effects of music on humanity: "If music is found to have a significant effect on the immune system's ability to fight disease, it will have a profound impact on its incorporation into health care settings including hospital waiting rooms; procedures such as surgery; and treatments such as chemotherapy and psychotherapy; as well as placing a larger significance and responsibility on our day-to-day consumption of music."[11] And of course it should have a special place in the field of preventative medicine. Overall it is clear that music is a resource not yet fully utilized; there is a need for even more prospective, randomized long-term trials with appropriate control groups especially for neurological conditions affecting cognition, behavior, and psychological health, and for rehabilitation programs used to treat neurodegenerative disease, or following surgery or neurotrauma of various kinds. As Lauren Stewart wrote: "When used appropriately, music is ethically acceptable, side-effect free, can be intricately tailored to personal preferences and tastes, and in some cases may provide a cost-effective alternative to pharmacological sedation."[208] Music clearly has the capacity to improve our sense of mental well-being and reduce feelings of isolation and vulnerability. Music has a holistic impact on individuals adversely affected by a variety of specific medical/psychological conditions, and to ignore the diagnostic and therapeutic power of music in situations where normal function is impaired in some way seems to me to be indefensible, especially when investigating mood and affective disorders.

One final comment: for many of the reasons discussed in this chapter, others believe music can be used as "therapeutic resource" to support children in conflict zones and in post-conflict situations where children (and adults) may suffer from post-traumatic stress disorder.[208,209] This disorder has many psychiatric symptoms as well as diverse physiological manifestations that can affect the autonomic, cardiovascular, respiratory, and immune systems. As we have seen, and as Nigel Osborne summarizes in his account, music can have beneficial effects on all these systems, and can also help in regulating movement and reducing anxiety in traumatized children: "it is reasonable to propose that children with symptoms of avoidance, numbing, or hyperarousal, or associated feelings of detachment, estrangement, anger, fear, lack of trust, distress, or simply unhappiness, may indeed (as they and their carers so often tell us) find a measure of physical and mental release in joyful shared experiences of musical expression."[209] With this goes not only the rehabilitation of self-respect and self-belief, but at the social level "music may be effective in facilitating social communication, collective creativity... and the expression of social identity."[209] And there, in a nutshell, is just one more reason why music, so important throughout our evolutionary history, remains important today, for our children, and for our children's children.

Chapter 9

Coda: *Homo sapientior*?

Musical training is a more potent instrument than any other, because rhythm and harmony find their way into the secret places of the soul.

—Plato's *Republic*

Codas (the Italian word for tails) are passages of music that bring a composition to an end. They can be of varying length and mood—sometimes energetic, sometimes bombastic, sometimes peaceful or melancholic—and they can sometimes be used as a retrospective, summing up much of what has gone before. In modern popular music songs often repeat and fade a phrase or musical "lick" into gradual silence, but in the classical repertoire the end of a piece of music is important; they are the last notes an audience hears. I wonder how much time composers need to take in order to be satisfied with those last few bars? Personally I like all sorts of codas, but that last impression is so, so important! So if you have come this far with me, how do I adequately sum up the previous chapters—leave the best impression?

As I said at the very beginning of this book, my primary aim has been to describe what we currently know (or think we know) about the origin and neuroscientific basis of music. In so doing I hoped to put forward a persuasive hypothesis as to why all of humanity evolved, and uniquely continues to possess, two complementary but distinct communication systems—language and music—and why music continues to be crucially important for the health and well-being of human society in the twenty-first century.

When talking to people about their private lives and personal experiences, almost all will agree that music is a wonderful thing—of emotional or psychological importance in one way or another. Yet in the domain of public policy, when prioritizing budgets, preparing curricula, or developing therapeutic strategies, the people that need to be convinced about the importance of music are the politicians, the educators, the neurologists and psychiatrists, and so on, most of whom in their leisure time probably *do* appreciate music and the positive contribution it makes to their lives. I suggest that this private/public dichotomy of thought and action, in the modern western world at least, has arisen because music is usually labeled as an "art," separated from "science" and quarantined from the 24/7 work and economic/financial issues that dominate our existence. This was not always the case. Ethnomusicologists know that music was (and is) a core part of daily life in indigenous societies. In ancient Greece there was no clear distinction between non-science and science disciplines, but there was a separation of knowledge/understanding for its own sake (*epistêmê*) and knowledge of crafts and skills needed for making or doing practical things (*technê*). What I find interesting is that the latter "crafts" included diverse activities such as house-building, weaving, cookery, geometry, politics, and prophecy, but *technê* also included medicine *and* music![1]

In the western world the separation of natural philosophy into science and art gathered pace about 400–500 years ago, driven by scholars such as Vesalius, Copernicus, and later Galileo,[2] each sphere becoming more and more specialized with its own discrete knowledge and vocabulary, once described as a separation into two cultures.[3] We now think of "science" as hypothesis and experiment, prediction and quantifiable observation, classification and statistics … and "art" as introspection, freedom of expression, beauty … Science underpins technology, industry, wealth generation, the health of our environment, while music "neither ploughs, sows, weaves nor feeds."[4] But the modern-day marginalization of music into the "arts" sector is to the detriment of our species. People who one way or another engage in the "arts" for at least 100 hours a year report a greater sense of mental well-being.[5] As I quoted much earlier in this book: "Many people assume that the arts are luxuries rather than necessities … they consider it a gloss upon the surface of life; a harmless indulgence rather than a necessity, of no great importance to our species."[6] Placing music into a silo is a grave mistake because music of whatever origin or quality is neither an art nor a science; it is a core and fundamental element of what it is to be human. This is something that John Blacking came to understand in Africa—the fundamental role of music in all aspects of life, and the fact that technology now artificially and improperly separates people that are, from those that are not, "musical."

I have argued that, early in our history, our sense of self and knowledge of our impermanence was intensified and focused through the lens of spoken language. Music's communal, socializing power acted as an essential counterweight to the individualization experienced by increasingly intelligent and articulate members of "*Homo sapientior.*" Music was able to maintain—as the title of this book suggests—a harmony of souls during the emergence of a "society of selves."[7] I believe that, in the modern age, it is more important than ever to place music and its physiological and behavioral effects on people into a more "scientific" context, to understand exactly where it is processed in the brain and how it impacts on life, and thereby reveal—as the ancients knew—that music has clear relationships with medicine and with mental health.

There is a nonverbal, empathic communication between people when playing or singing in a group; each individual does his/her own thing but the greater significance lies in how each person's contribution fits within the bigger communal structure. And of course, the resulting product is much more than the sum of its parts. Anyone who has played in an orchestra or a band, or sung in a choir, knows how that organism feels—you are an individual while at the same time part of this cohesive architecture—all for one and one for all. Music is in partnership with speech; it has essential elements that seem to spill over into language, elements that are underlying components of all human communication systems. Music is associated with altruism and prosocial behavior. Moreover, it evokes memories and stirs our emotions, and is a critical part of our mental well-being. While articulate speech chatters away in intersecting, turn-taking lines of individual counterpoint, music acts like a chorale, an "ice-breaker"[8] helping to build and maintain communal interactions. Social cooperativity and trust, facilitated and enhanced by music-making and dance, are what make humans special.

For whatever reasons, suicide rates have increased over the past 30 years; in a 1999 article in the *Medical Journal of Australia* it was estimated that the rate of suicide in the 15- to 24-year age group during that period had increased from 10 per 100,000 to 30 per 100,000 during that period—the rate had tripled. The rate also increased in the 25- to 34-year age group. Is this related to an increased sense of isolation and futility, with difficulty in dealing with the realities of life, in the young? People no longer understand where they belong, what it all means—there is a loss of a belief in the gods and in an afterlife. Was the realization of our impermanence something that needed to be dealt with, something perceived as a threat to the newly sentient *"Homo sapientior"* from the very beginning? Was it the case that the smarter we got, the lonelier we got? To quote Walter Freeman: "As knowledge increases by learning, brains of individuals grow progressively apart."[9] Music is a force that binds us together with others, in dance, in joy, in mourning, in war, in love; momentarily we forget our isolation, our mortality, and we step beyond the confines of our own individuality. Is this why our founder population survived, perhaps at the expense of other small pockets of evolving hominins, because it possessed this great gift? Was this what Nietzsche meant when he said "we possess art lest we perish from the truth?"

We do not produce huge numbers of offspring, but we do live for a relatively long time, allowing us to continually learn and adapt to life's challenges. Most scholars and writers would agree that, because of language—the ability to symbolize and organize information, to use generational/abstract thought, and pass on accrued knowledge to future generations—and more recently because of rapid advances in information technology, our evolutionary trajectory continues to quicken. If you accept that our generation time (the average age at which each generation produces the next) has, over our history, been about 20–25 years, and that we are perhaps 75,000–80,000 years old, then *"Homo sapientior"* has been around for only about 4,000–4,500 generations. Most of us will meet people who span about five generations—grandparents to grandchildren—less than a thousandth of the generations that have existed! Culturally, the first pictorial art and evidence of music emerged about halfway through our hypothetical time-line; from the first symbolic written notation to Shakespeare spanned about 400–500 generations, and from Shakespeare to the world-wide web and Google about 15–20 generations. We are in information overload. Biological acceleration may also be important—we are now at the technological stage where in-vitro fertilization and gene selection/engineering provide the potential means for our selfish genes to take over once more in the selection of the type of individuals who will constitute the next and future generations of *Homo sapientior*, or should that be *Homo sapientissimus*? Perhaps even more than ever, we will continue to need music as a "de-isolator," something to overcome individual differences and foster social cohesion, sharing common states of experience and arousal.

In this book I have attempted to provide a broad, multidisciplinary scientific rationale to explain why, during the evolution of the modern mind, we have retained music as an indelible form of communication in parallel to language—complementary in many ways, yet distinct, central to the human experience. "The basic premise of music is communication: communication which can leap across centuries and oceans; and communication of values and pleasures—intellectual, aesthetic, perhaps 'spiritual' but certainly physiological—which seem expressible best by music or possibly even only by music."[10] To quote my colleagues, music is perhaps "the most important thing we ever did"[11] and "a fundamental component of what makes human societies possible."[12] Luther regarded music as one of God's greatest gifts. Is the relatively recent separation of art from science in modern human life, so often the source of philosophical discussion and rationale for guileful political decisions, one of the most unfortunate things our species has ever done? Music is surely as important as reading and writing, and again needs to be integrated into our educational system; music should be accepted as a conventional and efficacious therapy by our medical and allied health communities. Given the rapidity of recent technological and social change we cannot afford to wait another generation to convince the politicians, bean counters, teachers, and clinicians that music remains essential for our psychological health and the social well-being of our society.

Far, far back in human history, there were times when music stood in the center of life, when it was an intermediary between natural and supernatural phenomena, when it was the sister of religion, the corner stone of all education. And, ah, they were happy times.[13]

References

Foreword

1. **Shapiro N** (1978) *An Encyclopedia of Quotations about Music*. Da Capo Press, New York.
2. **Bolhuis JJ, Tattersall I, Chomsky N, Berwick RC** (2014) How could language have evolved? PLoS Biol **12**: e1001934.
3. **Brewster D** (1855) *Memoirs of the Life, Writings, and Discoveries of Sir Isaac Newton*. T Constable and Company, Vol **2**, Ch 27.
4. **Haig D** (2007) "The gene meme," in **A. Grafen** and **M. Ridley**, eds, *Richard Dawkins: How a Scientist Changed the Way We Think* (Oxford University Press, Oxford), 50–65.
5. **Critchley M, Henson RA** (1977) *Music and the Brain: Studies in the Neurology of Music*. Heinemann Medical Books Ltd, London.
6. **Storr A** (1992) *Music and the Mind*. Harper Collins Publishers, London.
7. **Harvey AR** (2011) "Evolution, music and neurotherapy," in **A. Poiani**, ed., *Pragmatic Evolution: Applications of Revolutionary Theory* (Cambridge University Press, Cambridge UK), 150–163.
8. **Blacking J** (1976) *How Musical is Man?* Faber and Faber, London.

Chapter One

1. **Blacking J** (1976) *How Musical is Man?* Faber and Faber, London.
2. **Blacking J** (1995) *Music, Culture and Experience*. University of Chicago Press, London.
3. **Brown S, Merker B, Wallin NL** (2000) "An introduction to evolutionary musicology," in **N.L. Wallin, B. Merker** and **S. Brown**, eds, *The Origins of Music* (MIT Press, Cambridge MA), 3–24.
4. **Peretz I** (2006) The nature of music from a biological perspective. Cognition **100**: 1–32.
5. **Morley I** (2013) *The Prehistory of Music: Human Evolution, Archaeology, and the Origins of Musicality*. Oxford University Press, Oxford.
6. **Savage PE, Brown S, Sakai E, Currie TE** (2015) Statistical universals reveal the structures and functions of human music. Proc Natl Acad Sci USA **112**: 8987–8992.
7. **Sacks O** (2008) *Musicophilia*. Vintage Books, New York.
8. **Shapiro N** (1978) *An Encyclopedia of Quotations About Music*. Da Capo Press, New York.
9. **Kivy P** (1959) Charles Darwin on music. J Am Mus Soc **12**: 42–48.
10. **Darwin C** (1897) *The Descent of Man, and Selection in Relation to Sex* (2nd edition).
11. **Spencer H** (1891) "The origin and function of music," in *Essays: Scientific, Political, and Speculative*, Vol **2** (Williams and Norgate, London), 400–451.
12. **Kivy P** (1971) *Music, Language, and Cognition*. Oxford University Press, Oxford.
13. **Huxley A** (1931) *Music at Night*. Chatto and Windus, London.
14. **Bernstein L** (1976) *The Unanswered Question: Six Talks at Harvard*. Harvard University Press, Cambridge MA and London.
15. **Morgenstern S** (1956) *Composers on Music* (2nd edition). Pantheon Books, New York.
16. **Harrer G, Harrer H** (1977) "Music, emotion and autonomic function," in **M. Critchley** and **R. A. Henson**, eds, *Music and the Brain: Studies on the Neurology of Music* (Heinemann Medical Books Ltd, London), 202–216.

17. **Sloboda J** (1991) Music structure and emotional response: some empirical findings. Psych Music **19**: 110–120.
18. **Bernardi L, Porta C, Casucci G, Balsamo R, Bernardi NF, Fogari R,** et al. (2009) Dynamic interactions between musical, cardiovascular, and cerebral rhythms in humans. Circulation **119**: 3171–3180.
19. **Harrison L, Loui P** (2014) Thrills, chills, frissons, and skin orgasms: toward an integrative model of transcendent psychophysiological experiences in music. Front Psychol **5**: 790.
20. **Koelsch S** (2012) *Brain and Music*. Wiley Blackwell, Chichester, UK.
21. **Brown S, Martinez MJ, Parsons LM** (2006) The neural basis of dance. Cereb Cortex **16**: 1157–1167.
22. **Sievers B, Polansky L, Casey M, Wheatley T** (2013) Music and movement share a dynamic structure that supports universal expressions of emotion. Proc Natl Acad Sci U S A **110**: 70–75.
23. **Morley I** (2014) A multi-disciplinary approach to the origins of music: perspectives from anthropology, archaeology, cognition and behavior. J Anthrop Sci **92**: 147–177.
24. **Novembre G, Keller PE** (2014) A conceptual review on action-perception coupling in the musician's brain: what is it good for? Front Hum Neurosci **8**: 603.
25. **Fitch TW** (2006) The biology and evolution of music: a comparative perspective. Cognition **100**: 173–215.
26. **Brown S, Jordania J** (2011) Universals in the world's music. Psych Music: 1–20.
27. **Fischer R, Callander R, Reddish P, Bulbulia J** (2013) How do rituals affect cooperation? An experimental field study comparing nine ritual types. Hum Nat **24**: 115–125.
28. **Whitehouse H, Lanmann JA** (2014) The ties that bind us: ritual, fusion, and identification. Curr Anthrop **55**: 674–695.
29. **Hagen EH, Hammerstein P** (2009) Did Neanderthals and other early humans sing? Seeking the biological roots of music in the territorial advertisements of primates, lions, hyenas and wolves. Music Sci **13**: 292.
30. **Jordania J** (2011) *Why Do People Sing? Music in Human Evolution*. Logos, Tbilisi.
31. **Bannan N, Montgomery-Smith C** (2008) "Singing for the brain": reflections on the human capacity for music arising from a pilot study of group singing with Alzheimer's patients. J R Soc Promot Health **128**: 73–78.
32. **Pearce E, Launay J, Dunbar RIM** (2015) The ice-breaker effect: singing mediates fast social bonding. R Soc Open Sci **2**: 150221.
33. **Osborne N** (2012) Neuroscience and "real world" practice: music as a therapeutic resource for children in zones of conflict. Ann NY Acad Sci **1252**: 69–76.
34. **Storr A** (1992) *Music and the Mind*. Harper Collins, London.
35. **Cross I** (2001) Music, mind and evolution. Psych Music **29**: 95–102.
36. **Pinker S** (1997) *How the Mind Works*. W W Norton, New York.
37. **Huron D** (2003) "Is music an evolutionary adaptation?" in **I. Peretz** and **R. L. Zatorre,** eds, *The Cognitive Neuroscience of Music* (Oxford University Press, Oxford), 57–75.
38. **Zentner MR, Kagan J** (1996) Perception of music in infants. Nature **383**: 29.
39. **Trehub S** (2003) The developmental origins of musicality. Nat Neurosci **6**: 669–673.
40. **Perani D, Saccuman MC, Scifo P, Spada D, Andreolli G,** et al. (2010) Functional specializations for music processing in the human newborn brain. Proc Natl Acad Sci USA **107**: 4758–4763.
41. **Moerel M, De Martino F, Santoro R, Uqurbil K, Goebel R,** et al. (2013) Processing of natural sounds: characterization of multipeak spectral tuning in human auditory cortex. J Neurosci **33**: 11888–11898.
42. **McDermott JH, Lehr AJ, Oxenham AJ** (2010) Individual differences reveal the basis of consonance. Curr Biol **20**: 1035–1041.

43. Blasi A, Mercure E, Lloyd-Fox S, Thomson A, Brammer M, et al. (2011) Early specialization for voice and emotion processing in the infant brain. Curr Biol **21**: 1220–1224.

44. Ilie G, Thompson WF (2011) Experiential and cognitive changes following seven minutes exposure to music and speech. Music Percept **28**: 247–264.

45. Corbeil M, Trehub SE, Peretz I (2013) Speech vs. singing: infants choose happier sounds. Front Psychol **4**: 372.

46. Fritz T, Jentschke S, Gosselin N, Sammler D, Peretz I, et al. (2009) Universal recognition of three basic emotions in music. Curr Biol **19**: 573–576.

47. Cross I (1999) "Is music the most important thing we ever did? Music, development and evolution," in **S. W. Yi**, ed., *Music, Mind and Science* (Seoul National University Press, Seoul), 10–39.

48. Esch T, Guarna M, Bianchi E, Zhu W, Stefano GB (2004) Commonalities in the central nervous system's involvement with complementary medical therapies: limbic morphinergic processes. Med Sci Monit **10**: MS6–17.

49. Bardia A, Barton DL, Prokop LJ, Bauer BA, Moynihan TJ (2006) Efficacy of complementary and alternative medicine therapies in relieving cancer pain: a systematic review. J Clin Oncol **24**: 5457–5464.

50. Williams PD, Piamjariyakul U, Ducey K, Badura J, Boltz KD, et al. (2006) Cancer treatment, symptom monitoring, and self-care in adults: pilot study. Cancer Nurs **29**: 347–355.

51. Kozak LE, Kayes L, McCarty R, Walkinshaw C, Congdon S, et al. (2008) Use of complementary and alternative medicine (CAM) by Washington State hospices. Am J Hosp Palliat Care **25**: 463–468.

52. Baranowsky J, Klose P, Musial F, Haeuser W, Dobos G, Langhorst J (2009) Qualitative systemic review of randomized controlled trials on complementary and alternative medicine treatments in fibromyalgia. Rheumatol Int **30**: 1–21.

53. Brauer JA, El Sehamy A, Metz JM, Mao JJ (2010) Complementary and alternative medicine and supportive care at leading cancer centers: a systematic analysis of websites. J Altern Complement Med **16**: 183–186.

Chapter Two

1. Lewis J (2013) "A cross-cultural perspective on the significance of music and dance to culture and society," in **M. A. Arbib**, ed., *Language, Music and the Brain: A Mysterious Relationship* (MIT Press, Cambridge MA), 45–65.

2. Crystal D (2006) *How Language Works*. Penguin, London.

3. Pinker S (1994) *The Language Instinct*. Penguin, London, New York.

4. Fiebach CJ, Schlesewsky M, Lohmann G, von Cramon DY, Friederici AD (2005) Revisiting the role of Broca's area in sentence processing: syntactic integration versus syntactic working memory. Hum Brain Mapp **24**: 79–91.

5. Penhune VB, Cismaru R, Dorsaint-Pierre R, Petitto L-A, Zatorre RJ (2003) The morphometry of auditory cortex in the congenitally deaf measured using MRI. Neuroimage **20**: 1215–1225.

6. Fitch TW (2006) The biology and evolution of music: a comparative perspective. Cognition **100**: 173–215.

7. McCrone J (2003) Feral children. Lancet Neurol **2**: 132.

8. Harlow HF, Dodsworth RO, Harlow MK (1965) Total social isolation in monkeys. Proc Natl Acad Sci **54**: 90–97.

9. Highley JR, Esiri MM, McDonald B, Cortina-Borja M, Herron BM, Crow TJ (1999) The size and fibre composition of the corpus callosum with respect to gender and schizophrenia: a post-mortem study. Brain **122**: 99–110.

10. **Azevedo FAC, Carvalho LRB, Grinberg LT, Farfel JM, Ferretti REL,** et al. (2009) Equal numbers of neuronal and nonneuronal cells make the human brain an isometrically scaled-up primate brain. J Comp Neurol **513**: 532–541.

11. **Walløe S, Pakkenberg B, Fabricius K** (2014) Stereological estimation of total cell numbers in the human cerebral cortex and cerebellum. Front Hum Neurosci **8**: 508.

12. **Bernardi L, Porta C, Casucci G, Balsamo R, Bernardi NF,** et al. (2009) Dynamic interactions between musical, cardiovascular, and cerebral rhythms in humans. Circulation **119**: 3171–3180.

13. **Strait D, Kraus N, Skoe E, Ashley R** (2009) Musical experience and neural efficiency—effects of training on subcortical processing of vocal expressions of emotion. Eur J Neurosci **29**: 661–668.

14. **Brimijoin WO, Akeroid MA** (2012) The role of head movements and signal spectrum in an auditory front/back illusion. Iperception **3**: 179–182.

15. **Moore BCJ** (2003) *An Introduction to the Psychology of Hearing* (5th edition). Academic Press, London, San Diego.

16. **Robertson D** (2009) Centrifugal control in mammalian hearing. Clin Exp Pharmacol Physiol **36**: 603–611.

17. **Todd N, Paillard PM, Kluk AC, Whittle E, Colebatch JG** (2014) Vestibular receptors contribute to cortical auditory evoked potentials. Hearing Res **309**: 63–74.

18. **Koelsch S** (2014) Brain correlates of music-evoked emotions. Nat Rev Neurosci **15**: 170–180.

19. **Woods DL, Alain C** (2009) Functional imaging of human auditory cortex. Curr Opin Otolaryngol Head Neck Surg **17**: 407–411.

20. **Da Costa S, van der Zwaag W, Marques JP, Frackowiak RSJ, Clarke S, Saenz M** (2011) Human primary auditory cortex follows the shape of Heschl's gyrus. J Neurosci **31**: 14067–14075.

21. **Moerel M, De Martino F, Formisano E** (2014) An anatomical and functional topography of human auditory cortical areas. Front Neurosci **8**: 225.

22. **Woods DL, Herron TJ, Cate AD, Yund EW, Steckler GC,** et al. (2010) Functional properties of human auditory cortical fields. Front Syst Neurosci **4**: 155.

23. **Clarke S, Morosan P** (2012) "Architecture, connectivity and transmitter receptors in human auditory cortex," in **D. Poeppel** et al., eds, *The Human Auditory Cortex* (Springer-Verlag, New York), 11–38.

24. **Leaver AM, Rauschecker JP** (2016) Functional topography of human auditory cortex. J Neurosci **36**: 1416–1428.

25. **Humphries C, Liebenthal E, Binder JR** (2010) Tonotopic organization of human auditory cortex. Neuroimage **50**: 1202–1211.

26. **Striem-Amit E, Hertz U, Amedi A** (2011) Extensive cochleotopic mapping of human auditory cortical fields obtained with phase-encoding fMRI. PLoS One **6**: e17832.

27. **Dick F, Taylor Tierney A, Lutti A, Josephs O, Sereno MI, Weiskopf N** (2012) In vivo functional and myeloarchitectonic mapping of human primary auditory areas. J Neurosci **32**: 16095–16105.

28. **Moerel M, De Martino F, Formisano E** (2012) Processing of natural sounds in human auditory cortex: tonotopy, spectral tuning, and relation to voice sensitivity. J Neurosci **32**: 14205–14216.

29. **Norman-Haignere S, Kanwisher N, McDermott JH** (2013) Cortical pitch regions in humans respond primarily to resolved harmonics and are located in specific tonotopic regions of anterior auditory cortex. J Neurosci **33**: 19451–19469.

30. **Da Costa S, Saenz M, Clarke S, van der Zwaag W** (2015) Tonotopic gradients in human primary auditory cortex: concurring evidence from high-resolution 7 T and 3 T fMRI. Brain Topogr **28**: 66–69.

31. **Patterson RD, Johnsrude IS** (2008) Functional imaging of the auditory processing applied to speech sounds. Philos Trans R Soc Lond B Biol Sci **363**: 1023–1035.

32. Liégeois-Chauvel C, Giraud K, Badier J-M, Marquis P, Chauvel P (2003) "Intracerebral evoked potentials in pitch perception reveal a functional asymmetry of human auditory cortex," in I. Peretz and R. L. Zatorre, eds, *The Cognitive Neuroscience of Music* (Oxford University Press, Oxford), 152–167.

33. Zatorre RJ, Gandour JT (2008) Neural specializations for speech and pitch: moving beyond the dichotomies. Philos Trans R Soc Lond B Biol Sci **363**: 1087–1104.

34. Saccuman MC, Scifo P (2009) "Using MRI to characterize the anatomy and function of the auditory cortex in infancy," in S. Dalla Bella et al., eds, *The Neurosciences and Music III— Disorders and Plasticity*, Ann NY Acad Sci **1169**: 297–307 (Wiley-Blackwell, Boston).

35. Zatorre RJ, Zarate JM (2012) "Cortical processing of music," in D. Poeppel, ed., *The Human Auditory Cortex* (Springer-Verlag, New York), 261–294.

36. Leaver AM, Rauschecker JP (2010) Cortical representation of natural complex sounds: effects of acoustic features and auditory object category. J Neurosci **30**: 7604–7612.

37. Santoro R, Moerel M, de Martino F, Goebel R, Ugurbil K, et al. (2014) Encoding of natural sounds at multiple spectral and temporal resolutions in the human auditory cortex. PLoS Comput Biol **10**: e10003412.

38. Rauschecker JP, Tian B (2000) Mechanisms and streams for processing "what" and "where" in auditory cortex. Proc Natl Acad Sci USA **97**: 11800–11808.

39. Humphries C, Sabri M, Lewis K, Liebenthal E (2014) Heirarchical organization of speech perception in human auditory cortex. Front Neurosci **8**: 406.

40. Mesgarani N, Cheung C, Johnson K, Chang EF (2014) Phonetic feature encoding in human superior temporal gyrus. Science **343**: 1006–1010.

41. Overath T, McDermott JH, Zarate JM, Poeppel D (2015) The cortical analysis of speech-specific temporal structure revealed by responses to sound quilts. Nat Neurosci **18**: 903–911.

42. DeWitt I, Rauschecker JP (2012) Phoneme and word recognition in the auditory ventral stream. Proc Natl Acad Sci USA **109**: E505–E514.

43. Lolli SL, Lewenstein AD, Basurto J, Winnik S, Loui P (2015) Sound frequency affects speech emotion perception: results from congenital amusia. Front Psychol **6**: 1340.

44. Rauschecker JP (2012) Ventral and dorsal streams in the evolution of speech and language. Front Evol Neurosci **4**: 7.

45. Norman-Haignere S, Kanwisher NG, McDermott JH (2015) Distinct cortical pathways for music and speech revealed by hypothesis-free voxel decomposition. Neuron **88**: 1281–1296.

46. Powell J (2010) *How Music Works*. Particular Books, London.

47. Savage PE, Brown S, Sakai E, Currie TE (2015) Statistical universals reveal the structures and functions of human music. Proc Natl Acad Sci USA **112**: 8987–8992.

48. Patel AD, Iversen JR (2014) The evolutionary neuroscience of musical beat perception: the Action Simulation for Auditory Prediction (ASAP) hypothesis. Front Syst Neurosci **8**: 57.

49. Oxenham AJ (2012) Pitch perception. J Neurosci **32**: 13335–13338.

50. Moerel M, De Martino F, Santoro R, Uqurbil K, Goebel R, et al. (2013) Processing of natural sounds: characterization of multipeak spectral tuning in human auditory cortex. J Neurosci **33**: 11888–11898.

51. Moerel M, De Martino F, Santoro R, Yacoub E, Formisano E (2015) Representation of pitch chroma by multi-peak spectral tuning in human auditory cortex. Neuroimage **106**: 161–169.

52. Wright AA, Rivera JJ, Hulse SH, Shyan M, Neiworth JJ (2000) Music perception and octave generalization in rhesus monkeys. J Exp Psychol Gen **129**: 291–307.

53. London J (2004) *Hearing in Time: Psychological Aspects of Musical Meter*. Oxford University Press, Oxford.

54. **Nozaradan S, Peretz I, Missal M, Mouraux A** (2011) Tagging the neuronal entrainment to beat and meter. J Neurosci **31**: 10234–10240.

55. **Patil K, Pressnitzer D, Shamma S, Elhilali M** (2012) Music in our ears: the biological basis of musical timbre perception. PLoS Comput Biol **8**: e1002759.

56. **Bigand E, Delbé C, Poulin-Charronnat B, Leman M, Tillmann B** (2014) Empirical evidence for musical syntax processing? Computer simulations reveal the contribution of auditory short-term memory. Front Syst Neurosci **8**: 94.

57. **Von Kriegstein K, Smith DRR, Patterson RD, Kiebel SJ, Griffiths TD** (2010) How the human brain recognizes speech in the context of changing speakers. J Neurosci **30**: 629–638.

58. **Meyer A** (1977) "The search for a morphological substrate in the brains of eminent persons including musicians: a historical review," in **M. Critchley** and **R. A. Henson**, eds, *Music and the Brain: Studies on the Neurology of Music* (Heinemann Medical Books Ltd, London), 255–282.

59. **Geschwind N, Levitsky W** (1968) Human brain: left-right asymmetries in temporal speech region. Science **161**: 186–187.

60. **Scheid P, Eccles JC** (1975) Music and speech: artistic functions of the human brain. Psych Music **3**: 21–35.

61. **Nelken I** (2011) Music and the auditory brain: where is the connection? Front Hum Neurosci **5**: 106.

62. **Sergent J, Zuck E, Terriah S, MacDonald B** (1992) Distributed neural network underlying musical sight-reading and keyboard performance. Science **257**: 106–109.

63. **Sacks O** (2008) *Musicophilia.* Vintage Books, New York.

64. **Scott DF** (1977) "Musicogenic epilepsy. (2) the later story: its relation to auditory hallucinatory phenomena," in **M. Critchley** and **R. A. Henson**, eds, *Music and the Brain: Studies on the Neurology of Music* (Heinemann Medical Books Ltd, London), 354–364.

65. **Peretz I, Cummings S, Dubé MP** (2007) The genetics of congenital amusia (tone deafness): a family aggregation study. Am J Hum Genet **81**: 582–588.

66. **Johnson JK, Graziano AB** (2003) August Knoblauch and amusia: a nineteenth-century cognitive model of music. Brain Cogn **51**: 102–114.

67. **Milner B** (1971) Interhemispheric differences in the localization of psychological processes in man. Br Med Bull **27**: 272–277.

68. **Liégeois-Chauvel C, Peretz I, Babaï M, Laguitton V, Chauvel P** (1998) Contribution of different cortical areas in the temporal lobes to music processing. Brain **121**: 1853–1867.

69. **Kohlmetz C, Müller SV, Nager W, Münte TF, Altenmüller E** (2003) Selective loss of timbre perception for keyboard and percussion instruments following a right temporal lesion. Neurocase **9**: 86–93.

70. **Damásio AR, Damásio H** (1977) "Musical faculty and cerebral dominance," in **M. Critchley** and **R. A. Henson**, eds, *Music and the Brain: Studies on the Neurology of Music* (Heinemann Medical Books Ltd, London), 141–155.

71. **Henson RA** (1977) "Neurological aspects of musical experience," in **M. Critchley** and **R. A. Henson**, eds, *Music and the Brain: Studies on the Neurology of Music* (Heinemann Medical Books Ltd, London), 3–21.

72. **Zatorre RJ** (1984) Musical perception and cerebral function: a critical review. Music Percept **2**: 196–221.

73. **Stewart L, von Kriegstein K, Warren JD, Griffiths TD** (2006) Music and the brain: disorders of musical listening. Brain **129**: 2533–2553.

74. **Benton AL** (1977) "The amusias," in **M. Critchley** and **R. A. Henson**, eds, *Music and the Brain: Studies on the Neurology of Music* (Heinemann Medical Books Ltd, London), 398–422.

75. **Ruiz E, Montañés P** (2005) "Music and the brain: Gershwin and Shebalin," in **J. Bogousslavsky** and **F. Boller,** eds, *Neurological Disorders in Famous Artists*, Front Neurol Neurosci **19**: 172–178 (Karger, Basel).

76. **Baeck E** (2005) "The terminal illness and last compositions of Maurice Ravel," in **J. Bogousslavsky** and **F. Boller,** eds, *Neurological Disorders in Famous Artists*, Front Neurol Neurosci **19**: 132–140 (Karger, Basel).

77. **Finke C, Esfahani NE, Ploner CJ** (2012) Preservation of musical memory in an amnesic professional cellist. Curr Biol **22**: R591–R592.

78. **Lanteaume L, Khalfa S, Régis J, Marquis P, Chauvel P, Bartolomei F** (2007) Emotion induction after direct intracerebral stimulation of human amygdala. Cereb Cortex **17**: 1307–1313.

79. **Jin J, Zelano C, Gottfired JA, Mohanty A** (2015) Human amygdala represents the complete spectrum of subjective valence. J Neurosci **35**: 15145–15156.

80. **Penfield W, Roberts L** (1959) *Speech and Brain Mechanisms.* Princeton University Press, Princeton NJ.

81. **Engel AK, Moll CKE, Fried I, Ojemann GA** (2005) Invasive recordings from the human brain: clinical insights and beyond. Nat Rev **6**: 35–47.

82. **Penfield W, Perot P** (1963) The brain's record of auditory and visual experience. Brain **86**: 595–696.

83. **Kanai R, Rees G** (2011) The structural basis of inter-individual differences in human behaviour and cognition. Nat Rev Neurosci **12**: 231–242.

84. **Van Essen DC, Glasser MF, Dierker DL, Harwell J, Coalson T** (2012) Parcellations and hemispheric asymmetries of human cerebral cortex analyzed on surface-based atlases. Cereb Cortex **22**: 2241–2262.

85. **Schwarzkopf DS, Song C, Rees G** (2011) The surface area of human V1 predicts the subjective experience of object size. Nat Neurosci **14**: 28–30.

86. **Schwarzkopf DS, Rees G** (2013) Subjective size perception depends on central visual cortical magnification in human v1. PLoS One **8**: e60550.

87. **Button KS, Ioannidis JPA, Mokrysz C, Nosel BA, Flint J,** et al. (2013) Power failure: why small sample size undermines the reliability of neuroscience. Nat Neurosci **14**: 365–376.

88. **Chen JL, Kumar S, Williamson VJ, Scholz J, Griffiths TD, Stewart L** (2015) Detection of the arcuate fasciculus in congenital amusia depends on the tractography algorithm. Front Psychol **6**: 9.

89. **Buckner RL, Krienen FM, Yeo BTT** (2013) Opportunities and limitations of intrinsic functional connectivity MRI. Nat Neurosci **16**: 832–837.

90. **Wang D, Buckner RL, Liu H** (2014) Functional specialization in the human brain estimated by intrinsic hemispheric interaction. J Neurosci **34**: 12341–12352.

91. **Yakunina N, Kang EK, Kim TS, Min JH, Kim SS, Nam EC** (2015) Effects of scanner acoustic noise on intrinsic brain activity during auditory stimulation. Neuroradiology **57**: 1063–1073.

92. **Kocak M, Ulmer JL, Biswal BB, Aralasmak A, Daniels DL, Mark LP** (2005) The influence of gender on auditory and language cortical activation patterns: preliminary data. AJNR Am J Neuroradiol **26**: 2248–2255.

93. **Schleim S, Roiser JP** (2009) fMRI in translation: the challenges facing real-world applications. Front Hum Neurosci **3**: 63.

94. **Ojemann GA, Corina DP, Corrigan N, Schoenfield-McNeill J, Poliakov A,** et al. (2010) Neuronal correlates of functional magnetic resonance imaging in human temporal cortex. Brain **133**: 46–59.

95. **Conner CR, Ellmore TM, Pieters TA, DiSano MA, Tandon N** (2011) Variability of the relationship between electrophysiology and BOLD-fMRI across cortical regions in humans. J Neurosci **31**: 12855–12865.

96. Mishra AM, Ellens DJ, Schridde U, Motelow JE, Purcaro MJ, et al. (2011) Where fMRI and electrophysiology agree to disagree: corticothalamic and striatal activity patterns in the WAG/Rij rat. J Neurosci **31**: 15053–15064.

97. Griffiths TD, Hall DA (2012) Mapping pitch representation in neural ensembles with fMRI. J Neurosci **32**: 13343–13347.

98. Soares JM, Marques P, Alves V, Sousa N (2013) A hitchhiker's guide to diffusion tensor imaging. Front Neurosci **7**: 31.

99. Swettenham JB, Muthukumaraswamy SD, Singh KD (2013) BOLD responses in human primary visual cortex are insensitive to substantial changes in neural activity. Front Cell Neurosci **7**: 76.

100. Stelzer J, Lohmann G, Mueller K, Buschmann T, Turner R (2014) Deficient approaches to human neuroimaging. Front Hum Neurosci **8**: 462.

101. Logothetis NK (2008) What we can do and what we cannot do with fMRI. Nature **453**: 869–878.

102. Vanzetta I, Slovine H (2010) A BOLD assumption. Front Neuroenergetics **2**: 1–4.

103. Vartiainen J, Liljeström M, Koskinen M, Renvall H, Salmelin R (2011) Functional magnetic resonance imaging blood oxygenation level-dependent signal and magnetoencephalography evoked responses yield different neural functionality in reading. J Neurosci **31**: 1048–1058.

104. Gurden H (2013) Astrocytes: can they be the missing stars linking neuronal activity to neurofunctional imaging signals? Front Cell Neurosci **7**: 21.

105. Caggiano V, Pomper JK, Fleischer F, Fogassi L, Giese M, Their P (2013) Mirror neurons in monkey F5 do not adapt to the observation of repeated actions. Nat Commun **4**: 1433.

106. Angenstein F, Kammerer E, Scheich H (2009) The BOLD response in the rat hippocampus depends rather on local processing of signals than on the input or output activity. A combined functional MRI and electrophysiological study. J Neurosci **29**: 2428–2439.

107. Carp J (2012) The secret lives of experiments: methods reporting in the fMRI literature. Neuroimage **63**: 289–300.

108. David SP, Ware JJ, Chu IM, Loftus PD, Fusar-Poli P, et al. (2013) Potential reporting bias in fMRI studies of the brain. PLoS One **8**: e70104.

109. Hupé J-M, Dojat M (2015) A critical review of the neuroimaging literature on synesthesia. Front Hum Neurosci **9**: 103.

110. Peretz I, Coltheart (2003) Modularity of music processing. Nat Neurosci **6**: 688–691.

111. Koelsch S (2011) Towards a neural basis of music perception—a review and updated model. Front Psychol **2**: 1–20.

112. Koelsch S (2012) *Brain and Music*. Wiley Blackwell, Chichester, UK.

113. Janata P, Tomic ST, Rakowski SK (2007) Characterization of music-evoked autobiographical memories. Memory **15**: 845–860.

114. Janata P (2009) The neural architecture of music-evoked autobiographical memories. Cereb Cortex **19**: 2579–2594.

115. Sloboda J (2008) Science and music: the ear of the beholder. Nature **454**: 32–33.

116. Levitin DJ, Tirovolas AK (2009) Current advances in the cognitive neuroscience of music. Ann N Y Acad Sci **1156**: 211–231.

117. Schmithorst VJ, Holland SK (2003) The effect of musical training on music processing: a functional magnetic resonance imaging study in humans. Neurosci Lett **348**: 65–68.

118. Schlaug G, Jäncke L, Huang Y, Staiger JF, Steinmetz H (1995) Increased corpus callosum size in musicians. Neuropsychologia **33**: 1047–1055.

119. Schlaug G, Jäncke L, Huang Y, Steinmetz H (1995) In vivo evidence of structural brain asymmetry in musicians. Science **267**: 699–701.

120. **Ohnishi T, Matsuda H, Asada T, Aruga M, Hirakata M**, et al. (2001) Functional anatomy of musical perception in musicians. Cereb Cortex **11**: 754–760.

121. **Bermudez P, Lerch JP, Evans AC, Zatorre RJ** (2009) Neuroanatomical correlates of musicianship as revealed by cortical thickness and voxel-based morphometry. Cereb Cortex **19**: 1583–1596.

122. **Oechslin MS, Imfeld A, Loenneker T, Meyer M, Jäncke L** (2010) The plasticity of the superior longitudinal fasciculus as a function of musical expertise: a diffusion tensor imaging study. Front Hum Neurosci **3**: 76.

123. **Wilson SJ, Abbott DF, Lusher D, Gentle EC, Jackson GD** (2011) Finding your voice: a singing lesson from functional imaging. Hum Brain Mapp **32**: 2115–2130.

124. **Platel H, Price C, Baron JC, Wise R, Lambert J**, et al. (1997) The structural components of music perception: a functional anatomical study. Brain **120**: 229–243.

125. **Patterson RD, Uppenkamp S, Johnsrude IS, Griffiths T** (2002) The processing of temporal pitch and melody information in auditory cortex. Neuron **36**: 767–776.

126. **Peretz I, Zatorre RL** (2003) *The Cognitive Neuroscience of Music*. Oxford University Press, Oxford.

127. **Peretz I, Zatorre RL** (2005) Brain organization for music processing. Annu Rev Psychol **56**: 89–114.

128. **Janata P, Parsons LM** (2013) "Neural mechanisms of music, singing and dancing," in **M. A. Arbib**, ed., *Language, Music and the Brain: A Mysterious Relationship* (MIT Press, Cambridge MA), 307–328.

129. **Lappe C, Steinsträter O, Pantev C** (2013) Rhythmic and melodic deviations in musical sequences recruit different cortical areas for mismatch detection. Front Hum Neurosci **7**: 260.

130. **Tramo MJ, Cariani PA, Koh CK, Makris N, Braida LD** (2005) Neurophysiology and neuroanatomy of pitch perception: auditory cortex. Ann N Y Acad Sci **1060**: 148–174.

131. **Johnsrude IS, Penhune VB, Zatorre RJ** (2000) Functional specificity in the right human auditory cortex for perceiving pitch direction. Brain **123**: 155–163.

132. **Griffiths TD** (2012) Cortical mechanisms for pitch representation. J Neurosci **32**: 13333–13334.

133. **Wang X, Walker KMM** (2012) Neural mechanisms for the abstraction and use of pitch information in auditory cortex. J Neurosci **32**: 13339–13342.

134. **Norman-Haignere SV, Albouy P, Caclin A, McDermott JH, Kanwisher NG, Tillmann B** (2016) Pitch-responsive cortical regions in congenital amusia. J Neurosci **36**: 2986–2994.

135. **Pantev C, Hoke M, Lütkenhöner B, Lehnertz K** (1989) Tonotopic organization of the auditory cortex: pitch versus frequency representation. Science **246**: 486–488.

136. **Penagos H, Melcher JR, Oxenham AJ** (2004) A neural representation of pitch salience in nonprimary human auditory cortex revealed with functional magnetic resonance imaging. J Neurosci **24**: 6810–6815.

137. **Hall DA, Edmonson-Jones AM, Fridriksson J** (2006) Periodicity and frequency coding in human auditory cortex. Eur J Neurosci **24**: 3601–3610.

138. **Barker D, Plack CJ, Hall DA** (2012) Reexamining the evidence for a pitch sensitive region: a human fMRI study using iterated ripple noise. Cereb Cortex **22**: 745–753.

139. **Bendor D, Osmanski MS, Wang X** (2012) Dual-pitch processing mechanisms in primate auditory cortex. J Neurosci **32**: 16149–16161.

140. **Song X, Osmanski MS, Guo Y, Wang X** (2015) Complex pitch perception mechanisms are shared by humans and a New World monkey. Proc Natl Acad Sci USA **113**: 781–786.

141. **Warren JD, Uppenkamp S, Patterson R, Griffiths T** (2003) Separating pitch chroma and pitch height in the human brain. Proc Natl Acad Sci USA **100**: 10038–10042.

142. **Hyde KL, Peretz I, Zatorre RJ** (2008) Evidence for the role of the right auditory cortex in fine pitch discrimination. Neuropsychologia **46**: 632–639.

143. **Foster NEV, Zatorre RJ** (2010) Cortical structure predicts success in performing musical transformational judgements. Neuroimage **53**: 26–36.

144. **Peretz I, Gosselin N, Belin P, Zatorre RJ, Plailly J, Tillmann B** (2009) "Musical lexical networks: the cortical organization of music recognition," in **S. Dalla Bella** et al., eds, *The Neurosciences and Music III—Disorders and Plasticity*, Ann NY Acad Sci **1169**: 256–265 (Wiley-Blackwell, Boston).

145. **Menon V, Levitin DJ, Smith BK, Lembke A, Krasnow BD**, et al. (2002) Neural correlates of timbre change in harmonic sounds. Neuroimage **17**: 1742–1754.

146. **Keenan J, Thangarai V, Halpern A, Schlaug G** (2001) Absolute pitch and planum temporale. Neuroimage **14**: 1402–1408.

147. **Zatorre RJ** (2003) Absolute pitch: a model for understanding the influence of genes and development on neural and cognitive function. Nat Neurosci **6**: 692–695.

148. **Loui P, Li HC, Hohmann A, Schlaug G** (2011) Enhanced cortical connectivity in absolute pitch musicians: a model for local hyperconnectivity. J Cogn Neurosci **23**: 1015–1026.

149. **Baddeley A** (2003) Working memory: looking back and looking forward. Nat Rev Neurosci **4**: 29–39.

150. **Gaab N, Schulz K, Ozdemir E, Schlaug G** (2006) Neural correlates of absolute pitch differ between blind and sighted musicians. Neuroreport **17**: 1853–1857.

151. **Cameron DJ, Bentley J, Grahn JA** (2015) Cross-cultural influences on rhythm processing: reproduction, discrimination, and beat tapping. Front Psychol **6**: 366.

152. **Felix II RA, Fridberger A, Leijon S, Berrebi AS, Magnusson AK** (2011) Sound rhythms are encoded by postinhibitory rebound spiking in the superior paraolivary nucleus. J Neurosci **31**: 12566–12578.

153. **Tierney A, Kraus N** (2013) The ability to move to a beat is linked to the consistency of neural responses to sound. J Neurosci **33**: 14981–14988.

154. **Hove MJ, Schwartze M** (2014) Deconstructing the ability to move to a beat. J Neurosci **34**: 2403–2405.

155. **Geiser E, Ziegler E, Jancke L, Meyer M** (2009) Early electrophysiological correlates of meter and rhythm processing in music perception. Cortex **45**: 93–102.

156. **Thaut MH, Trimarchi PD, Parsons LM** (2014) Human brain basis of musical rhythm perception: common and distinct neural substrates for meter, tempo, and pattern. Brain Sci **4**: 428–452.

157. **Grahn JA, Rowe JB** (2013) Finding and feeling the musical beat: striatal dissociations between detection and prediction of regularity. Cereb Cortex **23**: 913–921.

158. **Konoike N, Kotozaki Y, Miyachi S, Miyauchi CM, Yomogida Y**, et al. (2012) Rhythm information represented in the fronto-parieto-cerebellar motor system. Neuroimage **63**: 328–338.

159. **Zatorre RJ, Chen JL, Penhune VB** (2007) When the brain plays music: auditory-motor interactions in music perception and production. Nat Rev **8**: 547–558.

160. **Chen JL, Penhune VB, Zatorre RJ** (2008) Listening to musical rhythms recruits motor regions of the brain. Cereb Cortex **18**: 2844–2854.

161. **Bengtsson SL, Ullén F, Ehrsson HH, Hashimoto T, Kito T**, et al. (2009) Listening to rhythms activates motor and premotor cortices. Cortex **45**: 62–71.

162. **Grahn JA, Rowe JB** (2009) Feeling the beat: premotor and striatal interactions in musicians and nonmusicians during beat perception. J Neurosci **29**: 7540–7548.

163. **Thaut MH, Stephan KM, Wunderlich G, Schicks W, Tellman L**, et al. (2009) Distinct cortico-cerebellar activations in rhythmic auditory motor synchronization. Cortex **45**: 44–53.

164. **Kung SJ, Chen JL, Zatorre RJ, Penhune VB** (2013) Interacting cortical and basal ganglia networks underlying finding and tapping to the musical beat. J Cogn Neurosci **25**: 401–420.

165. Angulo-Perkins A, Aubé W, Peretz I, Barios FA, Armony JL, Concha L (2014) Music listening engages specific cortical regions within the temporal lobes: differences between musicians and non-musicians. Cortex **59**: 126–137.

166. Ellis RJ, Bruijn B, Norton AC, Winner E, Schlaug G (2013) Training-mediated leftward asymmetries during music processing: a cross-sectional and longitudinal fMRI analysis. Neuroimage **75**: 97–107.

167. Leonard CM, Puranik C, Kuldau JM, Lombardino LJ (1998) Normal variation in the frequency and location of human auditory cortex landmarks. Heschl's gyrus: where is it? Cereb Cortex **8**: 397–406.

168. Wong PCM, Warrier CM, Penhune VB, Roy AK, Sadehh A, et al. (2008) Volume of left Heschl's gyrus and linguistic pitch learning. Cereb Cortex **18**: 828–836.

169. Warrier C, Wong P, Penhune V, Zatorre R, Parrish T, et al. (2009) Relating structure to function: Heschl's gyrus and acoustic processing. J Neurosci **29**: 61–69.

170. Hill J, Dierker D, Neil J, Inder T, Knutsen A, et al. (2010) A surface-based analysis of hemispheric asymmetries and folding of cerebral cortex in term-born human infants. J Neurosci **30**: 2268–2276.

171. Glasel H, Leroy F, Dubois J, Hertz-Pannier L, Mangin JF, Dehaene-Lambertz G (2011) A robust asymmetry in the infant brain: the rightward superior temporal sulcus. Neuroimage **58**: 716–723.

172. Seither-Preisler A, Parncutt R, Schneider P (2014) Size and synchronization of auditory cortex promotes musical, literacy and attentional skills in children. J Neurosci **34**: 10937–10949.

173. Gu J, Kanai R (2014) What contributes to individual differences in brain structure? Front Hum Neurosci **8**: 262.

174. Omar R, Hailstone JC, Warren JE, Crutch SJ, Warren JD (2010) The cognitive organization of music knowledge: a clinical analysis. Brain **133**: 1200–1213.

175. Peretz I (2006) The nature of music from a biological perspective. Cognition **100**: 1–32.

176. Hyde KL, Zatorre RJ, Griffiths TD, Lerch JP, Peretz I (2006) Morphometry of the amusic brain: a two-site study. Brain **129**: 2562–2570.

177. Hyde KL, Lerch JP, Zatorre RJ, Griffiths TD, Evans AC, Peretz I (2007) Cortical thickness in congenital amusia: when less is better than more. J Neurosci **21**: 13028–13032.

178. Albouy P, Mattout J, Bouet R, Maby E, Sanchez G, et al. (2013) Impaired pitch perception and memory in congenital amusia: the deficit starts in the auditory cortex. Brain **136**: 1639–1661.

179. Mandell J, Schulze K, Schlaug G (2007) Congenital amusia: an auditory-motor feedback disorder? Restor Neurol Neurosci **25**: 323–334.

180. Loui P, Alsop D, Schlaug G (2009) Tone deafness: a new disconnection syndrome? J Neurosci **29**: 10215–10220.

181. Zendel BR, Lagrois M-E, Robitaille N, Peretz I (2015) Attending to pitch information inhibits processing of pitch information: the curious case of amusia. J Neurosci **35**: 3815–3824.

182. Moreau P, Jolicœur P, Peretz I (2013) Pitch discrimination without awareness in congenital amusia: evidence from event-related potentials. Brain Cogn **81**: 337–344.

183. Williamson VJ, Stewart L (2010) Memory for pitch in congenital amusia: beyond a fine-grained pitch discrimination problem. Memory **18**: 657–669.

184. Peretz I, Brattico E, Järvenpää M, Tervaniemi M (2009) The amusic brain: in tune, out of key, and unaware. Brain **132**: 1277–1286.

185. Hutchins S, Peretz I (2012) Amusics can imitate what they cannot discriminate. Brain Lang **123**: 234–239.

186. **Thompson WF, Marin MM, Stewart L** (2012) Reduced sensitivity to emotional prosody in congenital amusia rekindles the musical protolanguage hypothesis. Proc Natl Acad Sci USA **109**: 19027–19032.

187. **Eyler LT, Pierce K, Courchesne E** (2012) A failure of left temporal cortex to specialize for language is an early emerging and fundamental property of autism. Brain **135**: 949–960.

188. **Lichtman JW, Sanes JR, Livet J** (2008) A technicolour approach to the connectome. Nat Rev Neurosci **9**: 417–422.

189. **Sörös P, Sokoloff LG, Bose A, McIntosh AR, Graham SJ, Stuss DT** (2006) Clustered functional MRI of overt speech production. Neuroimage **32**: 376–387.

190. **Guediche S, Holt LL, Laurent P, Lim S-J, Fiez JA** (2015) Evidence for cerebellar contributions to adaptive plasticity in speech perception. Cereb Cortex **25**: 1867–1877.

191. **Keren-Happuch E, Chen SH, Ho MH, Desmond JE** (2014) A meta-analysis of cerebellar contributions to higher cognition from PET and fMRI studies. Hum Brain Mapp **35**: 593–615.

192. **Buckner RL** (2013) The cerebellum and cognitive function: 25 years of insight from anatomy and neuroimaging. Neuron **80**: 807–815.

193. **Bogousslavsky J, Assal G** (2010) "Stendhal's aphasic spells: the first report of transient ischemic attacks followed by stroke," in H. **Bogousslavsky** and B. **Bäzner**, eds, *Neurological Disorders in Famous Artists—Part 3*, Front Neurol Neurosci **27**: 130–142 (Karger, Basel).

194. **Cogan GB, Thesen T, Carlson C, Doyle W, Devinsky O, Pesaran B** (2014) Sensory-motor transformations for speech occur bilaterally. Nature **507**: 94–98.

195. **Fadiga LK, Craighero L, D'Ausilio A** (2009) "Broca's area in language, action, and music," in S. **Dalla Bella** et al., eds, *The Neurosciences and Music III—Disorders and Plasticity*, Ann N Y Acad Sci **1169**: 448–458 (Wiley-Blackwell, Boston).

196. **Shtyrov Y, Osswald K, Pulvermüller F** (2008) Memory traces for spoken words in the brain as revealed by the hemodynamic correlate of the mismatch negativity. Brain **18**: 29–37.

197. **Perani D, Saccuman MC, Scifo P, Anwander A, Spada D,** et al. (2011) Neural language networks at birth. Proc Natl Acad Sci USA **108**: 16056–16061.

198. **Friederici AD** (2009) Pathways to language: fiber tracts in the human brain. Trends Cogn Sci **13**: 175–181.

199. **Rilling JK, Glasser MF, Preuss TM, Ma X, Zhao T,** et al. (2008) The evolution of the arcuate fasciculus revealed with comparative DTI. Nat Neurosci **11**: 426–428.

200. **Somers M, Ophoff RA, Aukes MF, Cantor RM, Boks MP,** et al. (2015) Linkage analysis in a Dutch population isolate shows no major gene for left-handedness or atypical language lateralization. J Neurosci **35**: 8730–8736.

201. **Kaiser A, Haller S, Schmitz S, Nitsch C** (2009) On sex/gender related similarities and differences in fMRI language research. Brain Res Rev **61**: 49–59.

202. **Ressel V, Pallier C, Ventura-Campos N, Díaz B, Roessler A,** et al. (2012) An effect of bilingualism on the auditory cortex. J Neurosci **32**: 16597–16601.

203. **O'Muircheartaigh J, Dean DC 3rd, Dirks H, Waskiewicz N, Lehman K,** et al. (2013) Interactions between white matter asymmetry and language during neurodevelopment. J Neurosci **33**: 16170–16177.

204. **Kovelman I, Shalinsky MH, White KS, Schmitt SN, Berens M,** et al. (2009) Dual language use in sign-speech bimodal linguals: fNIRS brain-imaging evidence. Brain Lang **109**: 112–123.

205. **Cao F, Tao R, Liu L, Perfetti CA, Booth JR** (2013) High proficiency in a second language is characterized by greater involvement of the first language network: evidence from Chinese learners of English. J Cogn Neurosci **25**: 1649–1663.

206. **Shannon RV** (2005) Speech and music have different requirements for spectral resolution. Int Rev Neurobiol **70**: 121–134.

207. **Shannon RV, Zeng F-G, Kamath V, Wygonski J, Ekelid M** (1995) Speech recognition with primarily temporal cues. Science **270**: 303–304.

208. **Warren JD, Jennings AR, Griffiths TD** (2005) Analysis of the spectral envelope of sounds by the human brain. Neuroimage **24**: 1052–1057.

209. **Zatorre RJ, Belin P** (2001) Spectral and temporal processing in human auditory cortex. Cereb Cortex **11**: 946–953.

210. **McDermott HJ** (2004) Music perception with cochlear implants: a review. Trends Amplif **8**: 49–82.

211. **Hopyan T, Peretz I, Chan LP, Papsin BC, Gordon KA** (2012) Children using cochlear implants capitalize on acoustical hearing for musical perception. Front Psychol **3**: 425.

212. **Asaridou SS, McQueen JM** (2013) Speech and music shape the listening brain: evidence for shared domain-general mechanisms. Front Psychol **4**: 321.

213. **Zarate JM** (2013) The neural control of singing. Front Hum Neurosci **7**: 237.

Chapter Three

1. **Pinker S** (1994) *The Language Instinct*. Penguin, London, New York.

2. **Collins CE, Leitch DB, Wong P, Kaas JH, Herculano-Houzel S** (2013) Faster scaling of visual neurons in cortical areas relative to subcortical structures in non-human primate brains. Brain Struct Funct **218**: 805–816.

3. **Wong P, Peebles JK, Asplund CL, Collins CE, Herculano-Houzel S, Kaas JH** (2013) Faster scaling of auditory neurons in cortical areas relative to subcortical structures in primate brains. Brain Behav Evol **81**: 209–218.

4. **Herculano-Houzel S, Kaas JH, de Oliveira-Souza R** (2016) Corticalization of motor control in humans is a consequence of brain scaling in primate evolution. J Comp Neurol **524**: 448–455.

5. **Herculano-Houzel S** (2012) The remarkable, yet not extraordinary, human brain as a scaled-up primate brain and its associated cost. Proc Natl Acad Sci USA **109**: 10661–10668.

6. **Deaner RO, Isler K, Burkart J, van Schaik C** (2007) Overall brain size, and not encephalization quotient, best predicts cognitive ability across non-human primates. Brain Behav Evol **70**: 115–124.

7. **Dunbar RIM, Shultz S** (2007) Understanding primate brain evolution. Philos Trans R Soc Lond B Biol Sci **362**: 649–658.

8. **Hublin JJ, Neubauer S, Gunz P** (2015) Brain ontogeny and life history in Pleistocene hominins. Philos Trans R Soc Lond B Biol Sci **370**: 20140062.

9. **DeFelipe J** (2011) The evolution of the brain, the human nature of cortical circuits, and intellectual creativity. Front Neuroanat **5**: 29.

10. **Walløe S, Pakkenberg B, Fabricius K** (2014) Stereological estimation of total cell numbers in the human cerebral cortex and cerebellum. Front Hum Neurosci **8**: 508.

11. **Gabi M, Collins CE, Wong P, Torres LB, Kaas JH, Herculano-Houzel S** (2010) Cellular scaling rules for the brains of an extended number of primate species. Brain Behav Evol **76**: 32–44.

12. **Buckner RL, Krienen FM** (2013) The evolution of distributed association networks in the human brain. Trends Cogn Sci **17**: 648–665.

13. **Herculano-Houzel S, Kaas J** (2011) Gorilla and orangutan brains conform to the primate cellular scaling rules: implications for human evolution. Brain Behav Evol **77**: 33–44.

14. **Pearce E, Stringer C, Dunbar RIM** (2013) New insights into differences in brain organization between Neanderthals and anatomically modern humans. Proc Roy Soc Lond B Biol Sci **280**: 2013.0168.

15. **Gil-de-Costa R, Hauser MD** (2006) Vervet monkeys and humans show brain asymmetries for processing conspecific vocalizations, but with opposite patterns of laterality. Proc Biol Sci 22: 2313–2318.

16. **Smaers JB, Steele J, Case CR, Cowper A, Maunts K, Zilles K** (2011) Primate prefrontal cortex evolution: human brains are the extreme of a lateralized ape trend. Brain Behav Evol 77: 67–78.

17. **Benitez-Burraco A, Longa VM** (2012) Right-handedness, lateralization and language in Neanderthals: a comment on Frayer et al. (2010). J Anthropol Sci 90: 1–6.

18. **Estalrrich A, Rosas A** (2013) Handedness in Neanderthals from the El Sidron (Asturias, Spain): evidence from instrumental striations with ontogenetic inferences. PLoS One 8: e62797.

19. **Frayer DW, Fiore I, Lalueza-Fox C, Radovcic J, Bondioli L** (2010) Right handed Neanderthals: Vindija and beyond. J Anthropol Sci 8: 113–127.

20. **Cogan GB, Thesen T, Carlson C, Doyle W, Devinsky O, Pesaran B** (2014) Sensory-motor transformations for speech occur bilaterally. Nature 507: 94–98.

21. **Simonyan K, Fuertinger S** (2015) Speech networks at rest and in action: interactions between functional brain networks controlling speech production. J Neurophysiol 113: 2967–2978.

22. **Good CD, Johnsrude I, Ashburner J, Henson RN, Friston KJ, Frackowiak RS** (2001) Cerebral asymmetry and the effects of sex and handedness on brain structure: a voxel-based morphometric analysis of 465 normal adult human brains. Neuroimage 14: 685–700.

23. **Lindenberg R, Fangerau H, Seitz RJ** (2007) "Broca's area" as a collective term? Brain Lang 102: 22–29.

24. **Van Essen DC, Glasser MF, Dierker DL, Harwell J, Coalson T** (2012) Parcellations and hemispheric asymmetries of human cerebral cortex analyzed on surface-based atlases. Cereb Cortex 22: 2241–2262.

25. **Sun T, Walsh CA** (2006) Molecular approaches to brain asymmetry and handedness. Nat Rev Neurosci 7: 655–662.

26. **Keller SS, Robert N, Hopkins W** (2009) A comparative magnetic resonance imaging study of the anatomy, variability, and asymmetry of Broca's area in the human and chimpanzee brain. J Neurosci 29: 14607–14616.

27. **Anderson B, Southern BD, Powers RE** (1999) Anatomic asymmetries of the posterior superior temporal lobes: a post-mortem study. Neuropsychiatry Neuropsychol Behav Neurol 12: 247–254.

28. **Loui P, Li HC, Hohmann A, Schlaug G** (2011) Enhanced cortical connectivity in absolute pitch musicians: a model for local hyperconnectivity. J Cogn Neurosci 23: 1015–1026.

29. **Penhune VB, Zatorre RJ, MacDonald JD, Evans AC** (1996) Interhemispheric anatomical differences in human primary auditory cortex: probabilistic mapping and volume measurement from magnetic resonance scans. Cereb Cortex 6: 661–672.

30. **Rilling JK, Glasser MF, Preuss TM, Ma X, Zhao T,** et al. (2008) The evolution of the arcuate fasciculus revealed with comparative DTI. Nat Neurosci 11: 426–428.

31. **Fonseca-Azevedo K, Herculano-Houzel S** (2012) Metabolic constraint imposes tradeoff between body size and number of brain neurons in human evolution. Proc Natl Acad Sci USA 109: 18571–18576.

32. **Navarrete A, van Schaik CP, Isler K** (2011) Energetics and the evolution of human brain size. Nature 480: 91–94.

33. **Stout D, Toth N, Schick K, Chaminade T** (2009) Neural correlates of Early Stone Age toolmaking: technology, language and cognition in human evolution. Philos Trans R Soc Lond B Biol Sci 363: 1939–1949.

34. **Herculano-Houzel S** (2015) Decreasing sleep requirement with increasing numbers of neurons as a driver for bigger brains and bodies in mammalian evolution. Proc Biol Sci 282: 20151853.

35. **Williams CL** (2008) Food for thought: brain, genes, and nutrition. Brain Res Bull **1237**: 1–4.

36. **Kuzawa CW, Chugani HT, Grossman LI, Lipovich L, Muzik O**, et al. (2014) Metabolic costs and evolutionary implications of human brain development. Proc Natl Acad Sci USA **111**: 13010–13015.

37. **Barnes SK, Ozanne SE** (2011) Pathways linking the early environment to long-term health and lifespan. Prog Biophys Mol Biol **106**: 323–336.

38. **Whitehouse AJO, Holt BJ, Serralha M, Holt PG, Kusel MMH, Hart PH** (2012) Maternal vitamin D levels during pregnancy and offspring neurocognitive development. Pediatrics **129**: 485–493.

39. **Stringer C** (2012) *Lone Survivors: How We Came to Be the Only Humans on Earth*. Griffin, New York.

40. **Sherwood CC, Subiaul F, Zawidzki TWl** (2008) A natural history of the human mind: tracing evolutionary changes in brain and cognition. J Anat **212**: 426–454.

41. **Rosenberg J, Tunney RJ** (2008) Human vocabulary use as display. Evol Psychol **6**: 538–549.

42. **Plotkin H** (1998) *Evolution in Mind: An Introduction to Evolutionary Psychology*. Harvard University Press, Cambridge MA.

43. **Noonan JP, Coop G, Kudaravalli S, Smith D, Krause J**, et al. (2006) Sequencing and analysis of Neanderthal genomic DNA. Science **314**: 1113–1118.

44. **Langergraber KE, Prüfer K, Rowney C, Boesch C, Crockford C**, et al. (2012) Generation times in wild chimpanzees and gorillas suggest earlier divergence times in great ape and human evolution. Proc Natl Acad Sci USA **109**: 15716–15721.

45. **Walter C** (2013) *Last Ape Standing*. Walker Publishing Company Inc, New York.

46. **Scharff C, Petri J** (2011) Evo-devo, deep homology and FoxP2: implications for the evolution of speech and language. Philos Trans R Soc Lond B Biol Sci **366**: 2124–2140.

47. **Dennett DC** (2006) *Kinds of Minds: Towards an Understanding of Consciousness*. Weidenfeld & Nicholson, London.

48. **Fisher SE** (2006) Tangled webs: tracing the connections between genes and cognition. Cognition **101**: 270–297.

49. **Xue Y, Wang Q, Long Q, Ng BL, Swerdlow H**, et al. (2009) Human Y chromosome base-substitution mutation rate measured by direct sequencing in a deep-rooting pedigree. Curr Biol **19**: 1453–1457.

50. **Gould SJ, Eldredge N** (1993) Punctuated equilibrium comes of age. Nature **366**: 223–227.

51. **Bateson P** (2006) "The Nests's Tale: affectionate disgreements with Richard Dawkins," in **A. Grafen** and **M. Ridley**, eds, *Richard Dawkins: How a Scientist Changed the Way We Think* (Oxford University Press, Oxford), 164–175.

52. **Chiaroni J, Underhill PA, Cavalli-Sforza LL** (2009) Y chromosome diversity, human expansion, drift, and cultural evolution. Proc Natl Acad Sci USA **106**: 20174–20179.

53. **Donald M** (1991) *Origins of the Modern Mind*. Harvard University Press, Cambridge MA.

54. **Finlay BL, Darlington RB** (1995) Linked regularities in the development and evolution of mammalian brains. Science **268**(5217): 1578–1584.

55. **de Winter W, Oxnard CE** (2001) Evolutionary radiations and convergences in the structural organization of mammalian brains. Nature **409**: 710–714.

56. **Sherwood CC, Stimpson CD, Raghanti MA, Wildman DE, Uddin M**, et al. (2006) Evolution of increased glia-neuron ratios in the human frontal cortex. Proc Natl Acad Sci USA **103**: 13606–13611.

57. **Van Essen DC, Glasser MF, Dierker DL, Harwell J** (2012) Cortical parcellation of the Macaque monkey analyzed on surface-based atlases. Cereb Cortex **22**: 2227–2240.

58. **Passingham RE, Smaers JB** (2014) Is the prefrontal cortex especially enlarged in the human brain? Allometric relations and remapping factors. Brain Behav Evol **84**: 156–166.

59. Semendeferi K, Teffer K, Buxhoeveden DP, Park MS, Bludau S, et al. (2011) Spatial organization of neurons in the frontal pole sets humans apart from great apes. Cereb Cortex **21**: 1485–1497.

60. Spocter MA, Hopkins WD, Barks SK, Bianchi S, Hehmeyer AE, et al. (2012) Neuropil distribution in the cerebral cortex differs between humans and chimpanzees. J Comp Neurol **520**: 2917–2929.

61. Bianchi S, Stimpson CD, Bauernfeind AL, Schapiro SJ, Baze WB, et al. (2013) Dendritic morphology of pyramidal neurons in the Chimpanzee neocortex: regional specializations and comparison to humans. Cereb Cortex **23**: 2429–2436.

62. Teffer K, Buxhoeveden DP, Stimpson CD, Fobbs AJ, Schapiro SJ, et al. (2013) Developmental changes in the spatial organization of neurons in the neocortex of humans and common chimpanzees. J Comp Neurol **521**: 4249–4259.

63. Hill J, Inder T, Neil J, Dierker D, Harwell J, Van Essen D (2010) Similar patterns of cortical expansion during human development and evolution. Proc Natl Acad Sci USA **107**: 13135–13140.

64. Petanjek Z, Judaš M, Šimić G, Rašin MR, Uylings HBM, et al. (2011) Extraordinary neotony of synaptic spines in the human prefrontal cortex. Proc Natl Acad Sci **108**: 13281–13286.

65. Glasser MF, Van Essen DC (2011) Mapping human cortical areas in vivo based on myelin content as revealed by T1- and T2-weighted MRI. J Neurosci **31**: 11597–11616.

66. Glasser MF, Goyal MS, Preuss TM, Raichle ME, Van Essen DC (2014) Trends and properties of human cerebral cortex: correlations with cortical myelin content. Neuroimage **93**: 165–175.

67. Song C, Schwarzkopf DS, Kanai R, Rees G (2009) Reciprocal anatomical relationship between primary sensory and prefrontal cortices in the human brain. J Neurosci **31**: 9472–9480.

68. Poeppel D, Emmorey K, Hickok G, Pylkkänen L (2012) Towards a new neurobiology of language. J Neurosci **32**: 14125–14131.

69. Schenker NS, Hopkins WD, Spocter MA, Garrison AR, Stimpson CD, et al. (2010) Broca's area homologue in chimpanzees (Pan troglodytes): probabilistic mapping, asymmetry, and comparison to humans. Cereb Cortex **20**: 730–742.

70. Gil-de-Costa R, Martin A, Lopes MA, Muños M, Fritz JB, Braun AR (2006) Species-specific calls activate homologs of Broca's and Wernicke's areas in the macaque. Nat Neurosci **9**: 1064–1070.

71. Marstaller L, Burianová H (2015) A common functional network for overt production of speech and gesture. Neuroscience **284**: 29–41.

72. Wakita M (2014) Broca's area processes the hierarchical organization of observed action. Front Hum Neurosci **7**: 937.

73. Fazio P, Cantagallo A, Craighero L, D'Ausilio A, Roy AC, et al. (2009) Encoding of human action in Broca's area. Brain **132**: 1980–1988.

74. Rauschecker JP (2012) Ventral and dorsal streams in the evolution of speech and language. Front Evol Neurosci **4**: 7.

75. Petrides M, Pandya DN (2009) Distinct parietal and temporal pathways to the homologues of Broca's area in the monkey. PLoS Biol **7**: e1000170.

76. Perani D, Saccuman MC, Scifo P, Anwander A, Spada D, et al. (2011) Neural language networks at birth. Proc Natl Acad Sci USA **108**: 16056–16061.

77. Brauer J, Anwander A, Perani D, Friederici AD (2013) Dorsal and ventral pathways in language development. Brain Lang **127**: 289–295.

78. Friederici AD, Gierhan SME (2013) The language network. Curr Opin Neurobiol **23**: 250–254.

79. Berwick RC, Friederici AD, Chomsky N, Bolhuis JJ (2013) Evolution, brain, and the nature of language. Trends Cogn Sci **17**: 89–96.

80. Axer H, Klingner CM, Prescher A (2013) Fiber anatomy of dorsal and ventral language streams. Brain Lang **127**: 192–204.

81. **Dick AS, Tremblay P** (2012) Beyond the arcuate fasciculus: consensus and controversy in the connectional anatomy of language. Brain **135**: 3529–3550.

82. **Fadiga LK, Craighero L, D'Ausilio A** (2009) "Broca's area in language, action, and music," in **S. Dalla Bella** et al., eds, *The Neurosciences and Music III—Disorders and Plasticity*, Ann N Y Acad Sci **1169**: 448–458. (Wiley-Blackwell, Boston).

83. **Skinner JL, Goldin-Meadow S, Nusbaum HC, Small SL** (2007) Speech-associated gestures, Broca's area, and the human mirror system. Brain Lang **101**: 260–277.

84. **Rizzolatti G, Sinigaglia C** (2010) The functional role of the parieto-frontal mirror circuit: interpretations and misinterpretations. Nat Rev Neurosci **11**: 264–274.

85. **Kuroshima H, Kaiser I, Fragaszy DM** (2014) Does own experience affect perception of others' actions in capuchin monkeys (Cebus apella)? Anim Cogn **17**: 1269–1279.

86. **Caggiano V, Fogassi L, Rizzolatti G, Casile A, Giese MA, Their P** (2013) Mirror neurons encode the subjective value of an observed action. Proc Natl Acad Sci USA **109**: 11848–11853.

87. **Coudé G, Festante F, Cilia A, Loiacono V, Bimbi M**, et al. (2016) Mirror neurons of ventral premotor cortex are modulated by social cues provided by others' gaze. J Neurosci **36**: 3145–3156.

88. **Kilner JN, Lemon RN** (2013) What we know currently about mirror neurons. Curr Biol **23**: R1057-R1062.

89. **Suddendorf T, Collier-Baker E** (2009) The evolution of primate visual self-recognition: evidence of absence in lesser apes. Proc Biol Sci **276**: 1671–1677.

90. **Macellini S, Ferrari PF, Bonini L, Fogassi L, Paukner AA** (2010) A modified mark test for own-body recognition in pig-tailed macaques (Macaca nemestrina). Anim Cogn 13: 631–639.

91. **De Waal FMB** (2008) Putting the altruism back into altruism: the evolution of empathy. Annu Rev Psychol **59**: 279–300.

92. **Rushworth MFS, Mars RB, Sallet J** (2013) Are there specialized circuits for social cognition and are they unique to humans? Curr Opin Neurobiol **23**: 436–442.

93. **Silk JB, House BR** (2011) Evolutionary foundations of human prosocial sentiments. Proc Natl Acad Sci USA **108**: 10910–10917.

94. **Boaz NT, Almquist AJ** (2002) *Biological Anthropology: A Synthetic Approach to Human Evolution* (2nd edition). Prentice Hall, New Jersey.

95. **Rizzolatti G, Craighero L** (2004) The mirror-neuron system. Annu Rev Neurosci **27**: 169–192.

96. **Gentilucci M, Corballis MC** (2006) From manual gesture to speech: a gradual transition. Neurosci Biobehav Rev **30**: 949–960.

97. **Okanoya K** (2007) Language evolution and an emergent property. Curr Opin Neurobiol **17**: 271–276.

98. **Arbib MA, Liebal K, Pika S** (2008) Primate vocalization, gesture, and the evolution of human language. Curr Anthropol **49**: 1053–1063.

99. **Corballis MC** (2010) Mirror neurons and the evolution of language. Brain Lang **112**: 35–45.

100. **Livingstone SR, Thompson WF** (2009) The emergence of music from the Theory of Mind. Music Sci (Special Issue 2009–2010): 83–115.

101. **Aziz-Zadeh L, Koski L, Zaidel E, Mazziotta J, Iacoboni M** (2006) Lateralization of the human mirror neuron system. J Neurosci **26**: 2964–2970.

102. **Kilner JM, Neal A, Weiskopf N, Friston KJ, Frith CD** (2009) Evidence of mirror neurons in human inferior frontal gyrus. J Neurosci **29**: 10153–10159.

103. **Bickerton D** (2007) Language evolution: a brief guide for linguists. Lingua **117**: 510–526.

104. **Aboitiz F, Garcia R** (2009) Merging of phonological and gestural circuits in early language evolution. Rev Neurosci **20**: 71–84.

105. Skipper JL, Goldin-Meadow S, Nusbaum HC, Small SL (2007) Speech-associated gestures, Broca's area, and the human mirror system. Brain Lang **101**: 260–277.

106. Rochas V, Gelmini L, Krolak-Salmon P, Poulet E, Saoud M, et al. (2013) Disrupting pre-SMA activity impairs facial happiness recognition: an event-related TMS study. Cereb Cortex **23**: 1517–1525.

107. Likowski KU, Muchlberger A, Gerdes ABM, Wieser MJ, Pauli P, Weyers P (2012) Facial mimicry and the mirror neuron system: simultaneous acquisition of facial electromyography and functional magnetic resonance imaging. Front Hum Neurosci **6**: 214.

108. Noordzij ML, Newman-Norlund SE, de Ruiter JP, Hagoort P, Levinson SC, Toni I (2009) Brain mechanisms underlying human communication. Front Hum Neurosci **3**: 14.

109. Kanai R, Bahrami B, Roylance R, Rees G (2012) Online social network size is reflected in human brain structure. Proc Biol Sci **279**: 1327–1334.

110. Ricciardi E, Bonin D, Sani L, Vecchi T, Guazzelli M, et al. (2009) Do we really need vision? How blind people "see" the actions of others. J Neurosci **29**: 9719–9724.

111. Peterson CC, Wellman HM (2009) From fancy to reason: scaling deaf and hearing children's understanding of theory of mind and pretence. Br J Dev Psychol **27**: 297–310.

112. Bedny M, Pascual-Leone A, Saxe RR (2009) Growing up blind does not change the neural bases of Theory of Mind. Proc Natl Acad Sci USA **106**: 11312–11317.

113. Friederici AD (2009) Pathways to language: fiber tracts in the human brain. Trends Cogn Sci **13**: 175–181.

114. Rilling JK, Glasser MF, Jbabdi S, Andersson J, Preuss TM (2012) Continuity, divergence, and the evolution of brain language pathways. Front Evol Neurosci **3**: 11.

115. Thiebaut de Schotten M, Dell'Acqua F, Valabregue R, Catani M (2012) Monkey to human comparative anatomy of the frontal lobe association tracts. Cortex **48**: 82–96.

116. Hecht EE, Gutman DA, Bradley BA, Preuss TM, Stout D (2015) Virtual dissection and comparative connectivity of the superior longitudinal fasciculus in chimpanzees and humans. Neuroimage **108**: 124–137.

117. Hickok G, Poeppel D (2007) The cortical organization of speech processing. Nat Rev Neurosci **8**: 393–402.

118. Karlsgodt KH, Kochunov P, Winkler AM, Laird AR, Almasy L, et al. (2010) A multimodal assessment of the genetic control over working memory. J Neurosci **30**: 8197–8202.

119. Raghanti MA, Stimpson CD, Marcinkiewicz JL, Erwin JM, Hof PR, Sherwood CC (2008) Differences in cortical serotonergic innervation among humans, chimpanzees, and macaque monkeys: a comparative study. Cereb Cortex **18**: 584–597.

120. Raghanti MA, Spocter MA, Stimpson CD, Erwin JM, Bonar CJ, et al. (2009) Species-specific distributions of tyrosine hydroxylase-immunoreactive neurons in the prefrontal cortex of anthropoid apes. Neuroscience **158**: 1551–1559.

121. Sherwood CC, Raghanti MA, Stimpson CD, Spocter MA, Uddin M, et al. (2010) Inhibitory interneurons of the human prefrontal cortex display conserved evolution of the phenotype and related genes. Proc Biol Sci **277**: 1011–1020.

122. Muntané G, Horvath JE, Hof PR, Ely JJ, Hopkins WD, et al. (2014) Analysis of synaptic gene expression in the neocortex of primates reveals evolutionary changes in glutamatergic neurotransmission. Cereb Cortex **25**: 1596–1607.

123. Kimelberg HK (2010) Functions of mature mammalian astrocytes: a current view. Neuroscientist **16**: 79.

124. Chung W-S, Welsh CA, Barres BA, Stevens B (2015) Do glia drive synaptic and cognitive impairment in disease? Nat Neurosci **18**: 1539–1545.

125. **Pereira Jr A, Furlan FB** (2010) Astrocytes and human cognition: modelling information integration and modulation of neuronal activity. Prog Neurobiol **92**: 405–420.

126. **Pannasch U, Rouach N** (2013) Emerging role for astroglial networks in information processing: from synapse to behaviour. Trends Neurosci **36**: 405–417.

127. **Perea G, Sur M, Araque A** (2014) Neuron-glia networks: integral gear of brain function. Front Cellular Neurosci **8**: 378.

128. **Perez-Alvarez A, Navarrete M, Covelo A, Martin ED, Araque A** (2014) Structural and functional plasticity of astrocytic processes and dendritic spine interactions. J Neurosci **34**: 12738–12744.

129. **Zorec R, Horvat A, Vardjan N, Verkhratsky A** (2015) Memory formation shaped by astroglia. Front Integr Neurosci **9**: 56.

130. **Oberheim NA, Tian GF, Han X, Peng W, Takano T**, et al. (2009) Uniquely hominid features of adult human astrocytes. J Neurosci **29**: 3276–3287.

131. **Oberheim NA, Wang X, Goldman S, Nedergaard M** (2006) Astrocytic complexity distinguishes the human brain. Trends Neurosci **29**: 547–553.

132. **Azevedo FAC, Carvalho LRB, Grinberg LT, Farfel JM, Ferretti REL**, et al. (2009) Equal numbers of neuronal and nonneuronal cells make the human brain an isometrically scaled-up primate brain. J Comp Neurol **513**: 532–541.

133. **Debanne D, Poo M-M** (2010) Spike-timing dependent plasticity beyond synapse—pre- and post-synaptic plasticity of intrinsic neuronal excitability. Front Synaptic Neurosci **2**: 21.

134. **Lamsa KP, Kullmann DM, Woodin MA** (2011) Spike-timing dependent plasticity in inhibitory circuits. Front Synaptic Neurosci **2**: 8.

135. **Testa-Silva G, Verhoog MB, Goriounova NA, Loebel A, Hjorth J**, et al. (2010) Human synapses show a wide temporal window for spike-timing-dependent plasticity. Front Synaptic Neurosci **2**: 1–11.

136. **Han X, Chen M, Wang F, Windrem M, Wang S**, et al. (2013) Forebrain engraftment by human glial progenitor cells enhances synaptic plasticity and learning in adult mice. Cell Stem Cell **12**: 342–353.

137. **Gilbert SL, Dobyns WB, Lahn BT** (2005) Opinion: genetic links between brain development and brain evolution. Nat Rev Genet **6**: 581–590.

138. **Boyd JL, Skove SL, Rouanet JP, Pilaz L-J, Bepler T**, et al. (2015) Human-chimpanzee differences in a FZD8 enhancer alter cell-cycle dynamics in the developing neocortex. Curr Biol **25**: 772–779.

139. **Luo XJ, Li M, Huang L, Nho K, Deng M**, et al. (2013) The interleukin 3 gene (IL3) contributes to human brain volume variation by regulating proliferation and survival of neural progenitors. PLoS One **7**: e50375.

140. **Li M, Huang L, Li K, Huo Y, Chen C, Wang J**, et al. (2016) Adaptive evolution of interleukin-3 (IL3), a gene associated with brain volume variation in general human populations. Hum Genet **135**: 377–392.

141. **Toga AW, Thompson PM** (2005) Genetics of brain structure and intelligence. Annu Rev Neurosci **28**: 1–23.

142. **Hulshoff Pol HE, Schnack HG, Posthuma D, Mandl RC, Baaré WF**, et al. (2006) Genetic contributions to human brain morphology and intelligence. J Neurosci **26**: 10235–10242.

143. **Chiang MC, Barysheva M, Shattuck DW, Lee AD, Madsen SK**, et al. (2009) Genetics of brain fiber architecture and intellectual performance. J Neurosci **29**: 2212–2224.

144. **Brans RG, Kahn RS, Schnack HG, van Baal GC, Posthuma D**, et al. (2010) Brain plasticity and intellectual ability are influenced by shared genes. J Neurosci **30**: 5519–5524.

145. **Bohlken MM, Brouwer RM, Mandl RC, van Haren NE, Brans RG**, et al. (2013) Genes contributing to subcortical volumes and intellectual ability implicate the thalamus. Hum Brain Mapp **35**: 2632–2642.

146. Prüfer K, Racimo F, Patterson N, Jay F, Sankararaman S, et al. (2014) The complete genome sequence of a Neanderthal from the Altai Mountains. Nature **505**: 43–49.

147. Wildman DE, Uddi M, Liu G, Grossman LI, Goodman M (2003) Implications of natural selection in shaping 99.4% nonsynonymous DNA identity between humans and chimpanzees: Enlarging genus Homo. PNAS **100**: 7181–7188.

148. Preuss TM, Cáceres M, Oldham MC, Geschwind DH (2004) Human brain evolution: insights from microarrays. Nat Rev Genet **5**: 850–860.

149. Dorus S Vallender EJ, Evans PD, Anderson JR, Gilbert SL, et al. (2004) Accelerated evolution of nervous system genes in the origin of Homo sapiens. Cell **119**: 1027.

150. Khaitovich P, Hellmann I, Enard W, Nowick K, Leinweber M, et al. (2005) Parallel patterns of evolution in the genomes and transcriptomes of humans and chimpanzees. Science **309**: 1850–1854.

151. Deary IJ, Spinath FM, Bates TC (2006) Genetics of intelligence. Eur J Hum Genet **14**: 690–700.

152. Burki F, Kaessmann H (2004) Birth and adaptation evolution of a hominoid gene that supports high neurotransmitter flux. Nat Genet **36**: 1061–1063.

153. Grossman LI, Wildman DE, Schmidt TR, Goodman M (2004) Accelerated evolution of the electron transport chain in anthropoid primates. Trends Genet **20**: 578–585.

154. Uddin M, Goodman M, Erez O, Romero R, Liu G, et al. (2008) Distinct genomic signatures of adaptation in pre- and postnatal environments during human evolution. Proc Natl Acad Sci USA **105**: 3215–3220.

155. Bozek K, Wei Y, Yan Z, et al. (2014) Exceptional evolutionary divergence of human muscle and brain metabolomes parallels human cognitive and physical uniqueness. PloS Biol **12**: 5e1001871.

156. Gilad Y, Oaslack A, Smyth GK, Speed TP, White KP (2006) Expression profiling in primates reveals a rapid evolution of human transcription factors. Nature **440**: 242–245.

157. Konopka G, Friedrich T, Davis-Turak J, Winden K, Oldham MC, et al. (2012) Human-specific transcriptional networks in the brain. Neuron **75**: 601–617.

158. Gittelman RM, Hun E, Ay F, Madeoy J, Pennacchio L, et al. (2015) Comprehensive identification and analysis of human accelerated regulatory DNA. Genome Res **25**: 1245–1255.

159. Pollard KS, Salama SR, King B, Kern AD, Dreszer T, et al. (2006) Forces shaping the fastest evolving regions in the human genome. PLoS Genet **2**: e168.

160. Burbano HA, Green RE, Maricic T, Lalueza-Fox C, de la Rasilla M, et al. (2012) Analysis of human accelerated DNA regions using archaic hominin genomes. PLoS One **7**: e32877.

161. Doan RN, Bae BI, Cubelos B, Chang C, Hossain AA, et al. (2016) Mutations in human accelerated regions disrupt cognition and social behaviour. Cell **167**: 341–354

162. Liu X, Somel M, Tang L, Yan Z, Jiang X, et al. (2012) Extension of cortical synaptic development distinguishes humans from chimpanzees and macaques. Genome Res **22**: 611–622.

163. Fu X, Giavalisco P, Liu X, Catchpole G, Fu N, et al. (2011) Rapid metabolic evolution in human prefrontal cortex. Proc Natl Acad Sci USA **108**: 6181–6186.

164. Teffer K, Semendeferi K (2012) Human prefrontal cortex: evolution, development, and pathology. Prog Brain Res **185**: 191–218.

165. Capra JA, Erwin GD, McKinsey G, Rubenstein JL, Pollard KS (2013) Many human accelerated regions are developmental enhancers. Philos Trans R Soc Lond B Biol Sci **368**: 20130025.

166. Valadkhan S, Nilsen TW (2010) Reprogramming of the non-coding transcriptome during brain development. J Biol **9**: 5.

167. Ezkurdia I, Juan D, Rodriguez JM, Frankish A, Diekhans M, et al. (2014) Multiple evidence strands suggest that there may be as few as 19,000 human protein-coding genes. Hum Mol Genet **23**: 5866–5878.

168. Mattick JS (2011) The central role of RNA in human development and cognition. FEBS Letters **585**: 1600–1616.

169. Somel M, Liu X, Tang L, Yan Z, Hu H, et al. (2011) MicroRNA-driven developmental remodeling in the brain distinguishes humans from other primates. PLoS Biol **9**: e1001214.

170. Follert P, Cremer H, Béclin C (2014) MicroRNAs in brain development and function: a matter of flexibility and stability. Front Mol Neurosci **7**: 5.

171. Griggs EM, Young EJ, Rumbaugh G, Miller CA (2013) MicroRNA-182 regulates amygdala-dependent memory formation. J Neurosci **33**: 1734–1740.

172. Lister R, Mukamel EA (2015) Turning over DNA methylation in the mind. Front Neurosci **9**: 252.

173. Feng J, Zhou Y, Campbell SL, Le T, Li E, et al. (2010) Dnmt1 and Dnmt3a maintain DNA methylation and regulate synaptic function in adult forebrain neurons. Nat Neurosci **13**: 423–430.

174. Gabel HW, Kinde B, Stroud H, Gilbert CS, Harmin DA, et al. (2015) Disruption of DNA-methylation-dependent long gene expression in Rett syndrome. Nature **522**: 89–93.

175. Zeng J, Konopka G, Hunt BG, Preuss TM, Geschind D, Yi SV (2012) Divergent whole-genome methylation maps of human and chimpanzee brains reveal epigenetic basis of human regulatory evolution. Am J Hum Genet **91**: 455–465.

176. Day JJ, Sweatt JD (2011) Epigenetic mechanisms in cognition. Neuron **70**: 813–829.

177. McQuown SC, Wood MA (2011) HDAC3 and the molecular brake pad hypothesis. Neurobiol Learn Mem **96**: 27–34.

178. Landry CD, Kandel ER, Rajasethuphathy P (2013) New mechanisms in memory storage: piRNAs and epigenetics. Trends Neurosci **36**: 535–542.

179. Shulha HP, Crisci JL, Reshetov D, Tushir JS, Cheung I, et al. (2012) Human-specific histone methylation signatures at transcription start sites in prefrontal neurons. PLoS Biol **10**: e1001427.

180. Paz-Yaacov N, Levanon EY, Nevo E, Kinar Y, Harmelin A, et al. (2010) Adenosine-to-inosine RNA editing shapes transcriptome diversity in primates. Proc Natl Acad Sci USA **107**: 12174–12179.

181. Deng W, Saxe MD, Gallina IS, Gage FH (2009) Adult-born hippocampal dentate granule cells undergoing maturation modulate learning and memory in the brain. J Neurosci **29**: 13532–13542.

182. Garrett L, Zhang J, Zimprich A, Niedermeier KM, Fuchs H, et al. (2015) Conditional reduction of adult born doublecortin-positive neurons reversibly impairs selective behaviors. Front Behav Neurosci **9**: 302.

183. Kempermann G, Fabel K, Ehninger D, Babu H, Leal-Galicia P, et al. (2010) Why and how physical activity promotes experience-dependent brain plasticity. Front Neurosci **4**: 189.

184. Lieberwirth C, Wang Z (2012) The social environment and neurogenesis in the adult mammalian brain. Front Hum Neurosci **6**: 118.

185. Cinini SM, Barnabe GF, Galváo-Coelho N, de Medeiros MA, Perez-Mendes P, et al. (2014) Social isolation disrupts hippocampal neurogenesis in young non-human primates. Front Neurosci **8**: 45.

186. Naninck EF, Hoeijmakers L, Kakava-Georgiadou N, Meesters A, Lazic SE, et al. (2015) Chronic early life stress alters developmental and adult neurogenesis and impairs cognitive function in mice. Hippocampus **25**: 309–328.

187. Eisch AJ, Petrik D (2012) Depression and hippocampal neurogenesis: a road to remission? Science **338**: 72–75.

188. Spalding KS, Bergmann O, Alkass K, Bernard S, Salehpour M, et al. (2013) Dynamics of hippocampal neurogenesis in adult humans. Cell **153**: 1219–1227.

189. Kempermann G (2013) What the bomb said about the brain. Science **340**: 1180–1181.

190. Maguire EA, Gadian DG, Johnsrude IS, Good CD, Ashburner J, et al. (2000) Navigation-related structural change in the hippocampi of taxi drivers. Proc Natl Acad Sci USA **97**: 4396–4403.

191. Sahay A, Wilson DA, Hen R (2011) Pattern separation: a common function for new neurons in hippocampus and olfactory bulb. Neuron **70**: 582–588.

192. Koelsch S, Skouras S, Jentschke S (2013) Neural correlates of emotional personality: a structural and functional magnetic resonance imaging study. PLoS One **8**: e77196.

193. Koelsch S (2014) Brain correlates of music-evoked emotions. Nat Rev Neurosci **15**: 170–180.

194. Muotri AR, Zhao C, Marchetto MCN, Gage FH (2009) Environmental influence on LI retrotransposons in the adult hippocampus. Hippocampus **19**: 1002–1007.

195. Singer T, McConnell MJ, Marchetto MC, Coufal NG, Gage FH (2010) LINE-1 retrotransposons: mediators of somatic variation in neuronal genomes? Trends Neurosci **33**: 345–354.

196. Chanda ML, Levitin DJ (2013) The neurochemistry of music. Trends Cogn Sci **17**: 179–193.

197. Fukui H, Toyoshima K (2008) Music facilitates the neurogenesis, regeneration and repair of neurons. Med Hypotheses **71**: 765–769.

198. Bae B-I, Jayaraman D, Walsh CA (2015) Genetic changes shaping the human brain. Dev Cell **32**: 423–434.

199. Preuss TM (2012) Human brain evolution: from gene discovery to phenotypic discovery. Proc Natl Acad Sci USA **109**: 10709–10716.

200. Koten JW Jr, Wood G, Hagoort P, Goebel R, Propping P, et al. (2009) Genetic contribution to variation in cognitive function: an fMRI study in twins. Science **323**: 1737–1740.

201. Blokland GAM, McMahon KL, Thompson PM, Martin NG, de Zubicaray GI, Wright MJ (2011) Heritability of working memory brain activation. J Neurosci **31**: 10882–10890.

202. Turkheimer E, Haley A, Waldron M, D'Onofrio B, Gottesman II (2003) Socioeconomic status modifies heritability of IQ in young children. Psychol Sci **14**: 623–628.

203. Rietveld CA, Medland SE, Derringer J, Yang J, Esko T, et al. (2013) GWAS of 126,559 individuals identifies genetic variants associated with educational attainment. Science **340**: 1467–1471.

204. Rietveld CA, Conley D, Eriksson N, Esko T, Medland SE, et al. (2014) Replicability and robustness of genome-wide-association studies for behavioral traits. Psychol Sci **25**: 1975–1986.

205. Davies G, Tenesa A, Payton A, Yang J, Harris SE, et al. (2011) Genome-wide association studies establish that human intelligence is highly heritable and polygenic. Mol Psychiatry **16**: 996–1005.

206. Plomin R, Deary IJ (2015) Genetics and intelligence differences: five special findings. Mol Psychiatry **20**: 98–108.

207. Schwarz F, Springer SA, Altheide TK, Varki NM, Gagneux P, Varki A (2016) Human-specific derived alleles of CD33 and other genes protect against postreproductive cognitive decline. Proc Natl Acad Sci **113**: 74–79.

208. Khaitovich P, Muetzel B, She X, Lachmann M, Hellmann I, et al. (2004) Regional patterns of gene expression in human and chimpanzee brains. Genome Res **14**: 1462–1473.

209. Newbury DF, Fisher SE, Monaco AP (2010) Recent advances in the genetics of language impairment. Genome Med **2**: 6.

210. Kang C, Drayna D (2011) Genetics of speech and language disorders. Annu Rev Genomics Hum Genet **12**: 5.1–5.20.

211. Spiteri E, Konopka G, Coppola G, Bomar J, Oldham M, et al. (2007) Identification of the transcriptional targets of FOXP2, a gene linked to speech and language, in developing human brain. Am J Hum Genet **81**: 1144–1157.

212. Vernes SC, Spiteri E, Nicod J, Groszer M, Taylor JM, et al. (2007) High-throughput analysis of promoter occupancy reveals direct neural targets of FOXP2, a gene mutated in speech and language disorders. Am J Hum Genet **81**: 1232–1250.

213. Konopka G, Bomar JM, Winden K, Coppola G, Jonsson ZO, et al. (2009) Human-specific transcriptional regulation of CNS development genes by FOXP2. Nature **462**: 213–218.

214. Enard W (2011) FOXP2 and the role of cortico-basal ganglia circuits in speech and language evolution. Curr Opin Neurobiol **21**: 415–424.

215. Murugan M, Harward S, Scharff C, Mooney R (2013) Diminished FoxP2 levels affect dopaminergic modulation of corticostriatal signaling important for song variability. Neuron **80**: 1464–1476.

216. Mozzi A, Forni D, Clerici M, Pozzoli U, Mascheretti S, et al. (2016) The evolutionary history of genes involved in spoken and written language: beyond FOXP2. Scientific Reports **6**: 22157.

217. Krause J, Lalueza-Fox C, Orlando L, Enard W, Green RE, et al. (2007) The derived FOXP2 variant of modern humans was shared with Neandertals. Curr Biol **17**: 1908–1912.

218. Reich D, Green RE, Kircher M, Krause J, Patterson N, et al. (2010) Genetic history of an archaic hominin group from Denisova cave in Siberia. Nature **468**: 1053–1060.

219. Maricic T, Günther V, Georgiev O, Gehre S, Curlin M, et al. (2013) A recent evolutionary change affects a regulatory element in the human FOXP2 gene. Mol Biol Evol **30**: 844–852.

220. Mukamel Z, Konopka G, Wexler E, Osborn GE, Dong H, et al. (2011) Regulation of MET by FOXP2: genes implicated in higher cognitive dysfunction and autism risk. J Neurosci **31**: 11437–11442.

221. Bates TC, Luciano M, Medland SE, Montgomery GW, Wright MJ, Martin NG (2011) Genetic variance in a component of the language acquisition device: ROBO1 polymorphisms associated with phonological buffer deficits. Behav Genet **41**: 50–57.

222. Shtyrov Y, Osswald K, Pulvermüller F (2008) Memory traces for spoken words in the brain as revealed by the hemodynamic correlate of the mismatch negativity. Brain **18**: 29–37.

223. Shtyrov Y, Nikulin VV, Pulvermüller F (2010) Rapid cortical plasticity underlying novel word learning. J Neurosci **30**: 16864–16867.

224. Alberini CM, Chen DY (2012) Memory enhancement: consolidation, reconsolidation and insulin-like growth factor 2. Trends Neurosci **35**: 274–283.

225. Pruunsild P, Sepp M, Orav E, Koppel I, Timmusk T (2011) Identification of cis-elements and transcription factors regulating neuronal activity-dependent transcription of human BDNF gene. J Neurosci **31**: 3295–3308.

226. Zeng Y, Tan M, Kohyama J, Sneddon M, Watson JB, et al. (2011) Epigenetic enhancement of BDNF signalling rescues synaptic plasticity in aging. J Neurosci **31**: 17800–17810.

227. Karpova NN (2014) Role of epigenetics in activity-dependent neuronal plasticity. Neuropharmacol **76**: 709–718.

228. Leal G, Comprido D, Duarte CB (2014) BDNF-induced local protein synthesis and synaptic plasticity. Neuropharmacol **76**: 639–656.

229. Erickson KI, Miller DL, Roecklein KA (2011) The aging hippocampus: interactions between exercise, depression, and BDNF. Neuroscientist **18**: 82–97.

230. Bekinschtein P, Kent BA, Oomen CA, Clemenson GD, Gage FH, et al. (2014) Brain-derived neurotrophic factor interacts with adult-born immature cells in the dentate gyrus during consolidation of overlapping memories. Hippocampus **24**: 905–911.

231. Hsiao Y-H, Hung H-C, Chen S-H, Gean P-W (2014) Social interaction rescues memory deficit in an animal model of Alzheimer's Disease by increasing BDNF-dependent hippocampal neurogenesis. J Neurosci **34**: 16207–16219.

232. Hong C-J, Liou Y-L, Tsai S-J (2011) Effects of BDNF polymorphisms on brain function and behavior in health and disease. Brain Res Bull **86**: 287–297.

233. Ninan I, Bath KG, Dagar K, Perez-Castro R, Plummer MR, et al. (2010) The BDNF val66met polymorphism impairs NMDA receptor-dependent synaptic plasticity in the hippocampus. J Neurosci **30**: 8866–8870.

234. Phillips C, Baktir MA, Srivatsan M, Salehi A (2014) Neuroprotective effects of physical activity on the brain: a closer look at trophic factor signaling. Front Cell Neurosci 8: 170.

235. Bath KG, Lee FS (2006) Variant BDNF (Val66Met) impact on brain structure and function. Cogn Affect Behav Neurosci 6: 79–85.

236. Thomason ME, Yoo DJ, Glover GH, Gotlib IH (2009) BDNF genotype modulates resting functional connectivity in children. Front Hum Neurosci 3: 55.

237. Yu H, Wang Y, Pattwell S, Jing D, Liu T, et al. (2009) Variant BDNF Val66Met polymorphism affects extinction of conditioned aversive memory. J Neurosci 29: 4056–4064.

238. Chen DY, Bambah-Mukku D, Pollonini G, Alberini CM (2012) Glucocorticoid receptors recruit the CaMKIIα-BDNF-CREB pathways to mediate memory consolidation. Nat Neurosci 15: 1707–1714.

239. Cordeira JW, Frank L, Sena-Esteves M, Pothos EM, Rios M (2010) Brain-derived neurotrophic factor regulated hedonic feeding by acting on the mesolimbic dopamine system. J Neurosci 30: 2533–2541.

240. Witte AV, Kürten J, Jansen S, Schirmacher A, Brand E, et al. (2012) Interaction of BDNF and COMT polymorphisms on paired-associative stimulation-induced cortical plasticity. J Neurosci 32: 4553–4561.

241. De Quervain DJ-F, Henke K, Aerni A, Coluccia D, Wollmer MA, et al. (2003) A functional genetic variation of the 5-HT2a receptor affects human memory. Nat Neurosci 6: 1141–1142.

242. de Quervain DJ-F, Papassotiropoulos A (2006) Identification of a genetic cluster influencing memory performance and hippocampal activity in humans. Proc Natl Acad Sci USA 103: 4270–4274.

243. Filippini N, Scassellati C, Boccardi M, Pievani M, Testa C, et al. (2006) Influence of serotonin receptor 2A His452Tyr polymorphism on brain temporal structures: a volumetric MR study. Eur J Hum Genet 14: 443–449.

244. Lemaitre H, Mattay VS, Sambataro F, Verchinski B, Straub RE, et al. (2010) Genetic variation in FGF20 modulates hippocampal biology. J Neurosci 30: 5992–5997.

245. Qiu S, Korwek KM, Weeber EJ (2006) A fresh look at an ancient receptor family: emerging roles for low density lipoprotein receptors in synaptic plasticity and memory formation. Neurobiol Learn Mem 85: 16–29.

246. Yau SY, Li A, Hoo RL, Ching YP, Christie BR, et al. (2014) Physical exercise-induced hippocampal neurogenesis and antidepressant effects are mediated by the adipocyte hormone adiponectin. Proc Natl Acad Sci USA 111: 15810–15815.

247. Schneider A, Huentelman MJ, Kremerskothen J, Duning K, Spoelgen R, Nikolich K (2010) KIBRA: a new gateway to learning and memory? Front Aging Neurosci 2: 4.

248. Wilbrecht L, Holtmaat A, Wright N, Fox K, Svoboda K (2010) Structural plasticity underlies experience-dependent functional plasticity of cortical circuits. J Neurosci 30: 4927–4932.

249. Papassotiropoulos A, Stephan DA, Huentelman MJ, Hoerndli FJ, Craig DW, et al. (2006) Common Kibra alleles are associated with human memory performance. Science 314: 475–478.

250. Bates TC, Price JF, Harris SE, Marioni RE, Fowkes FGR, et al. (2009) Association of KIBRA and memory. Neurosci Lett 458: 140–143.

251. Kauppi K, Nilsson L-G, Adolfsson R, Eriksson E, Nyberg L (2011) KIBRA polymorphism is related to enhanced memory and elevated hippocampal processing. J Neurosci 31: 14218–14222.

252. Franks KH, Summers MJ, Vickers JC (2014) KIBRA gene polymorphism has no association with verbal or visual episodic memory performance. Front Aging Neurosci 6: 270.

253. Palombo DJ, Amaral RSC, Olsen RK, Müller DJ, Todd RM, et al. (2013) KIBRA polymorphism is associated with individual differences in hippocampal subregions: evidence from anatomical segmentation using high-resolution MRI. J Neurosci 33: 13088–13093.

254. Gosso MF, de Geus EJ, van Belzen MJ, Polderman TJ, Heutink P, et al. (2006) SNAP-25 gene is associated with cognitive ability: evidence from a family-based study in two independent Dutch cohorts. Mol Psychiatry 11: 878–886.

255. Vogler C, Spalek K, Aerni A, Demougin P, Müller A, et al. (2009) CPEB3 is associated with human episodic memory. Front Behav Neurosci 3: 4.

256. Bhatt DH, Zhang S, Gan W-B (2009) Dendritic spine dynamics. Annu Rev Physiol 71: 261–282.

257. Chen B-S, Thomas EV, Sanz-Clement A, Roche KW (2011) NMDA receptor-dependent regulation of dendritic spine morphology by SAP102 splice variants. J Neurosci 31: 89–96.

258. Hill WD, Davies G, van de Lagemaat LN, Christoforou A, Marioni RE, et al. (2014) Human cognitive ability is influenced by genetic variation in components of postsynaptic signalling complexes assembled by NMDA receptors and MAGUK proteins. Transl Psychiatry 4: e341.

259. Newbury DF, Monaco AP (2010) Genetic advances in the study of speech and language disorders. Neuron 68: 309–320.

260. Whitehouse AJO, Bishop DVM, Ang QW, Pennell CE, Fisher SE (2011) CNTNAP2 variants affect early language development in the general population. Genes Brain Behav 10: 451–456.

261. Ramachandran VS (2003) *The Emerging Mind*. Profile Books, London.

262. McDougall I, Brown FH, Fleagle JG (2005) Stratigraphic placement and age of modern humans from Kibish, Ethiopia. Nature 433: 733–736.

263. Mellars P (2006) Why did modern human populations disperse from Africa ca. 60,000 years ago? A new model. Proc Natl Acad Sci USA 103: 9381–9386.

264. Liu W, Jin CZ, Zhang YQ, Cai YJ, Xing S, et al. (2010) Human remains from Zhirendong, South China, and modern human emergence in East Asia. Proc Natl Acad Sci USA 107: 19201–19206.

265. Armitage SJ, Jasim SA, Marks AE, Parker AG, Usik VI, Uerpmann H-P (2011) The southern route "out of Africa": evidence for an early expansion of modern humans into Arabia. Science 331: 453–456.

266. Bae CJ, Wang W, Zhao J, Huang S, Tian F, Shen G (2014) Modern human teeth from Late Pleistocene Luna Cave (Guangxi, China). Quart Internat 354: 169–183.

267. Reyes-Centeno H, Ghirotto S, Détroit F, Grimaud-Hervé D, Barbujani AG, Harvati K (2014) Genomic and cranial phenotype data support multiple modern human dispersals from Africa and a southern route into Asia. Proc Natl Acad Sci USA 111: 7248–7253.

268. Kuhlwilm M, Gronau I, Hubisz MJ, de Filippo C, Prado-Martinez J, et al. (2016) Ancient gene flow from early modern humans into Eastern Neanderthals. Nature 530: 429–433.

269. Osborne AH, Vance D, Rohling EJ, Barton N, Rogerson M, Fello N (2008) A humid corridor across the Sahara for the migration of early modern humans out of Africa 120,000 years ago. Proc Natl Acad Sci USA 105: 16444–16447.

270. Castañeda IS, Mulitza S, Schefuss E, Lopes dos Santos RA, Sinninghe Damsté JS, Schouten S (2009) Wet phases in the Sahara/Sahel region and human migration patterns in North Africa. Proc Natl Acad Sci USA 106: 20159–20163.

271. Reyes-Centeno H, Hubbe M, Hanihara T, Stringer C, Havarti K (2015) Testing modern human out-of-Africa dispersal models and implications for modern human origins. J Hum Evol 87: 95–106.

272. Rightmire GR (2009) Middle and later Pleistocene hominins in Africa and Southwest Asia. Proc Natl Acad Sci USA 106: 16046–16050.

273. Bolhuis JJ, Tattersall I, Chomsky N, Berwick RC (2014) How could language have evolved? PLoS Biol 12: e1001934.

274. **Relethford JH** (2008) Genetic evidence and the modern human origins debate. Heredity **100**: 555–563.

275. **Green RE, Krause J, Ptak SE, Briggs AW, Ronan MT**, et al. (2006) Analysis of one million base pairs of Neanderthal DNA. Nature **44**: 330–336.

276. **Belle EMS, Benazzo A, Ghirotto S, Colonna V, Barbujani G** (2009) Comparing models on the genealogical relationships among Neandertal, Cro-Magnoid and modern Europeans by serial coalescent simulations. Heredity **102**: 218–225.

277. **Green RE, Krause J, Briggs AW, Maricic T, Stenzel U**, et al. (2010) A draft sequence of the Neandertal genome. Science **328**: 710–722.

278. **Rieux A, Eriksson A, Li M, Sobkiowiak B, Weinert LA**, et al. (2014) Improved calibration of the human mitochondrial clock using ancient genomes. Mol Biol Evol **31**: 2780–2792.

279. **Mendez FL, Poznik GD, Castellano S, Bustamante CD** (2016) The divergence of Neandertal and modern human Y chromosomes. Am J Hum Genet **98**: 728–734.

280. **Oxnard CE** (2015) *The Scientific Bases of Human Anatomy* (**M. Cartmell** and **K. B. Brown**, eds). Wiley-Blackwell, Chichester UK.

281. **Chernigovskaya TV** (2004) Homo loquens: evolution of cerebral functions and language. J Evol Biochem Physiol **40**: 495–503.

282. **Masataka N** (2009) The origins of language and the evolution of music: a comparative perspective. Phys Life Rev **6**: 11–22.

283. **Tattersall I** (2002) *The Monkey in the Mirror: Essays on the Science of What Makes Us Human.* Harcourt Brace, New York.

284. **Oppenheimer S** (2012) Out-of-Africa, the peopling of continents and islands: tracing uniparental gene trees across the map. Philos Trans R Soc Lond B Biol Sci **367**: 770–784.

285. **Mellars P, Gori KC, Carr M, Soares PA, Richards MB** (2013) Genetic and archaeological perspectives on the initial modern human colonization of southern Asia. Proc Natl Acad Sci USA **110**: 10699–10704.

286. **Hershkovitz I, Marder O, Ayalon A, Bar-Matthews M, Yasur G**, et al. (2015) Levantine cranium from Manot Cave (Israel) foreshadows the first European modern humans. Nature **520**: 216–219.

287. **Racimo F, Sankararaman S, Nielsen R, Huerta-Sánchez E** (2015) Evidence for archaic adaptive introgression in humans. Nat Rev Genet **16**: 359–371.

288. **Mellars P** (2004) Neanderthals and the modern human colonization of Europe. Nature **432**: 461–465.

289. **Deshpande O, Batzoglou, Feldman MW, Cavalli-Sforza LL** (2009) A serial founder effect model for human settlement out of Africa. Proc Biol Sci **276**: 291–300.

290. **Behar DM, Villems R, Soodyall H, Blue-Smith J, Pereira L (Genographic Consortium)** (2008) The dawn of human matrilineal diversity. Am J Hum Genet **82**: 1130–1140.

291. **Tishkoff SA, Gonder MK, Henn BM, Mortensen H, Knight A**, et al. (2007) History of click-speaking populations of Africa inferred from mtDNA and Y chromosome genetic variation. Mol Biol Evol **24**: 2180–2195.

292. **Fu Q, Mittnik A, Johnson PLF, Bos K, Lari M**, et al. (2013) A revised timescale for human evolution based on ancient mitochondrial genomes. Curr Biol **23**: 553–559.

293. **Harpending HC, Batzer MA, Gurven M, Jorde LB, Rogers AR, Sherry ST** (1998) Genetic traces of ancient demography. Proc Natl Acad Sci USA **95**: 1961–1967.

294. **Brookfield JFY** (2000) Human evolution: how recent were the Y chromosome ancestors? Curr Biol **10**: R722-R723.

295. **Ambrose SH** (1998) Late Pleistocene human population bottlenecks, volcanic winter, and differentiation of modern humans. J Hum Evol **34**: 623–651.

296. Svensson A, Bigler M, Blunier T, Clausen HB, Dahl-Jensen D, et al. (2012) Direct linking of Greenland and Antarctic ice cores at the Toba eruption (74 kyr BP). Clim Past Discuss **8**: 5389–5427.

297. Lane CS, Chorn BT, Johnson TC (2013) Ash from the Toba supereruption in Lake Malawi shows no volcanic winter in East Africa at 75 ka. Proc Natl Acad Sci USA **110**: 8025–8029.

298. Rampino MR, Self S (1992) Volcanic winter and accelerated glaciation following the Toba super-eruption. Nature **359**: 50–52.

299. Acharyya SK, Basu PK (1992) Toba ash on the Indian subcontinent and its implications for correlation of late pleistocene alluvium. Quat Res **40**: 10–19.

300. Woillard GM, Mook WG (1982) Grande Pile peat bog: a continuous pollen record for the last 140000 years. Quat Res **215**: 1–21.

301. Pickrell JK, Reich D (2014) Toward a new history and geography of human genes informed by ancient DNA. Trends Genet **30**: 377–389.

302. Green RE, Shapiro B (2013) Human evolution: turning back the clock? Curr Biol **23**: R286.

303. Fu Q, Li H, Moorjani P, Jay F, Slepchenko SM, et al. (2014) Genome sequence of a 45,000-year-old modern human from western Siberia. Nature **514**: 445–450.

304. Thomas GWC, Hahn MW (2014) The human mutation rate is increasing, even as it slows. Mol Biol Evol **31**: 253–257.

305. Wang C-C, Gilbert MTP, Jin L, Li H (2014) Evaluating the Y chromosomal timescale in human demographic and lineage dating. Investig Genet **5**: 12.

306. Harris K (2015) Evidence for recent, population-specific evolution of the human mutation rate. Proc Natl Acad Sci USA **112**: 3439–3444.

307. Ségurel L, Wyman MJ, Przeworski M (2014) Determinants of mutation rate variation in the human germline. Annu Rev Hum Genet **15**: 47–70.

308. Jobling MA, Tyler-Smith C (2003) The human Y chromosome: an evolutionary marker comes of age. Nat Rev Genet **4**: 598–612.

309. Underhill PA, Shen P, Lin AA, Passarino G, Yang WH, et al. (2000) Y chromosome sequence variation and the history of human populations. Nat Genet **26**: 358–361.

310. Underhill PA, Kivisild T (2007) Use of Y chromosome and mitochondrial DNA population structure in tracing human migrations. Annu Rev Genet **41**: 539–564.

311. Templeton AR (2007) Genetics and recent human evolution. Evolution **61**: 1507–1519.

312. Wei W, Ayub Q, Xue Y, Tyler-Smith C (2013) A comparison of Y-chromosomal lineage dating using either resequencing or Y-SNP plus Y-STR genotyping. Forensic Sci Int Genet **7**: 568–572.

313. Endicott P, Ho P, Stringer C (2010) Using genetic evidence to evaluate four palaeoanthropological hypotheses for the timing of Neanderthal and modern human origins. J Hum Evol **59**: 87–95.

314. Rito T, Richards MB, Fernandes V, Alshamali F, Cerny V, et al. (2013) The first modern human dispersals across Africa. PLoS One **8**: e80031.

315. Atkinson QD, Gray RD, Drummond AJ (2009) Bayesian coalescent inference of major human mitochondrial DNA haplotype expansions in Africa. Proc Biol Sci **276**: 367–373.

316. Soares P, Alshamali F, Pereira JB, Fernandes V, Silva NM, et al. (2012) The expansion of mtDNA haplogroup L3 within and out of Africa. Mol Biol Evol **29**: 915–927.

317. Lohmueller KE, Indap AR, Schmidt S, Boyko AR, Hernandez RD, et al. (2008) Proportionally more deleterious genetic variation in European than in African populations. Nature **451**: 994–998.

318. Scally A, Durbin R (2012) Revising the human mutation rate: implications for understanding human evolution. Nat Rev Genet **13**: 745–753.

319. Posth C, Renaud G, Mittnik A, Drucker DG, Rougier H, et al. (2016) Pleistocene mitochondrial genomes suggest a single major dispersal of non-Africans and a late glacial population turnover in Europe. Curr Biol **26**: 827–833.

320. Rasmussen M, Guo X, Wang Y, Lohmueller KE, Rasmussen S, et al. (2011) An Aboriginal Australian genome reveals separate human dispersals into Asia. Science **334**: 94–98.

321. Linz B, Balloux F, Moodley Y, Manica A, Liu H, et al. (2007) An African origin for the intimate association between humans and Helicobacter pylori. Nature **445**: 915–918.

322. Moodley Y, Linz B, Bond RP, Nieuwoudt M, Soodyall H, et al. (2012) Age of the association between Helicobacter pylori and man. PLoS Pathog **8**: e1002693.

323. Reed DL, Smith VS, Hammond SL, Rogers AR, Clayton DH (2004) Genetic analysis of lice supports direct contact between modern and archaic humans. PLoS Biol **2**: e340.

324. Morriss-Kay GM (2010) The evolution of human artistic creativity. J Anat **216**: 158–176.

325. Jacobs Z, Roberts RG (2009) Catalysts for Stone Age innovations. Commun Integr Biol **2**: 191–193.

326. Wadley L (2014) South African middle and later stone age research: a retrospective. S Afr Archaeol Bull **69**: 208–212.

327. Henshilwood CS, d'Errico F, Yates R, Jacobs Z, Tribolo C, et al. (2002) Emergence of modern human behaviour: Middle Stone Age engravings from South Africa. Science **295**: 1278–1280.

328. Henshilwood CS, d'Errico F, Vanhaeren M, van Niekerk K, Jacobs Z (2004) Middle Stone Age shell beads from South Africa. Science **304**: 404.

329. Bouzouggar A, Barton N, Vanhaeren M, d'Errico F, Collcutt S, et al. (2007) 82,000-year-old shell beads from North Africa and implications for the origins of modern human behavior. Proc Natl Acad Sci USA **104**: 9964–9969.

330. Henshilwood CS, d'Errico F, van Nierkerk KL, Coquinot Y, Jacobs Z, et al. (2011) A 100,000-year-old ochre-processing workshop at Blombos Cave, South Africa. Science **334**: 219–222.

331. Jacobs Z, Roberts RG, Galbraith RF, Deacon HJ, Grün R, et al. (2008) Ages for the Middle Stone Age of southern Africa: implications for human behavior and dispersal. Science **322**: 733–735.

332. Peeters R, Simone L, Nelissen K, Fabbri-Destro M, Vanduffel W, et al. (2009) The representation of tool use in humans and monkeys: common and uniquely human features. J Neurosci **29**: 11523–11539.

333. D'Errico F, Henshilwood C, Lawson G, Vanhaeren M, Tillier A-M, et al. (2003) Archaeological evidence for the emergence of language, symbolism, and music—an alternative multidisciplinary perspective. J World Prehist **17**: 1–70.

334. Vanhaeren M, d'Errico F, van Nierkerk KL, Henshilwood CS, Erasmus RM (2013) Thinking strings: additional evidence for personal ornament use in the Middle Stone Age at Blombos Cave, South Africa. J Hum Evol **64**: 500–517.

335. Botha R (2008) Prehistoric shell beads as a window on language evolution. Lang Commun **28**: 197–212.

336. Powell A, Shennan S, Thomas MG (2009) Late Pleistocene demography and the appearance of modern human behaviour. Science **324**: 1298–1301.

337. Muthukrishna M, Shulman BW, Vasilescu V, Heinrich J (2013) Sociality influences cultural complexity. Proc Biol Soc **281**: 20132511.

338. Amati D, Shallice T (2007) On the emergence of modern humans. Cognition **103**: 358–385.

339. Pike AWG, Hoffmann DL, García-Diez M, Pettitt PB, Alcolea J, et al. (2012) U-series dating of Paleolithic art in 11 caves in Spain. Science **336**: 1409–1413.

340. González-Sainz C, Ruiz-Redondo A, Garate-Maidagan D, Iriarte-Avilés E (2013) Not only Chauvet: dating Aurignacian rock art in Altxerri B cave (northern Spain). J Hum Evol **65**: 457–464.

341. Aubert M, Brumm A, Ramli M, Sutikna T, Saptomo EW, et al (2014) Pleistocene cave art from Sulawesi, Indonesia. Nature **314**: 223–227.

342. **Mithen S** (1996) *The Prehistory of the Mind: The Cognitive Origins of Art, Religion and Science.* Thames and Hudson, London.

343. **Kunej D, Turk I** (2000) "New perspectives on the beginnings of music: archeological and musicological analysis of a Middle Paleolithic bone 'flute'," in **N. L. Wallin, B. Merker** and **S. Brown**, eds, *The Origins of Music* (MIT Press, Cambridge MA), 235–268.

344. **Bryson B** (2003) *A Short History of Nearly Everything.* Black Swan, London.

345. **Walker AC, Shipman P** (1996) *The Wisdom of the Bones.* Alfred E. Knopf, New York.

346. **Conard NJ, Malina M, Münzel SC** (2009) New flutes document the earliest musical tradition in southwestern Germany. Nature **460**: 737–740.

347. **Higham T, Basell L, Jacobi R, Wood R, Bronk Ramsey C, Conard NJ** (2012) Testing models for the beginnings of the Aurignacian and the advent of figurative art and music: the radiocarbon chronology of Geißenklösterle. J Hum Evol **62**: 664–676.

348. **Morley I** (2014) A multi-disciplinary approach to the origins of music: perspectives from anthropology, archaeology, cognition and behavior. J Anthropol Sci **92**: 147–177.

349. **Thaut MH** (2009) The musical brain—an artful biological necessity. *Karger Gazette* (Music and Medicine) No. 70: 2–4.

350. **Dutton D** (2009) *The Art Instinct.* Oxford University Press, Oxford.

351. **Haldane JBS** (1935) The rate of spontaneous mutation of a human gene. J Genet **31**: 317–326.

352. **Bergström A, Nagle N, Chen Y, McCarthy S, Pollard MO**, et al. (2016) Deep roots for Aboriginal Australian Y chromosomes. Curr Biol **26**: 809–813.

353. **Sankararaman S, Mallick S, Patterson N, Reich D** (2016) The combined landscape of Denisovan and Neanderthal ancestry in present-day humans. Curr Biol **26**: 1–7.

354. **Pääbo S** (2015) The diverse origins of the human gene pool. Nat Rev Genet **16**: 313–314.

355. **Vernot B, Akey JM** (2015) Complex history of admixture between modern humans and Neandertals. Am J Hum Genet **96**: 448–453.

356. **Lohsa K, Frantz LA** (2014) Neandertal admixture in Eurasia confirmed by maximum-likelihood analysis of three genomes. Genetics **196**: 1241–1251.

357. **Evans PD, Mekel-Bobrov N, Valender EJ, Hudson RR, Lahn BT** (2006) Evidence that the adaptive allele of the brain size gene microcephalin introgressed into Homo sapiens from an archaic Homo lineage. Proc Natl Acad Sci USA **103**: 18178–18183.

358. **Ségurel L, Quintana-Murci L** (2014) Preserving immune diversity through ancient inheritance and admixture. Curr Opin Immunol **30**: 79–84.

359. **Sankararaman S, Mallick S, Dannemann M, Prüfer K, Kelso J**, et al. (2014) The genomic landscape of Neanderthal ancestry in present-day humans. Nature **507**: 354–357.

360. **Villa P, Roebroeks W** (2014) Neandertal demise: an archaeological analysis of the modern human superiority complex. PLoS One **9**: e96424.

361. **Tattersall I** (2010) Human evolution and cognition. Theory Biosci **129**: 193–201.

362. **de Chardin PT** (1955) *The Phenomenon of Man.* Harper Perennial, New York, London.

363. **Gilpin W, Feldman MW, Aoki K** (2015) An ecocultural model predicts Neanderthal extinction through competition with modern humans. Proc Natl Acad Sci USA **113**: 2134–2139.

364. **Gould SJ, Vrba ES** (1982) Exaptation: a missing term in the science of form. Paleobiology **8**: 4–15.

365. **Calvin WH** (1996) *How Brains Think: Evolving intelligence, Then and Now.* Weidenfeld & Nicholson, London.

366. **Hauser MD, Chomsky N, Fitch WT** (2002) The faculty of language: what is it, who has it, and how did it evolve? Science **298**: 1569–1579.

367. **Wynn T, Coolidge FL** (2011) The implications of the working memory model for the evolution of modern cognition. Int J Evol Biol **2011**: 741357.

368. **Pinker S** (2013) *Language, Cognition, and Human Nature: Selected Articles*. Oxford University Press, Oxford.

369. **Nowak MA, Karakauer DC** (1999) The evolution of language. Proc Natl Acad Sci USA **96**: 8028–8033.

370. **Suddendorf Y, Corballis MC** (2007) The evolution of foresight: what is mental time travel, and is it unique to humans? Behav Brain Sci **30**: 299–351.

371. **Mengham R** (1994) *On Language: Descent from the Tower of Babel*. Little Brown & Company.

372. **Chomsky N** (2006) *Language and Mind* (3rd edition). Cambridge University Press, Cambridge, New York.

373. **Fitch TW** (2006) The biology and evolution of music: a comparative perspective. Cognition **100**: 173–215.

374. **Pinker S** (1997) *How the Mind Works*. W W Norton, New York.

375. **Everett DL** (2005) Cultural constraints on grammar and cognition in Pirahã. Curr Anthropol **46**: 621–646.

376. **Fitch TW, Hauser MD, Chomsky N** (2005) The evolution of the language faculty: clarifications and implications. Cognition **97**: 179–210.

377. **Jackendoff R, Pinker S** (2005) The nature of the language faculty and its implications for evolution of language (reply to Fitch, Hauser, and Chomsky). Cognition **97**: 211–225.

378. **Campbell BG** (1985) *Humankind Emerging* (4th edition). Little Brown, Boston, Toronto.

379. **Fay N, Arbib M, Garrod S** (2013) How to bootstrap a human communication system. Cogn Sci **37**: 1356–1367.

380. **Fay N, Lister CJ, Ellison TM, Goldin-Meadow S** (2014) Creating a communication system from scratch: gesture beats vocalization hands down. Front Psychol **5**: 354.

381. **Dawkins CR** (1998) *Unweaving the Rainbow*. The Penguin Press, London.

382. **Bargary G, Mitchell KJ** (2009) Synaesthesia and cortical connectivity. Trends Neurosci **31**: 335–342.

383. **Weiss PH, Fink GR** (2009) Grapheme-colour synaesthetes show increased grey matter volumes of parietal and fusiform cortex. Brain **132**: 65–70.

384. **Rouw R, Scholte HS** (2010) Neural basis of individual differences in synesthetic experiences. J Neurosci **30**: 6205–6213.

385. **Dovern A, Fink GR, Fromme AC, Wohlschläger AM, Weiss PH, Reidl V** (2012) Intrinsic network connectivity reflects consistency of synesthetic experiences. J Neurosci **32**: 7614–7621.

386. **Neufeld J, Sinke C, Dillo W, Emrich HM, Szycik GR**, et al. (2012) The neural correlates of coloured music: a functional MRI investigation of auditory-visual synaesthesia. Neuropsychologia **50**: 85–89.

387. **Zamm A, Schlaug G, Eagleman DM, Loui P** (2013) Pathways to seeing music: enhanced structural connectivity in colored-music synaesthesia. Neuroimage **74**: 359–366.

388. **Hupé J-M, Dojat M** (2015) A critical review of the neuroimaging literature on synesthesia. Front Hum Neurosci **9**: 103.

389. **Beeli G, Esslen M, Jäncke L** (2005) Synaesthesia: when coloured sounds taste sweet. Nature **434**: 38.

390. **Brang D, Williams LE, Ramachandran VS** (2012) Grapheme-color synesthetes show enhanced crossmodal processing between auditory and visual modalities. Cortex **48**: 630–637.

391. **Mulvenna CM** (2007) "Synaesthesia, the arts and creativity: a neurological connection," in **H. Bogousslavsky**, ed., *Neurological Disorders in Famous Artists—Part 2*, Front Neurol Neurosci **22**: 206–222 (Karger, Basel).

392. **Barnett KJ, Finucane C, Asher JE, Bargary G, Corvin AP**, et al. (2008) Familial patterns and the origins of individual differences in synaesthesia. Cognition **106**: 871–893.

393. Tomson SN, Avidan N, Lee K, Sarma AK, Tushe R, et al. (2011) The genetics of colored sequence synesthesia: suggestive evidence of linkage to 16q and genetic heterogeneity for the condition. Behav Brain Res **223**: 48–52.

394. Kayser C, Petkov CI, Augath M, Logothetis NK (2007) Functional imaging reveals visual modification of specific fields in auditory cortex. J Neurosci **27**: 1824–1835.

395. Kayser C, Petkov CI, Logothetis NK (2008) Visual modulation of neurons in auditory cortex. Cereb Cortex **18**: 1560–1574.

396. Naue N, Rach S, Strüber D, Huster RJ, Zaehle T, et al. (2011) Auditory event-related response in visual cortex modulates subsequent visual responses in humans. J Neurosci **31**: 7729–7736.

397. Poirier C, Collignon O, Scheiber C, Renier L, Vanlierde A, et al. (2006) Auditory motion perception activates visual motion areas in early blind subjects. Neuroimage **31**: 279–285.

398. Driver J, Noesselt T (2008) Multisensory interplay reveals crossmodal influences on "sensory-specific" brain regions, neural responses, and judgements. Neuron **57**: 11–23.

399. Klinge C, Eippert F, Röder B, Büchel C (2010) Corticocortical connections mediate primary visual cortex responses to auditory stimulation in the blind. J Neurosci **30**: 12798–12805.

400. Wan CY, Wood AG, Reutens DC, Wilson SJ (2010) Congenital blindness leads to enhanced vibrotactile perception. Neuropsychologia **48**: 631–635.

401. Lane C, Kanjlia S, Omaki A, Bedni M (2015) "Visual" cortex of congenitally blind adults responds to syntactic movement. J Neurosci **35**: 12859–12868.

402. Collignon O, Vandewalle G, Voss P, Albouy G, Charbonneau G, et al. (2011) Functional specialization for auditory-spatial processing in the occipital cortex of congenitally blind humans. Proc Natl Acad Sci USA **108**: 4435–4440.

403. Deutsch D (2006) "Selfish genes and information flow," in A. Grafen and M. Ridley, eds, *Richard Dawkins: How a Scientist Changed the Way We Think* (Oxford University Press, Oxford), 125–129.

404. Whiten A, Mesoudi A (2008) Establishing an experimental science of culture: animal social diffusion experiments. Philos Trans R Soc Lond B Biol Sci **363**: 3477–3488.

405. Szathmáry E, Számadó S (2008) Language: a social history of words. Nature **456**: 40–41.

406. Portin P (2015) A comparison of biological and cultural evolution. J Genet **94**: 155–168.

407. Ross CT, Richerson PJ (2014) New frontiers in the study of human cultural and genetic evolution. Curr Opin Genet Devel **29**: 103–109.

408. House BR, Silk JB, Henrich J, Barrett HC, Scelza BA, et al. (2013) Ontogeny of prosocial behaviour across diverse societies. Proc Natl Acad Sci USA **110**: 14586–14591.

409. Henrich J, Heine SJ, Norenzayan A (2010) The weirdest people in the world? Behav Brain Sci **33**: 61–135.

410. Muthukrishna M, Henrich J (2016) Innovation in the collective brain. Philos Trans R Soc Lond B Biol Sci **371**: 1690.

411. Fritz T, Jentschke S, Gosselin N, Sammler D, Peretz I, et al. (2009) Universal recognition of three basic emotions in music. Curr Biol **19**: 573–576.

412. Sievers B, Polansky L, Casey M, Wheatley T (2013) Music and movement share a dynamic structure that supports universal expressions of emotion. Proc Natl Acad Sci USA **110**: 70–75.

413. Egermann H, Fernando N, Chuen L, McAdams S (2015) Music induces universal emotion-related psychophysiological responses: comparing Canadian listeners to Congolese Pygmies. Front Psychol **5**: 1341.

414. Castro L, Toro MA (2014) Cumulative cultural evolution: the role of teaching. J Theor Biol **347**: 74–83.

415. Deutscher G (2005) *The Unfolding of Language: The Evolution of Mankind's Greatest Invention*. Arrow Books, London.

416. **Kaelin WG Jr, McKnight SL** (2013) Influence of metabolism on epigenetics and disease. Cell **153**: 56–69.

417. **Hawks J, Wang ET, Cochran GM, Harpending HC, Moyzis RK** (2007) Recent acceleration of human adaptive evolution. Proc Natl Acad Sci USA **104**: 20753–20758.

418. **Laland KN, Odling-Smee J, Myles S** (2010) How culture shaped the human genome: bringing genetics and the human sciences together. Nat Rev Genet **11**: 137–148.

419. **Perreault C** (2012) The pace of cultural evolution. PLoS One **7**: e45150.

420. **West-Eberhard MJ** (1979) Sexual selection, social competition and evolution. Proc Am Phil Soc **123**: 222–234.

421. **Boyd R, Richerson PJ** (2009) Culture and the evolution of human cooperation. Philos Trans R Soc Lond B Biol Sci **364**: 3281–3288.

422. **Henrich J, Chudek M, Boyd R** (2015) The Big Man Mechanism: how prestige fosters cooperation and creates prosocial leaders. Philos Trans R Soc Lond B Biol Sci **370**: 1683.

423. **Lichtman JW** (2009) Connectomics in the developing nervous system. Neurorehabil Neural Repair **23**: 958.

424. **Molino J** (2000) "Toward an evolutionary theory of music and language," in **N. L. Wallin, B. Merker** and **S. Brown**, eds, *The Origins of Music* (MIT Press, Cambridge MA), 165–176.

425. **Huron D** (2003) "Is music an evolutionary adaptation?" in **I. Peretz** and **R. L. Zatorre**, eds, *The Cognitive Neuroscience of Music* (Oxford University Press, Oxford), 57–75.

426. **Jablonka E, Lamb MJ** (2007) Précis of evolution in four dimensions. Behav Brain Sci **30**: 353–365.

427. **Gash DM, Deane AS** (2015) Neuron-based heredity and human evolution. Front Neurosci **9**: 209.

Chapter Four

1. **Kivy P** (1959) Charles Darwin on music. J Am Mus Soc **12**: 42–48.

2. **Tifferet S, Gaziel O, Baram Y** (2012) Guitar increases male facebook attractiveness: preliminary support for the sexual selection theory of music. LEBS **3**: 4–6.

3. **Guégeun N, Meineri S, Fischer-Lokou J** (2013) Men's music ability and attractiveness to women in a real-life courtship context. Psych Music **42**: 545–549.

4. **Lie HC, Rhodes G, Simmons LW** (2008) Genetic diversity revealed in human faces. Evolution **62**: 2473–2486.

5. **Plomin R, Deary IJ** (2015) Genetics and intelligence differences: five special findings. Mol Psychiatry **20**: 98–108.

6. **Mosing MA, Pedersen NL, Madison G, Ullén F** (2014) Genetic pleiotropy explains associations between musical auditory discrimination and intelligence. PloS One **9**: e113874.

7. **Fitch TW** (2006) The biology and evolution of music: a comparative perspective. Cognition **100**: 173–215.

8. **Merker B** (2012) "The vocal learning constellation: imitation, ritual culture, encephalization," in **N. Bannan**, ed., *Music, Language and Human Evolution* (Oxford University Press, Oxford), 215–260.

9. **Noonan JP, Coop G, Kudaravalli S, Smith D, Krause J**, et al. (2006) Sequencing and analysis of Neanderthal genomic DNA. Science **314**: 1113–1118.

10. **Green RE, Krause J, Briggs AW, Maricic T, Stenzel U**, et al. (2010) A draft sequence of the Neandertal genome. Science **328**: 710–722.

11. **Langergraber KE, Prüfer K, Rowney C, Boesch C, Crockford C**, et al. (2012) Generation times in wild chimpanzees and gorillas suggest earlier divergence times in great ape and human evolution. Proc Natl Acad Sci USA **109**: 15716–15721.

12. **Prüfer K, Racimo F, Patterson N, Jay F, Sankararaman S**, et al. (2014) The complete genome sequence of a Neanderthal from the Altai Mountains. Nature **505**: 43–49.

13. **Kuhlwilm M, Gronau I, Hubisz MJ, de Filippo C, Prado-Martinez J,** et al. (2016) Ancient gene flow from early modern humans into Eastern Neanderthals. Nature **530**: 429–433.

14. **Mendez FL, Poznik GD, Castellano S, Bustamante CD** (2016) The divergence of Neandertal and modern human Y chromosomes. Am J Hum Genet **98**: 728–734.

15. **Hauser MD, McDermott J** (2003) The evolution of the music faculty: a comparative perspective. Nat Neurosci **6**: 663–668.

16. **Scherer KR** (2013) "Emotion in action, interaction, music, and speech," in **M. A. Arbib,** ed., *Language, Music and the Brain: A Mysterious Relationship* (MIT Press, Cambridge MA), 107–139.

17. **Scharff C, Petri J** (2011) Evo-devo, deep homology and FoxP2: implications for the evolution of speech and language. Philos Trans R Soc Lond B Biol Sci **366**: 2124–2140.

18. **Rohrmeier M, Zuidema W, Wiggins GA, Scharff C** (2015) Principles of structure building in music, language and animal song. Philos Trans R Soc Lond B Biol Sci **370**: 20140097.

19. **Patel AD, Iversen JR, Bregman MR, Schulz I** (2009) Experimental evidence for synchronization to a musical beat in a nonhuman animal. Curr Biol **19**: 827–830.

20. **Konoike N, Kotozaki Y, Miyachi S, Miyauchi CM, Yomogida Y,** et al. (2012) Rhythm information represented in the fronto-parieto-cerebellar motor system. Neuroimage **63**: 328–338.

21. **Large EW, Gray PM** (2015) Spontaneous tempo and rhythmic entrainment in a bonobo (Pan paniscus). J Comp Psychol **129**: 317–328.

22. **Merchant H, Grahn J, Trainor L, Rohrmeier M, Fitch WT** (2015) Finding the beat: a neural perspective across humans and non-human primates. Philos Trans R Soc Lond B Biol Sci **370**: 20140093.

23. **Zarco W, Merchant H, Prado L, Mendez JC** (2009) Subsecond timing in primates: comparisons of interval production between human subjects and Rhesus monkeys. J Neurophysiol **102**: 3191–3202.

24. **Tierney A, Kraus N** (2013) The ability to tap to a beat relates to cognitive, linguistic and perceptual skills. Brain Lang **124**: 225–231.

25. **Patel AD, Iversen JR** (2014) The evolutionary neuroscience of musical beat perception: the Action Simulation for Auditory Prediction (ASAP) hypothesis. Front Syst Neurosci **8**: 57.

26. **Dalla Bella S, Berkowska M, Sowiński J** (2015) Moving to the beat and singing are linked in humans. Front Hum Neurosci **9**: 663.

27. **Felix II RA, Fridberger A, Leijon S, Berrebi AS, Magnusson AK** (2011) Sound rhythms are encoded by postinhibitory rebound spiking in the superior paraolivary nucleus. J Neurosci **31**: 12566–12578.

28. **Tierney A, Kraus N** (2013) The ability to move to a beat is linked to the consistency of neural responses to sound. J Neurosci **33**: 14981–14988.

29. **Hove MJ, Schwartze M** (2014) Deconstructing the ability to move to a beat. J Neurosci **34**: 2403–2405.

30. **Huang J, Gamble D, Sarnlertsophon K, Wang X, Hsiao S** (2012) Feeling music: integration of auditory and tactile inputs in musical meter perception. PLoS One **7**: e48496.

31. **Boaz NT, Almquist AJ** (2002) *Biological Anthropology: A Synthetic Approach to Human Evolution* (2nd edition). Prentice Hall, New Jersey.

32. **Clarke E, Reichard UH, Zuberbühler K** (2006) The syntax and meaning of wild gibbon songs. PLoS One **1**: e73.

33. **Fishman YI, Volkov IO, Noh MD, Garell PC, Bakken H,** et al. (2001) Consonance and dissonance of musical chords: neural correlates in auditory cortex of monkeys and humans. J Neurophysiol **86**: 2761–2788.

34. **Fishman YI, Micheyl C, Steinschneider M** (2013) Neural representation of harmonic complex tones in primary auditory cortex of the awake monkey. J Neurosci **33**: 10312–10323.

35. **Wright AA, Rivera JJ, Hulse SH, Shyan M, Neiworth JJ** (2000) Music perception and octave generalization in rhesus monkeys. J Exp Psychol Gen **129**: 291–307.

36. **Hauser MD** (2000) "The sound and the fury: primate vocalizations as reflections of emotion and thought," in **N. L. Wallin, B. Merker** and **S. Brown**, eds, *The Origins of Music* (MIT Press, Cambridge MA), 77–102.

37. **Richman B** (2000) "How music fixed 'nonsense' into significant formulas: on rhythm, repetition, and meaning," in **N. L. Wallin, B. Merker** and **S. Brown**, eds, *The Origins of Music* (MIT Press, Cambridge MA), 301–314.

38. **Wilson B, Petkov CI** (2011) Communication and the primate brain: insights from neuroimaging studies in humans, chimpanzees and macaques. Hum Biol **83**: 175–189.

39. **Remedios R, Logothetis NK, Kayser C** (2009) Monkey drumming reveals common networks for perceiving vocal and nonvocal communication sounds. Proc Natl Acad Sci USA **106**: 18010–18015.

40. **Kirschner S, Tomasello M** (2009) Joint drumming: social context facilitates synchronization in preschool children. J Exp Child Psychol **102**: 299–314.

41. **Fancourt D, Perkins R, Ascenso S, Carvalho LA, Steptoe A, Williamon A** (2016) Effects of group drumming interventions on anxiety, depression, social resilience and inflammatory immune response among mental health service users. PloS One **11**: e0151136.

42. **King SL, Janki VM** (2013) Bottlenose dolphins can use learned vocal labels to address each other. Proc Natl Acad Sci USA **110**: 13216–13221.

43. **King SL, Sayigh LS, Wells RS, Fellner W, Janik VM** (2013) Vocal copying of individually distinctive signature whistles in bottlenose dolphins. Proc Biol Sci **280**: 20130053.

44. **Ujhelyi M** (2000) "Social organization as a factor in the origins of language and music," in **N. L. Wallin, B. Merker** and **S. Brown**, eds, *The Origins of Music* (MIT Press, Cambridge MA), 125–134.

45. **Geissmann T** (2000) "Gibbon songs and human music from an evolutionary perspective," in **N. L. Wallin, B. Merker** and **S. Brown**, eds, *The Origins of Music* (MIT Press, Cambridge MA), 103–124.

46. **Takahashi DY, Fenley AR, Teramoto Y, Narayanam DZ, Borjon JI**, et al. (2015) The developmental dynamics of marmoset monkey vocal production. Science **349**: 734–738.

47. **Chow CP, Mitchell JF, Miller CT** (2015) Vocal turn-taking in a non-human primate is learned during ontogeny. Proc Biol Sci **282**: 20150069.

48. **Kato M, Okanoya K, Koike T, Sasaki E, Okano H**, et al. (2014) Human speech- and reading-related genes display partially overlapping expression patterns in the marmoset brain. Brain Lang **133**: 26–38.

49. **Worley KC, Warren WC, Rogers J, Locke D, Muzny DM**, et al. (2014) The common marmoset genome provides insight into primate biology and evolution. Nat Genet **46**: 850–860.

50. **Borjon JI, Ghazanfar AA** (2014) Convergent evolution of vocal cooperation without convergent evolution of brain size. Brain Behav Evol **84**: 93–102.

51. **Ghazanfar AA, Takahashi DY** (2014) The evolution of speech: vision, rhythm and cooperation. Trends Cogn Sci **18**: 543–553.

52. **Levinson SC** (2016) Turn-taking in human communication—origins and implications for language processing. Trends Cogn Sci **20**: 6–14.

53. **Rukstalis M, French JA** (2005) Vocal buffering of the stress response: exposure to conspecific vocalizations moderates urinary cortisol excretion in isolated marmosets. Horm Behav **47**: 1–7.

54. **Bannan N** (2012) "Harmony and its role in human evolution," in **N. Bannan**, ed., *Music, Language and Human Evolution* (Oxford University Press, Oxford), 288–339.

55. **Behroozmand R, Oya H, Nourski KV, Kawasaki H, Larson CR**, et al. (2016) Neural correlates of vocal production and motor control in human Heschl's gyrus. J Neurosci **36**: 2302–2315.

56. **Wilson SJ, Abbott DF, Lusher D, Gentle EC, Jackson GD** (2011) Finding your voice: a singing lesson from functional imaging. Hum Brain Mapp **32**: 2115–2130.

57. **Berwick RC, Beckers GJ, Okanoya K, Bolhuis JJ** (2012) A bird's eye view of human language evolution. Front Evol Neurosci **4**: 5.

58. **Pfenning AR, Hara E, Whitney O, Rivas MV, Wang R,** et al. (2014) Convergent transcriptional specializations in the brains of humans and song-learning birds. Science **346**: 1256846.

59. **Hoeschele M, Merchant H, Kikuchi Y, Hattori Y, ten Cate C** (2015) Searching for the origins of musicality across species. Philos Trans Roy Soc B Biol Sci **370**: 20140094.

60. **Kanduri C, Kuusi T, Ahvenainen M, Philips AK, Lähdesmäki H, Järvelä I** (2015) The effect of music performance on the transcriptome of professional musicians. Sci Rep **5**: 9506.

61. **Moorman S, Gobes SM, Kuijpers M, Kerkhofs A, Zandbergen MA, Bolhuis JJ** (2012) Human-like brain hemispheric dominance in birdsong learning. Proc Natl Acad Sci USA **109**: 12782–12787.

62. **Earp SE, Maney DL** (2012) Birdsong: is it music to their ears? Front Evol Neurosci **4**: 14.

63. **Bencivelli S** (2011) *Why We Like Music: Ear, Emotion, Evolution.* Music World Media, Hudson NY.

64. **Snowdon CT, Teie D** (2010) Affective responses in tamarins elicited by species-specific music. Biol Lett **23**: 30–32.

65. **Koelsch S** (2014) Brain correlates of music-evoked emotions. Nat Rev Neurosci **15**: 170–180.

66. **Gil-de-Costa R, Hauser MD** (2006) Vervet monkeys and humans show brain asymmetries for processing conspecific vocalizations, but with opposite patterns of laterality. Proc Natl Acad Sci USA **22**: 2313–2318.

67. **Savage PE, Brown S, Sakai E, Currie TE** (2015) Statistical universals reveal the structures and functions of human music. Proc Natl Acad Sci USA **112**: 8987–8992.

68. **Crystal D** (2006) *How Language Works.* Penguin, London.

69. **Lieberman P** (2016) The evolution of language and thought. J Anthropol Sci **94**: 127–146.

70. **Bolhuis JJ, Tattersall I, Chomsky N, Berwick RC** (2014) How could language have evolved? PLoS Biol **12**: e1001934.

71. **Stravinsky I** (1936) *Chronicle of My Life.* Victor Gollancz, London.

72. **Shapiro N** (1978) *An Encyclopedia of Quotations About Music.* Da Capo Press, New York.

73. **Arbib MA** (2013) "Five terms in search of a synthesis," in **M. A. Arbib,** ed., *Language, Music and the Brain: A Mysterious Relationship* (MIT Press, Cambridge MA), 3–44.

74. **Nelken I** (2011) Music and the auditory brain: where is the connection? Front Hum Neurosci **5**: 106.

75. **Blacking J** (1976) *How Musical is Man?* Faber and Faber, London.

76. **Demorest SM, Morrison SJ, Stambaugh LA, Beken M, Richards TL, Johnson C** (2010) An fMRI investigation of the cultural specificity of music memory. Soc Cogn Affect Neurosci **5**: 282–291.

77. **Merker B** (2000) "Synchronous chorusing and human origins," in **N. L. Wallin, B. Merker** and **S. Brown,** eds, *The Origins of Music* (MIT Press, Cambridge MA), 315–328.

78. **Sievers B, Polansky L, Casey M, Wheatley T** (2013) Music and movement share a dynamic structure that supports universal expressions of emotion. Proc Natl Acad Sci USA **110**: 70–75.

79. **Morley I** (2014) A multi-disciplinary approach to the origins of music: perspectives from anthropology, archaeology, cognition and behavior. J Anthropol Sci **92**: 147–177.

80. **Lieberman P, Crelin ES** (1971) On the speech of Neanderthal Man. Linguistic Inquiry **11**: 203–222.

81. **Lieberman P** (1975) *On the Origins of Language: An Introduction to the Evolution of Speech.* Macmillan, New York.

82. **Fitch TW** (2000) The evolution of speech: a comparative review. Trends Cogn Sci **4**: 258–267.

83. **Stoessel A, David R, Gunz P, Schmidt T, Spoor F, Hublin JJ** (2016) Morphology and function of Neandertal and modern human ear ossicles. Proc Natl Acad Sci USA **113**: 11489–11494.

84. **D'Anastasio R, Wroe S, Tuniz C, Mancini L, Cesana DT,** et al. (2013) Micro-biomechanics of the Kebara 2 hyoid and its implications for speech in Neanderthals. PLoS One **8**: e82261.

85. **Campbell BG** (1985) *Humankind Emerging* (4th edition). Little Brown, Boston, Toronto.

86. **MacLarnon A, Hewitt G** (1999) The evolution of human speech: the role of enhanced breathing control. Am J Phys Anthropol **109**: 341–363.

87. **Frayer DW, Nicolay C** (2000) "Fossil evidence for the origin of speech sounds," in **N. L. Wallin, B. Merker** and **S. Brown,** eds, *The Origins of Music* (MIT Press, Cambridge MA), 217–234.

88. **Zarate JM** (2013) The neural control of singing. Front Hum Neurosci **7**: 237.

89. **Walter C** (2013) *Last Ape Standing*. Walker Publishing Company Inc, New York.

90. **De Gusta D, Gilbert WH, Turner SP** (1999) Hypoglossal canal size and hominid speech. Proc Natl Acad Sci USA **96**: 1800–1804.

91. **Kumar V, Croxson PL, Simonyan K** (2016) Structural organization of the laryngeal motor cortical network and its implication for evolution of speech production. J Neurosci **36**: 4170–4181.

92. **Pisanski K, Cartei V, McGettigan C, Raine J, Reby D** (2016) Voice modulation: a window into the origins of human vocal control? Trends Cogn Sci **20**: 304–318.

93. **Brown S, Laird AR, Pfordresher PQ, Thelen SM, Turkeltaub P, Liotti M** (2009) The somatotopy of speech: phonation and articulation in the human motor cortex. Brain Cogn **70**: 31–41.

94. **Simonyan K, Ostuni J, Ludlow CL, Horwitz B** (2009) Functional but not structural networks of the human laryngeal motor cortex show left hemispheric lateralization during syllable but not breathing production. J Neurosci **29**: 14912–14923.

95. **Liégeois-Chauvel C, Giraud K, Badier J-M, Marquis P, Chauvel P** (2003) "Intracerebral evoked potentials in pitch perception reveal a functional asymmetry of human auditory cortex," in **I. Peretz** and **R. L. Zatorre,** eds, *The Cognitive Neuroscience of Music* (Oxford University Press, Oxford), 152–167.

96. **Xueqin L, Harbottle G, Zhang J, Wang C** (2003) The earliest writing? Sign use in the seventh millennium BC at Jiahu, Henan Province, China. Antiquity **77**: 31–45.

97. **Rasmussen M, Guo X, Wang Y, Lohmueller KE, Rasmussen S,** et al. (2011) An Aboriginal Australian genome reveals separate human dispersals into Asia. Science **334**: 94–98.

98. **Renfrew C** (2008) Neuroscience, evolution and the sapient paradox: the factuality of value and of the sacred. Philos Trans R Soc Lond B Biol Sci **363**: 2041–2047.

99. **Renfrew C, Frith C, Malafouris L** (2008) Introduction. The sapient mind: archaeology meets neuroscience. Philos Trans R Soc Lond B Biol Sci **363**: 1935–1938.

100. **Richardson FM, Seghier ML, Leff AP, Thomas MSC, Price CJ** (2011) Multiple routes from occipital to temporal cortices during reading. J Neurosci **31**: 8239–8247.

101. **Clegg B** (2003) *The First Scientist: A Life of Roger Bacon*. Constable, London.

102. **Scott JT** (1998) The harmony between Rousseau's musical theory and his philosophy. J Hist Ideas **59**: 287–308.

103. **Brown S** (2000) "The 'musilanguage' model of human evolution," in **N. L. Wallin, B. Merker** and **S. Brown,** eds, *Origins of Music* (MIT Press, Cambridge MA), 271–300.

104. **Masataka N** (2009) The origins of language and the evolution of music: a comparative perspective. Phys Life Rev **6**: 11–22.

105. **Thompson WF, Marin MM, Stewart L** (2012) Reduced sensitivity to emotional prosody in congenital amusia rekindles the musical protolanguage hypothesis. Proc Natl Acad Sci USA **109**: 19027–19032.

106. **Mithen S** (2005) *The Singing Neanderthals: The Origins of Music, Language, Mind, and Body*. Orion, London.

107. **Simon J** (2005) Rousseau and aesthetic modernity: music's power of redemption. Eighteenth-Century Music **2**: 41–56.

108. **Blank H, Anwander A, von Kriegstein K** (2011) Direct structural connections between voice- and face-recognition areas. J Neurosci **31**: 12906–12915.

109. **Fazio P, Cantagallo A, Craighero L, D'Ausilio A, Roy AC, et al.** (2009) Encoding of human action in Broca's area. Brain **132**: 1980–1988.

110. **Marstaller L, Burianová H** (2015) A common functional network for overt production of speech and gesture. Neuroscience **284**: 29–41.

111. **Frayer DW, Fiore I, Lalueza-Fox C, Radovcic J, Bondioli L** (2010) Right handed Neanderthals: Vindija and beyond. J Anthropol Sci **8**: 113–127.

112. **Estalrrich A, Rosas A** (2013) Handedness in Neanderthals from the El Sidron (Asturias, Spain): evidence from instrumental striations with ontogenetic inferences. PLoS One **8**: e62797.

113. **Stout D, Chaminade T** (2012) Stone tools, language and the brain in human evolution. Philos Trans R Soc Lond B Biol Sci **367**: 75–87.

114. **Hubbard Al, Wilson SM, Callan DE, Dapretto M** (2009) Giving speech a hand: gesture modulates activity in auditory cortex during speech perception. Hum Brain Mapp **30**: 1028–1037.

115. **Holle H, Obleser J, Rueschemeyer SA, Gunter TC** (2010) Integration of iconic gestures and speech in left superior temporal areas boosts speech comprehension under adverse listening conditions. Neuroimage **49**: 875–884.

116. **Skipper JL, Goldin-Meadow S, Nusbaum HC, Small SL** (2007) Speech-associated gestures, Broca's area, and the human mirror system. Brain Lang **101**: 260–277.

117. **Kircher T, Straube B, Luebe D, Weis S, Sachs O, et al.** (2009) Neural interaction of speech and gesture: differential activations of metaphoric co-verbal gestures. Neuropsychologia **47**: 169–179.

118. **Straube B, Green A, Weis S, Chatterjee A, Kircher T** (2009) Memory effects of speech and gesture binding: cortical and hippocampal activation in relation to subsequent memory performance. J Cogn Neurosci **21**: 821–836.

119. **Straube B, Green A, Weis S, Kircher T** (2012) A supramodal neural network for speech and gesture semantics: and fMRI study. PLoS One **11**: e51207.

120. **Good A, Reed MJ, Russo FA** (2014) Compensatory plasticity in the deaf brain: effects on perception of music. Brain Sci **4**: 560–574.

121. **Wan CY, Wood AG, Reutens DC, Wilson SJ** (2010) Congenital blindness leads to enhanced vibrotactile perception. Neuropsychologia **48**: 631–635.

122. **Lane C, Kanjlia S, Omaki A, Bedni M** (2015) "Visual" cortex of congenitally blind adults responds to syntactic movement. J Neurosci **35**: 12859–12868.

123. **Bedny M, Richardson H, Saxe R** (2015) "Visual" cortex responds to spoken language in blind children. J Neurosci **35**: 11674–11681.

124. **Poeppel D, Emmorey K, Hickok G, Pylkkänen L** (2012) Towards a new neurobiology of language. J Neurosci **32**: 14125–14131.

125. **Kayser C, Petkov CI, Augath M, Logothetis NK** (2007) Functional imaging reveals visual modification of specific fields in auditory cortex. J Neurosci **27**: 1824–1835.

126. **Kayser C, Petkov CI, Logothetis NK** (2008) Visual modulation of neurons in auditory cortex. Cereb Cortex **18**: 1560–1574.

127. **Perrodin C, Kayser C, Logothetis NK, Petkov CI** (2014) Auditory and visual modulation of temporal lobe neurons in voice-sensitive and association cortices. J Neurosci **34**: 2524–2537.

128. **Goldin-Meadow S, Brentari D** (2015) Gesture, sign and language: the coming of age of sign language and gesture studies. Behav Brain Sci Oct **5**:1–82 [Epub ahead of print].

129. **Petitto LA, Marentette PF** (1991) Babbling in the manual mode: evidence for the ontogeny of language. Science **251**: 1493–1496.

130. **Petitto LA, Zatorre RL, Gauna K, Nikelski EJ, Dostie D, Evans AC** (2000) Speech-like cerebral activity in profoundly deaf people processing sign languages: implications for the neural basis of human language. Proc Natl Acad Sci USA **97**: 13961–13966.

131. **Capek CM, Grossi G, Newman AJ, McBurney SL, Corina D, et al.** (2009) Brain systems mediating semantic and syntactic processing in deaf native signers: Biological invariance and modality specificity. Proc Natl Acad Sci USA **106**: 8784–8789.

132. **Hill J, Dierker D, Neil J, Inder T, Knutsen A, et al.** (2010) A surface-based analysis of hemispheric asymmetries and folding of cerebral cortex in term-born human infants. J Neurosci **30**: 2268–2276.

133. **Glasel H, Leroy F, Dubois J, Hertz-Pannier L, Mangin JF, Dehaene-Lambertz G** (2011) A robust asymmetry in the infant brain: the rightward superior temporal sulcus. Neuroimage **58**: 716–723.

134. **Penhune VB, Cismaru R, Dorsaint-Pierre R, Petitto L-A, Zatorre RJ** (2003) The morphometry of auditory cortex in the congenitally deaf measured using MRI. Neuroimage **20**: 1215–1225.

135. **Allen JS, Emmorey K, Bruss J, Damasio H** (2008) Morphology of the insula in relation to hearing status and sign language experience. J Neurosci **28**: 11900–11905.

136. **Ruytjens L, Albers F, van Dijk P, Wit H, Willemsen A** (2007) Activation in primary auditory cortex during silent lipreading is determined by sex. Audiol Neurootol **12**: 371–377.

137. **Good CD, Johnsrude I, Ashburner J, Henson RN, Friston KJ, Frackowiak RS** (2001) Cerebral asymmetry and the effects of sex and handedness on brain structure: a voxel-based morphometric analysis of 465 normal adult human brains. Neuroimage **14**: 685–700.

138. **Blacking J** (1990) *A Commonsense View of All Music.* Cambridge University Press, Cambridge.

139. **Stringer C** (2012) *Lone Survivors: How We Came to Be the Only Humans on Earth.* St Martin's Griffin, New York.

140. **Mithen S** (2009) "The music instinct: the evolutionary basis of musicality," in **S. Dalla Bella** et al., *The Neurosciences and Music III—Disorders and Plasticity*, in Ann NY Acad Sci **1169**: 3–12 (Wiley-Blackwell, Boston).

141. **Jaubert J, Verheyden S, Genty D, Soulier M, Cheng H, et al.** (2016) Early Neanderthal constructions deep in Bruniquel Cave in southwestern France. Nature **534**: 111–114.

142. **Freeman W** (2000) "A neurological role of music in social bonding," in **N. L. Wallin, B. Merker** and **S. Brown**, eds, *The Origins of Music* (MIT Press, Cambridge MA), 411–424.

143. **Olson S** (2002) *Mapping Human History.* Bloomsbury Publishing, London.

144. **Scott BH, Mishkin M, Yin P** (2012) Monkeys have a limited form of short-term memory in audition. Proc Natl Acad Sci USA **109**: 12237–12241.

145. **Wynn T, Coolidge FL** (2011) The implications of the working memory model for the evolution of modern cognition. Int J Evol Biol **2011**: 741357.

146. **Amati D, Shallice T** (2007) On the emergence of modern humans. Cognition **103**: 358–385.

147. **Bickerton D** (2007) Language evolution: a brief guide for linguists. Lingua **117**: 510–526.

148. **Perlovsky L** (2010) Musical emotions: functions, origins, evolution. Phys Life Rev **7**: 2–27.

149. **Sacks O** (2008) *Musicophilia.* Vintage Books, New York.

150. **Özdemir E, Norton A, Schlaug G** (2006) Shared and distinct neural correlates of singing and speaking. Neuroimage **33**: 628–635.

151. **Schön D, Gordon R, Campagne A, Magne C, Astésano C, et al.** (2010) Similar cerebral networks in language, music and song perception. Neuroimage **52**: 450–461.

152. **Fedorenko E, Behr MK, Kanwisher N** (2011) Functional specificity for high-level linguistic processing in the human brain. Proc Natl Acad Sci USA **108**: 16428–16433.

153. Fedorenko E, McDermott JH, Norman-Haignere S, Kanwisher N (2012) Sensitivity to musical structure in the human brain. J Neurophysiol **108**: 3289–3300.

154. Honey CJ, Thompson CR, Lerner Y, Hasson U (2012) Not lost in translation: neural responses shared across languages. J Neurosci **32**: 15277–15283.

155. Merrill J, Sammler D, Bangert M, Goldhahn D, Lohmann G, et al. (2012) Perception of words and pitch patterns in song and speech. Front Psychol **3**: 76.

156. Rauschecker JP (2012) Ventral and dorsal streams in the evolution of speech and language. Front Evol Neurosci **4**: 7.

157. Asaridou SS, McQueen JM (2013) Speech and music shape the listening brain: evidence for shared domain-general mechanisms. Front Psychol **4**: 321.

158. Nan Y, Friederici AD (2013) Differential roles of right temporal cortex and Broca's area in pitch processing: evidence from music and Mandarin. Hum Brain Mapp **34**: 2045–2054.

159. Sammler D, Koelsch S, Ball T, Brandt A, Grigutsch M, et al. (2013) Co-localizing linguistic and musical syntax with intracranial EEG. Neuroimage **64**: 134–146.

160. Royal I, Lidji P, Théoret H, Russo FA, Peretz I (2015) Excitability of the motor system: a transcranial magnetic stimulation study on singing and speaking. Neuropsychologia **75**: 525–532.

161. Simonyan K, Fuertinger S (2015) Speech networks at rest and in action: interactions between functional brain networks controlling speech production. J Neurophysiol **113**: 2967–2978.

162. Abrams DA, Bhatara A, Ryali S, Balaban E, Levitin DJ, Menon V (2011) Decoding temporal structure in music and speech relies on shared brain resources but elicits different fine-scale spatial patterns. Cereb Cortex **21**: 1507–1518.

163. Farbood MM, Heeger DJ, Marcus G, Hasson U, Lerner Y (2015) The neural processing of hierarchical structure in music and speech at different timescales. Front Neurosci **9**: 157.

164. Norman-Haignere S, Kanwisher NG, McDermott JH (2015) Distinct cortical pathways for music and speech revealed by hypothesis-free voxel decomposition. Neuron **88**: 1281–1296.

165. Zatorre RJ, Zarate JM (2012) "Cortical processing of music," in D. Poeppel et al., eds, *The Human Auditory Cortex* (Springer, New York), 261–294.

166. Patel AD (2008) *Music, Language, and the Brain*. Oxford University Press, New York.

167. Perry DW, Zatorre RJ, Petrides M, Alivisatos B, Meyer E, Evans AC (1999) Localization of cerebral activity during simple singing. Neuroreport **10**: 3453–3458.

168. Zarate JM, Zatorre RJ (2008) Experience-dependent neural substrates involved in vocal pitch regulation during singing. Neuroimage **40**: 1871–1887.

169. Callan DE, Tsytsarev V, Hanakawa T, Callan AM, Katsuhara M, et al. (2006) Song and speech: brain regions involved with perception and covert production. Neuroimage **31**: 1327–1342.

170. Halwani GF, Loui P, Rüber T, Schlaug G (2011) Effects of practice and experience on the arcuate fasciculus: comparing singers, instrumentalists, and non-musicians. Front Psychol **2**: 156.

171. Loui P (2015) A dual-stream neuroanatomy of singing. Music Percept **32**: 232–241.

172. Jungblut M, Huber W, Pustelniak M, Schnitker R (2012) The impact of rhythm complexity on brain activation during simple singing: an event-related fMRI study. Restor Neurol Neurosci **30**: 39–53.

173. Alonso I, Davachi L, Valabrègue R, Lambrecq V, Dupont S, Samson S (2016) Neural correlates of binding lyrics and melodies for the encoding of new songs. Neuroimage **127**: 333–345.

174. Le Bomin S, Lecointre G, Heyer E (2016) The evolution of musical diversity: the key role of vertical transmission. PLoS One **11**: e0151570.

175. Brown S, Martinez MJ, Parsons LM (2006) Music and language side by side in the brain: a PET study of the generation of melodies and sentences. Eur J Neurosci **23**: 2791–2803.

176. Levitin DJ, Menon V (2003) Musical structure is processed in "language" areas of the brain: a possible role for Brodmann Area 47 in temporal coherence. Neuroimage **20**: 2142–2152.

177. Perrachione TK, Fedorenko EG, Vinke L, Gibson E, Dilley LC (2013) Evidence for shared cognitive processing of pitch in music and language. PLoS One **8**: e73372.

178. Rogalsky C, Rong F, Saberi K, Hickok G (2011) Functional anatomy of language and music perception: temporal and structural factors investigated using functional magnetic resonance imaging. J Neurosci **31**: 3843–3852.

179. Bidelman GM, Hutka S, Moreno S (2013) Tone language speakers and musicians share enhanced perceptual and cognitive abilities for musical pitch: evidence for bidirectionality between the domains of language and music. PLoS ONE **8**: e60676.

180. Sachs C (1962) *The Wellsprings of Music*. Da Capo Press, New York.

181. Patel AD, Foxton J, Griffiths TD (2005) Musically tone-deaf individuals have difficulty discriminating intonation contours extracted from speech. Brain Cogn **59**: 310–313.

182. Jiang C, Hamm JP, Lim VK, Kirk IJ, Yang Y (2010) Processing melodic contour and speech intonation in congenital amusics with Mandarin Chinese. Neuropsychologia **48**: 2630–2639.

183. Nan Y, Sun Y, Peretz I (2010) Congenital amusia in speakers of a tone language: association with lexical tone agnosia. Brain **133**: 2635–2642.

184. Tillmann B, Burnham D, Nguyen S, Grimault N, Gosselin N, Peretz I (2011) Congenital amusia (or tone-deafness) interferes with pitch processing in tone languages. Front Psychol **2**: 120.

185. Liu F, Jiang C, Pfordresher PQ, Mantell JT, Xu Y, et al. (2013) Individuals with congenital amusia imitate pitches more accurately in singing than in speaking: implications for music and language processing. Atten Percept Psychophys **75**: 1783–1798.

186. Jiang C, Hamm JP, Lim VK, Kirk IJ, Chen X, Yang Y (2012) Amusia results in abnormal brain activity following inappropriate intonation during speech comprehension. PLoS One **7**: e41411.

187. Koelsch S, Kasper E, Sammler D, Schulze K, Gunter T, Friederici AD (2004) Music, language and meaning: brain signatures of semantic processing. Nat Neurosci **7**: 302–307.

188. Jäncke L (2008) Music, memory and emotion. J Biol **7**: 21.

189. Steinbeis N, Koelsch S (2008) Comparing the processing of music and language meaning using EEG and fMRI provides evidence for similar and distinct neural representations. PLoS One **3**(5): e2226.

190. Fedorenko E, Patel A, Casasanto D, Winawer J, Gibson E (2009) Structural integration in language and music: evidence for a shared system. Mem Cognit **37**: 1–9.

191. Gordon RL, Magne CL, Large EW (2011) EEG correlates of song prosody: a new look at the relationship between linguistic and musical rhythm. Front Psychol **2**: 352.

192. Sammler D, Koelsch S, Friederici AD (2011) Are left fronto-temporal brain areas a prerequisite for normal music-syntactic processing? Cortex **47**: 659–673.

193. Yasui T, Kaga K, Sakai KL (2009) Language and music: differential hemispheric dominance in detecting unexpected errors in the lyrics and melody of memorized songs. Hum Brain Mapp **30**: 588–601.

194. Carreiras M, Lopez J, Rivero F, Corina D (2005) Neural processing of a whistled language. Nature **433**: 31–32.

195. Patel AD (2003) Language, music, syntax and the brain. Nat Neurosci **6**: 674–681.

196. Bigand E, Delbé C, Poulin-Charronnat B, Leman M, Tillmann B (2014) Empirical evidence for musical syntax processing? Computer simulations reveal the contribution of auditory short-term memory. Front Syst Neurosci **8**: 94.

197. Maess B, Koelsch S, Gunter TC, Friederici AD (2001) Musical syntax is processed in Broca's area: a magnetoencephalography (MEG) study. Nat Neurosci 4: 540–545.

198. Koelsch S, Gunter TC, v Cramon DY, Zysset S, Lohmann G, Friederici AD (2002) Bach speaks: a cortical "language-network" serves the processing of music. Neuroimage 17: 956–966.

199. Minati L, Rosazza C, D'Incerti L, Pietrocini E, Valentini L, et al. (2008) FMRI/ERP of musical syntax: comparison of melodies and unstructured note sequences. Neuroreport 19: 1381–1385.

200. Koelsch S, Fritz T, Schulze K, Alsop D, Schlaug G (2005) Adults and children processing music: an fMRI study. Neuroimage 25: 1068–1076.

201. Koelsch S, Rohrmeier M, Torrecuso R, Jentschke S (2013) Processing of hierarchical syntactic structure in music. Proc Natl Acad Sci USA 110: 15443–15448.

202. Wakita M (2014) Broca's area processes the heirarchical organization of observed action. Front Hum Neurosci 7: 937.

203. Musso M, Weiller C, Horn A, Glauche V, Umarova R, et al. (2015) A single dual-stream framework for syntactic computations in music and language. Neuroimage 117: 267–283.

204. Kunert R, Willems RM, Casasanto D, Patel AD, Hagoort P (2015) Music and language syntax interact in Broca's area: an fMRI study. PLoS One 10: e0141069.

205. Koelsch S, Fritz T, Schlaug G (2008) Amygdala activity can be modulated by unexpected chord functions during music listening. Neuroreport 19: 1815–1819.

206. Stefanics G, Háden GP, Sziller I, Balázs L, Beke A, Winkler I (2009) Newborn infants process pitch intervals. Clin Neurophysiol 120: 304–308.

207. Batterink L, Neville HJ (2013) The human brain processes syntax in the absence of conscious awareness. J Neurosci 33: 8528–8533.

208. Slevc LR, Faroqi-Shah Y, Saxena S, Okada BM (2016) Preserved processing of musical structure in a person with agrammatic aphasia. Neurocase 26: 1–7.

209. LaCroix AN, Diaz AF, Rogalsky C (2015) The relationship between the neural computations for speech and music perception is context-dependent: an activation likelihood estimate study. Front Psychol 6: 1138.

210. Slevc LR, Okada BM (2015) Processing structure in language and music: a case for shared reliance on cognitive control. Psychon Bull Rev 22: 637–652.

211. Angulo-Perkins A, Aubé W, Peretz I, Barios FA, Armony JL, Concha L (2014) Music listening engages specific cortical regions within the temporal lobes: differences between musicians and non-musicians. Cortex 59: 126–137.

212. Mesgarani N, Cheung C, Johnson K, Chang EF (2014) Phonetic feature encoding in human superior temporal gyrus. Science 343: 1006–1010.

213. Overath T, McDermott JH, Zarate JM, Poeppel D (2015) The cortical analysis of speech-specific temporal structure revealed by responses to sound quilts. Nat Neurosci 18: 903–911.

214. Smolders JW, Aertsen AM, Johannesma PI (1979) Neural representation of the acoustic biotope. A comparison of the response of auditory neurons to tonal and natural stimuli in the cat. Biol Cybern 35: 11–20.

215. Johannesma P, Aertsen A (1982) Statistical and dimensional analysis of the neural representation of the acoustic biotope in frog. J Med Syst 6: 399–421.

216. Fritz J, Poeppel D, Trainor L, Schlaug G, Patel AD, et al. (2013) "The neurobiology of language, speech, and music," in M. A. Arbib, ed., *Language, Music and the Brain:A Mysterious Relationship* (MIT Press, Cambridge MA), 417–459.

217. Cross I, Fitch WT, Aboitiz F, Iriki A, Jarvis ED, et al. (2013) "Culture and evolution," in M. A. Arbib, ed., *Language, Music and the Brain: A Mysterious Relationship* (MIT Press, Cambridge MA), 541–562.

218. **Meyer LB** (1956) *Emotion and Meaning in Music*. Chicago University Press, Chicago and London.

219. **Juslin PN, Västfäll D** (2008) Emotional responses to music: the need to consider underlying mechanisms. Behav Brain Sci **31**: 559–621.

220. **Zentner M, Grandjean D, Scherer K** (2008) Emotions evoked by the sound of music: characterization, classification and measurement. Emotion **8**: 494–521.

221. **Koelsch S** (2010) Towards a neural basis of music-evoked emotions. Trends Cogn Sci **14**: 131–137.

222. **Rose S** (2005) *The 21st Century Brain: Explaining, Mending and Manipulating the Mind*. Jonathan Cape, London.

223. **Peretz I** (2006) The nature of music from a biological perspective. Cognition **100**: 1–32.

224. **Hornby N** (2003) *31 Songs*. Penguin, New York.

225. **Salimpoor VN, Benovoy M, Longo G, Cooperstock JR, Zatorre RJ** (2009) The rewarding aspects of music listening are related to degree of emotional arousal. PLoS One **4**: e7487.

226. **Harrison L, Loui P** (2014) Thrills, chills, frissons, and skin orgasms: toward an integrative model of transcendent psychophysiological experiences in music. Front Psychol **5**: 790.

227. **D'Hondt F, Lassonde M, Collignon O, Dubarry A-S, Robert M**, et al. (2010) Early brain-body impact of emotional arousal. Front Hum Neurosci **4**: 33.

228. **Button KS, Ioannidis JPA, Mokrysz C, Nosel BA, Flint J**, et al. (2013) Power failure: why small sample size undermines the reliability of neuroscience. Nat Neurosci **14**: 365–376.

229. **Leitman DI, Wolf DH, Ragland JD, Laukka P, Loughead J**, et al. (2010) "It's not what you say, but how you say it": a reciprocal temporo-frontal network for affective prosody. Front Hum Neurosci **4**: 19.

230. **Kocak M, Ulmer JL, Biswal BB, Aralasmak A, Daniels DL, Mark LP** (2005) The influence of gender on auditory and language cortical activation patterns: preliminary data. AJNR Am J Neuroradiol **26**: 2248–2255.

231. **Yakunina N, Kang EK, Kim TS, Min JH, Kim SS, Nam EC** (2015) Effects of scanner acoustic noise on intrinsic brain activity during auditory stimulation. Neuroradiology **57**: 1063–1073.

232. **Skouras S, Gray M, Critchley H, Koelsch S** (2013) fMRI scanner noise interaction with affective neural processes. PLoS One **8**: e80564.

233. **Blood AJ, Zatorre RL, Bermudez P, Evans AC** (1999) Emotional responses to pleasant and unpleasant music correlate with activity in paralimbic regions. Nat Neurosci **2**: 322–327.

234. **Blood AJ, Zatorre RL** (2001) Intensely pleasurable responses to music correlate with activity in brain regions implicated in reward and emotion. Proc Natl Acad Sci USA **98**: 11818–11823.

235. **Menon V, Levitin DJ** (2005) The rewards of music listening: response and physiological connectivity of the mesolimbic system. Neuroimage **28**: 175–184.

236. **Carter RM, MacInnes JJ, Huettel SA, Adcock RA** (2009) Activation of the VTA and nucleus accumbens increases in anticipation of both gains and losses. Front Behav Neurosci **3**: 21.

237. **Mannella F, Gurney K, Baldassarre G** (2013) The nucleus accumbens as a nexus between values and goals in goal-directed behaviour: a review and a new hypothesis. Front Behav Neurosci **7**: 135.

238. **Khant T, Chang LJ, Park SQ, Heinzle J, Haynes J-D** (2012) Connectivity-based parcellation of the human orbitofrontal cortex. J Neurosci **32**: 6240–6250.

239. **Mitterschiffthaler MT, Fu CHY, Dalton JA, Andrew CM, Williams SCR** (2007) A functional MRI study of happy and sad affective states induced by classical music. Hum Brain Mapp **28**: 1150–1162.

240. **Oelmann H, Laeng B** (2009) The emotional meaning of harmonic intervals. Cogn Process **10**: 113–131.

241. Pallesen KJ, Brattico E, Bailey C, Korvenoja A, Koivisto J, et al. (2005) Emotion processing of major, minor, and dissonant chords: a functional magnetic resonance imaging study. Ann NY Acad Sci **1060**: 450–453.

242. Koelsch S, Fritz T, v Cramon DY, Müller K, Friederici AD (2006) Investigating emotion with music: an fMRI study. Hum Brain Mapp **27**: 239–250.

243. Mueller K, Fritz T, Mildner T, Richter M, Schulze K, et al. (2015) Investigating the dynamics of the brain response to music: a central role of the ventral striatum/nucleus accumbens. Neuroimage **116**: 68–79.

244. Cox A (2001) The mimetic hypothesis and embodied musical meaning. Music Sci **2**: 195–212.

245. Kleber B, Birbaumer N, Veit R, Trevorrow T, Lotze M (2007) Overt and imagined singing of an Italian aria. Neuroimage **36**: 889–900.

246. Trost W, Ethofer T, Zentner M, Vuilleumier P (2012) Mapping aesthetic musical emotions in the brain. Cereb Cortex **22**: 2769–2783.

247. Brattico E, Bogert B, Alluri V, Tervaniemi M, Eerola T, Jacobsen T (2016) It's sad but I like it: the neural dissociation between musical emotions and liking in experts and laypersons. Front Hum Neurosci **9**: 676.

248. Eschrich S, Münte TF, Altenmüller EO (2008) Unforgettable film music: the role of emotion in episodic long-term memory of music. BMC Neurosci **9**: 48.

249. Koelsch S (2009) "A neuroscientific perspective on music therapy", in S. Dalla Bella et al., *The Neurosciences and Music III—Disorders and Plasticity*, Ann NY Acad Sci **1169**: 374–384. Wiley-Blackwell, Boston.

250. Blum K, Chen TJ, Chen AL, Madigan M, Downs BW, et al. (2010) Do dopaminergic gene polymorphisms affect mesolimbic reward activation of music listening response? Therapeutic impact on Reward Deficiency Syndrome (RDS). Med Hypotheses **74**: 513–520.

251. Klasen M, Kenworthy CA, Mathiak KA, Kircher TTJ, Mathiak K (2011) Supramodal representation of emotions. J Neurosci **31**: 13635–13643.

252. Eldar E, Ganor O, Admon R, Bleich A, Hendler T (2007) Feeling the real world: limbic response to music depends on related content. Cereb Cortex **17**: 2828–2840.

253. Bouhuys AL, Bloem GM, Groothuis TGG (1995) Induction of depressed and elated mood by music influences the perception of facial expressions in healthy subjects. J Affect Disord **33**: 215–226.

254. Vines BW, Krumhansl CL, Wanderley MM, Dalca IM, Levitin DJ (2011) Music to my eyes: cross-modal interactions in the perception of emotions in musical performance. Cognition **118**: 157–170.

255. Jeong J-W, Diwadkar VA, Chugani CD, et al. (2010) Congruence of happy and sad emotion in music and faces modifies cortical audiovisual activation. Neuroimage **54**: 2973–2982.

256. Dutton D (2009) *The Art Instinct*. Oxford University Press, Oxford, UK.

257. Boltz M, Schulkind M, Kantra S (1991) Effects of background music on the remembering of filmed events. Mem Cognit **19**: 593–606.

258. Baumgartner T, Esslen M, Jäncke L (2006) From emotion perception to emotion experience: emotions evoked by pictures and classical music. Int J Psychophysiol **60**: 34–43.

259. Griffiths TD, Warren JD, Dean JL, Howard D (2004) "When the feeling's gone": a selective loss of musical emotion. J Neurol Neurosurg Psychiatry **75**: 344–345.

260. Gosselin N, Peretz I, Noulhiane M, Hasboun D, Beckett C, et al. (2005) Impaired recognition of scary music following unilateral temporal lobe excision. Brain **128**: 628–640.

261. Gosselin N, Peretz I, Johnsen E, Adolphs R (2007) Amygdala damage impairs emotional recognition of music. Neuropsychologia **45**: 236–244.

262. Khalfa S, Guye M, Peretz I, Chapon F, Girard N, et al. (2008) Evidence of lateralized anteromedial temporal structures involvement in musical emotion processing. Neuropsychologia **46**: 2485–2493.

263. Lerner Y, Papo D, Zhdanov A, Belozersky L, Hendler T (2009) Eyes wide shut: amygdala mediates eyes-closed effect on emotional experience with music. PLoS One **4**: e6230.

264. Chanda ML, Levitin DJ (2013) The neurochemistry of music. Trends Cogn Sci **17**: 179–193.

265. Pereira CS, Teixeira J, Figueiredo P, Xavier J, Castro SL, Brattico E (2011) Music and emotions in the brain: familiarity matters. PLoS One **6**: e27241.

266. Salimpoor VN, Benovoy M, Larcher K, Dagher A, Zatorre RJ (2011) Anatomically distinct dopamine release during anticipation and experience of peak emotion in music. Nat Neurosci **14**: 257–264.

267. Salimpoor VN, van den Bosch, Kovacevic N, McIntosh AR, Dagher A, Zatorre RJ (2013) Interactions between the nucleus accumbens and auditory cortices predict music reward value. Science **340**: 216–219.

268. Zatorre RJ, Salimpoor VN (2013) From perception to pleasure: music and its neural substrates. Proc Natl Acad Sci USA **110**: 10430–10437.

269. Gold BP, Frank MJ, Bogert B, Brattico E (2013) Pleasurable music affects reinforcement learning according to the listener. Front Psychol **4**: 541.

270. Leaver AM, Van Lare J, Zielinski B, Halpern AR, Rauschecker JP (2009) Brain activation during anticipation of sound sequences. J Neurosci **29**: 2477–2485.

271. Keeler JR, Roth EA, Neuser BL, Spitsbergen JM, Waters DJ, Vianney JM (2015) The neurochemistry and social flow of singing: bonding and oxytocin. Front Hum Neurosci **9**: 518.

272. Nilsson U (2009) Soothing music can increase oxytocin levels during bed rest after open-heart surgery: a randomised control trial. J Clin Nurs **18**: 2153–2161.

273. Kosfeld M, Heinrichs M, Zak PJ, Fischbacher U, Fehr E (2005) Oxytocin increases trust in humans. Nature **435**: 673–676.

274. Baumgartner T, Heinrichs M, Vonlanthen A, Fischbacher U, Fehr E (2008) Oxytocin shapes the neural circuitry of trust and adaptation in humans. Neuron **58**: 639–650.

275. Israel S, Lerer E, Shalev I, Uzefovsky F, Riebold M, et al. (2009) The oxytocin receptor (OXTR) contributes to prosocial fund allocations in the dictator game and the social value orientations task. PLoS One **4**: e5535.

276. Strathearn L, Fonagy P, Amico J, Montague PR (2009) Adult attachment predicts maternal brain and oxytocin response to infant cues. Neuropsychopharmacology **34**: 2655–2666.

277. Hurlemann R, Patin A, Onur OA, Cohen MX, Baumgartner T, et al. (2010) Oxytocin enhances amygdala-dependent, socially reinforced learning and emotional empathy in humans. J Neurosci **30**: 4999–5007.

278. Rilling JK, Demarco AC, Hackett PD, Thompson R, Ditzen B, et al. (2011) Effects of oxytocin and vasopressin on cooperative behaviour and associated brain activity in men. Psychoneuroendocrinology **37**: 447–461.

279. Bethlehem RAI, Baron-Cohen S, Van Honk J, Auyeung B, Bos PA (2014) The oxytocin paradox. Front Behav Neurosci **8**: 48.

280. Lieberwirth C, Wang Z (2014) Social bonding: regulation by neuropeptides. Front Neurosci **8**: 171.

281. Preckel K, Scheele D, Kendrick KM, Maier W, Hurlemann R (2014) Oxytocin facilitates social approach behaviour in women. Front Behav Neurosci **8**: 191.

282. Marsh N, Scheele D, Gerhardt H, Strang S, Enax L, et al. (2015) The neuropeptide oxytocin induces a social altruism bias. J Neurosci **35**: 15696–15701.

283. **Ulmer-Yaniv A, Avitsur R, Kanat-Maymon Y, Schneiderman I, Zagoory-Sharon O, Feldman R** (2016) Affiliation, reward, and immune biomarkers coalesce to support social synchrony during periods of bond formation in humans. Brain Behav Immun **56**: 130–139.

284. **Le Merrer J, Becker JA, Befort K, Kieffer BL** (2009) Reward processing by the opioid system in the brain. Physiol Rev **89**: 1379–1412.

285. **Dunbar RIM, Kaskatis K, MacDonald I, Barra V** (2012) Performance of music elevates pain threshold and positive affect: implications for the evolutionary function of music. Evol Psych **10**: 688–702.

286. **Tarr B, Launay J, Dunbar RIM** (2014) Music and social bonding: "self-other" merging and neurohormonal mechanisms. Front Psychol **5**: 1096.

287. **Tarr B, Launay J, Cohen E, Dunbar R** (2015) Synchrony and exertion during dance independently raise pain threshold and encourage social bonding. Biol Lett **11**: 20150767.

288. **Weinstein D, Launay J, Pearce E, Dunbar RI, Stewart L** (2016) Group music performance causes elevated pain thresholds and social bonding in small and large groups of singers. Evol Hum Behav **37**: 152–158.

289. **McKinney CH, Tims FC, Kumar AM, Kumar M** (1997) The effect of selected classical music and spontaneous imagery on plasma beta-endorphin. J Behav Med **20**: 85–99.

290. **Stefano GB, Zhu W, Cadet P, Salamon E, Mantione KJ, et al.** (2004) Music alters constitutively expressed opiate and cytokine processes in listeners. Med Sci Monit **10**: MS18-MS27.

291. **Hu H, Real E, Takamiya K, Kang M-G, Ledoux J, et al.** (2007) Emotion enhances learning via nor-epinephrine regulation of AMPA-receptor trafficking. Cell **131**: 160–173.

292. **Tang J, Dani JA** (2009) Dopamine enables in vivo synaptic plasticity associated with the addictive drug nicotine. Neuron **63**: 673–682.

293. **Bancroft J** (2005) The endocrinology of sexual arousal. J Endocrinol **186**: 411–427.

294. **Sabatinelli D, Bradley MM, Lang PJ, Costa VD, Versace F** (2007) Pleasure rather than salience activates human nucleus accumbens and medial prefrontal cortex. J Neurophysiol **98**: 1374–1379.

295. **Sescousse G, Caldú X, Segura B, Dreher JC** (2013) Processing of primary and secondary rewards: a quantitative meta-analysis and review of human functional neuroimaging studies. Neurosci Biobehav Rev **37**: 681–696.

296. **Mas-Herrero E, Zatorre RJ, Rodriguez-Fornella A, Marco-Pallerés J** (2014) Dissociation between musical and monetary reward responses in specific musical anhedonia. Curr Biol **24**: 1–6.

297. **Krüger TH, Hartmann U, Schedlowski M** (2005) Prolactinergic and dopaminergic mechanisms underlying sexual arousal and orgasm in humans. World J Urol **23**: 130–138.

298. **Goldstein JM, Seidman LJ, Horton NJ, Makris N, Kennedy DN, et al.** (2001) Normal sexual dimorphism of the adult human brain assessed by in vivo magnetic resonance imaging. Cereb Cortex **11**: 490–497.

299. **Cosgrove KP, Mazure CM, Staley JK** (2007) Evolving knowledge of sex differences in brain structure, function and chemistry. Biol Psychiatry **62**: 847–855.

300. **Luders E, Gaser C, Narr KL, Toga AW** (2009) Why sex matters: brain size independent differences in gray matter distributions between men and women. J Neurosci **29**: 14265–14270.

301. **Henson RA** (1977) "Neurological aspects of musical experience," in M. Critchley and R. A. Henson, eds, *Music and the Brain: Studies on the Neurology of Music* (Heinemann Medical Books Ltd, London), 3–21.

302. **Park M, Gutyrchik E, Welker L, Carl P, Pöppel E, et al.** (2015) Sadness is unique: neural processing of emotions in speech prosody in musicians and non-musicians. Front Hum Neurosci **8**: 1049.

303. **Vuoskoski JK, Thompson WF, McIlwain D, Eerola T** (2011) Who enjoys listening to sad music and why? Music Percept **29**: 311–317.

304. **Taruffi L, Koelsch S** (2014) The paradox of music-evoked sadness: an online survey. PLoS One **9**: e110490.

305. **Sachs ME, Damasio A, Habibi A** (2015) The pleasures of sad music: a systematic review. Front Hum Neurosci **9**: 404.

306. **Fritz T, Jentschke S, Gosselin N, Sammler D, Peretz I,** et al. (2009) Universal recognition of three basic emotions in music. Curr Biol **19**: 573–576.

307. **Egermann H, Fernando N, Chuen L, McAdams S** (2015) Music induces universal emotion-related psychophysiological responses: comparing Canadian listeners to Congolese Pygmies. Front Psychol **5**: 1341.

308. **Tomasello M, Carpenter M, Call J, Behne T, Moll H** (2005) Understanding and sharing intentions: the origins of cultural cognition. Behav Brain Sci **28**: 675–691.

309. **Pearce E, Launay J, Dunbar RIM** (2015) The ice-breaker effect: singing mediates fast social bonding. R Soc Open Sci **2**: 150221.

310. **Trehub SE, Becker J, Morley I** (2015) Cross-cultural perspectives on music and musicality. Philos Trans R Soc Lond B Biol Sci **370**: 20140096.

311. **Huron D** (2003) "Is music an evolutionary adaptation?" in **I. Peretz** and **R. L. Zatorre**, eds, *The Cognitive Neuroscience of Music* (Oxford University Press, Oxford), 57–75.

312. **Fancourt D, Ockelford A, Belai A** (2014) The psychoneuroimmunological effects of music: a systematic review and a new model. Brain Behav Immun **36**: 15–26.

313. **Malm WP** (1967) *Music Cultures of the Pacific, the Near East, and Asia*. Prentice-Hall, New Jersey.

314. **Magowan F** (2007) *Melodies of Mourning: Music and Emotion in Northern Australia*. UWA Press, Crawley WA.

315. **Cross I** (2003) "Music, cognition, culture and evolution," in **I. Peretz** and **R. L. Zatorre**, eds, *The Cognitive Neuroscience of Music* (Oxford University Press, Oxford), 42–56.

316. **Pamjav H, Juhász Z, Zalán A, Németh E, Damdin B** (2012) A comparative phylogenetic study of genetics and folk music. Mol Genet Genomics **287**: 337–349.

317. **Brown S, Savage PE, Ko AM, Stoneking M, Ko YC,** et al. (2013) Correlations in the population structure of music, genes and language. Proc Biol Soc **281**(1774): 20132072.

318. **Cross I** (2009) The evolutionary nature of musical meaning. Music Sci (Special Issue "Music and evolution"): 179–200.

319. **Novembre G, Keller PE** (2014) A conceptual review on action-perception coupling in the musician's brain: what is it good for? Front Hum Neurosci **8**: 603.

320. **Cross I, Woodruff GE** (2009) "Music as a communicative medium," in **R. Botha** and **C. Knight**, eds, *The Prehistory of Language* (Oxford University Press, Oxford), 77–98.

321. **Trehub S** (2000) "Human processing dispositions and musical universals," in **N. L. Wallin, B. Merker** and **S. Brown**, eds, *The Origins of Music* (MIT Press, Cambridge MA), 427–448.

322. **Dissanayake E** (2000) "Antecedents of the temporal arts in early mother-infant interaction," in **N. L. Wallin, B. Merker** and **S. Brown**, eds, *The Origins of Music* (MIT Press, Cambridge MA), 389–410.

323. **Miall DS, Dissanayake E** (2003) The poetics of babytalk. Hum Nat **14**: 337–364.

324. **Falk D** (2004) Prelinguistic evolution in early hominids: whence motherese? Behav Brain Sci **27**: 491–503.

325. **Trevarthan C** (2008) The musical art of infant conversation: narrating in the time of sympathetic experience, without rational interpretation, before words. Music Sci 12(Suppl 1): 15–46.

326. **Dissanayake E** (2000) *Art and Intimacy: How the Arts Began* (McLellan Endowed Series). University of Washington Press, Seattle, London UK.

327. **Corbeil M, Trehub SE, Peretz I** (2013) Speech vs. singing: infants choose happier sounds. Front Psychol **4**: 372.

328. **Fernald A** (1989) Intonation and communicative intent in mother's speech to infants: is the melody the message? Child Dev **60**: 1497–1510.

329. **Trehub S** (2003) The developmental origins of musicality. Nat Neurosci **6**: 669–673.

330. **Cross I** (2009) Communicative development: neonate crying reflects patterns of native-language speech. Curr Biol **19**: R1078-R1079.

331. **Trainor LJ, Schmidt LA** (2003) "Processing emotions induced by music," in **I. Peretz** and **R. L. Zatorre**, eds, *The Cognitive Neuroscience of Music* (Oxford University Press, Oxford), 310–324.

332. **DeCasper AJ, Fifer WP** (1980) Of human bonding: newborns prefer their mothers' voices. Science **208**: 1174–1176.

333. **DeCasper AJ, Prescott PA** (1984) Human newborns' perception of male voices: preference discrimination and reinforcing value. Dev Psychobiol **17**: 481–491.

334. **Malloch S, Trevarthen C** (2008) *Communicative Musicality: Exploring the Basis of Human Companionship.* Oxford University Press, Oxford.

335. **Kliemann D, Dziobek I, Hatri A, Steimke R, Heekeren HR** (2010) Atypical reflexive gaze patterns on emotional faces in autism spectrum disorders. J Neurosci **30**: 12281–12287.

336. **Strathearn L, Li J, Fonagy P, Montague PR** (2008) What's in a smile? Maternal brain responses to infant facial cues. Pediatrics **122**: 40–51.

337. **Lenzi D, Trentini C, Pantanao P, Macaluso E, Iacobini M**, et al. (2009) Neural basis of maternal communication and emotional expression processing during infant preverbal stage. Cereb Cortex **19**: 1124–1133.

338. **Nummenmaa L, Calder AJ** (2009) Neural mechanisms of social attention. Trends Cogn Sci **13**: 135–143.

339. **Likowski KU, Muchlberger A, Gerdes ABM, Wieser MJ, Pauli P, Weyers P** (2012) Facial mimicry and the mirror neuron system: simultaneous acquisition of facial electromyography and functional magnetic resonance imaging. Front Hum Neurosci **6**: 214.

340. **Cross I** (1999) "Is music the most important thing we ever did? Music, development and evolution," in **S. W. Yi**, ed., *Music, Mind and Science* (Seoul National University Press, Seoul), 10–39.

341. **DeCasper AJ, Prescott PA** (2009) Lateralized processes constrain auditory reinforcement in human newborns. Hear Res **255**: 135–141.

342. **Granier-Deferre C, Ribeiro A, Jacquet AY, Bassereau S** (2011) Near-term foetuses process temporal features of speech. Dev Sci **14**: 336–352.

343. **Partanen E, Kujala T, Näätänen R, Liitola A, Sambeth A, Huotilainen M** (2013) Learning-induced neural plasticity of speech processing before birth. Proc Natl Acad Sci USA **110**: 15145–15150.

344. **Kisilevsky BS, Hains SMJ, Jacquet A-Y, Granier-Deferre C, Lecanuet JP** (2004) Maturation of fetal responses to music. Dev Sci **7**: 550–559.

345. **Kisilevsky BS, Hains SMJ, Brown CA, Lee CT, Cowperthwaite B**, et al. (2009) Fetal sensitivity to properties of maternal speech and language. Infant Behav Dev **32**: 59–71.

346. **Ullal-Gupta S, Vanden Bosch der Nederlanden CM, Tichko P, Lahav A, Hannon EE** (2013) Linking prenatal experience to the emerging musical mind. Front Syst Neurosci **7**: 48.

347. **Beauchemin M, González-Frankenberger B, Tremblay J, Vannasing P, Martínez-Montes E**, et al. (2011) Mother and stranger: an electrophysiological study of voice processing in newborns. Cereb Cortex **21**: 1705–1711.

348. **Trehub S** (2012) Behavioral methods in infancy: pitfalls of single measures. Ann NY Acad Sci **1252**: 37–42.

349. **Trehub S** (2003) "Musical predispositions in infancy," in **I. Peretz** and **R. L. Zatorre**, eds, *The Cognitive Neuroscience of Music* (Oxford University Press, Oxford), 3–20.

350. **Saccuman MC, Scifo P** (2009) "Using MRI to characterize the anatomy and function of the auditory cortex in infancy," in **S. Dalla Bella** et al., *The Neurosciences and Music III—Disorders and Plasticity*, Ann NY Acad Sci **1169**: 297–307 (Wiley-Blackwell, Boston).

351. **Winkler I, Háden GP, Ladinig O, Sziller I, Honing H** (2009) Newborn infants detect the beat of music. Proc Natl Acad Sci USA **106**: 2468–2471.

352. **He C, Trainor LJ** (2009) Finding the pitch of the missing fundamental in infants. J Neurosci **29**: 7718–7722.

353. **Grossman T** (2010) The development of emotion perception in face and voice during infancy. Restor Neurol Neurosci **28**: 219–236.

354. **Blasi A, Mercure E, Lloyd-Fox S, Thomson A, Brammer M**, et al. (2011) Early specialization for voice and emotion processing in the infant brain. Curr Biol **21**: 1220–1224.

355. **Ilie G, Thompson WF** (2011) Experiential and cognitive changes following seven minutes' exposure to music and speech. Music Percept **28**: 247–264.

356. **Koelsch S, Siebel WA** (2005) Towards a neural basis of music perception. Trends Cogn Sci **9**: 578–584.

357. **Koelsch S** (2012) *Brain and Music.* Wiley Blackwell, Chichester, UK.

358. **Fransson P, Skiold B, Horsch S, Nordell A, Blennow M**, et al. (2007) Resting-state networks in the infant brain. Proc Natl Acad Sci USA **104**: 15531–15536.

359. **Perani D, Saccuman MC, Scifo P, Spada D, Andreolli G**, et al. (2010) Functional specializations for music processing in the human newborn brain. Proc Natl Acad Sci USA **107**: 4758–4763.

360. **Sambeth A, Ruohio K, Alku P, Fellman V, Huotilainen M** (2008) Sleeping newborns extract prosody from continuous speech. Clin Neurophysiol **119**: 332–341.

361. **Saito Y, Aoyama S, Kondo T, Fukumoto R, Konishi N**, et al. (2007) Frontal cerebral blood flow change associated with infant-directed speech. Arch Dis Child Fetal Neonatal Ed **92**: F113-F116.

362. **Gómez DM, Berent I, Banavides-Varela S, Bion RA, Cattarossi L**, et al. (2014) Language universals at birth. Proc Natl Acad Sci USA **111**: 5837–5841.

363. **Berent I, Pan H, Zhao X, Epstein J, Bennett ML**, et al. (2014) Language universals engage Broca's area. PLoS One **9**: e95155.

364. **Peña M, Maki A, Kovačić D, Dehaene-Lambertz G, Kolzumi H**, et al. (2003) Sounds and silence: an optical topography study of language recognition at birth. Proc Natl Acad Sci USA **100**: 11702–11705.

365. **Alexandra PF, Ferguson M, Molfese DL, Peach K, Lehman C, Molfese VJ** (2007) Smoking during pregnancy affects speech-processing ability in newborn infants. Environ Health Perspect **115**: 623–629.

366. **Perani D, Saccuman MC, Scifo P, Anwander A, Spada D**, et al. (2011) Neural language networks at birth. Proc Natl Acad Sci USA **108**: 16056–16061.

367. **Hinkley LBN, Marco EJ, Brown EG, Bukshpun P, Gold J**, et al. (2016) The contribution of the corpus callosum to language lateralization. J Neurosci **36**: 4522–4533.

368. **Paus T, Collins DL, Evans AC, Leonard G, Pike B, Zijdenbos A** (2001) Maturation of white matter in the human brain: a review of magnetic resonance studies. Brain Res Bull **54**: 255–266.

369. **Dehaene-Lambertz G, Hertz-Pannier L, Dubois J, Meriaux S, Roche A**, et al. (2006) Functional organization of perisylvian activation during presentation of sentences in preverbal infants. Proc Natl Acad Sci USA **103**: 14240–14245.

370. Dehaene-Lambertz G, Montavont A, Jobert A, Allirol L, Dubois J, et al. (2010) Language or music, mother or Mozart? Structural and environmental influences on infants' language networks. Brain Lang 114: 53–65.

371. Leroy F, Glasel H, Dubois J, Hertz-Pannier L, Thirion B, et al. (2011) Early maturation of the linguistic dorsal pathway in human infants. J Neurosci 31: 1500–1506.

372. Holland SK, Vannest J, Mecoli M, Jacola LM, Tillema JM, et al. (2007) Functional MRI of language lateralization during development in children. Int J Audiol 46: 533–551.

373. Thiessen ED, Saffran JR (2009) "How the melody facilitates the message and vice versa in infant learning and memory," in S. Dalla Bella et al., *The Neurosciences and Music III—Disorders and Plasticity*, Ann NY Acad Sci 1169: 225–233 (Wiley-Blackwell, Boston).

374. Pujol J, Soriano-Mas C, Ortiz H, Sebastián-Gallés N, Losilla JM, Deus J (2006) Myelination of language-related areas in the developing brain. Neurology 66: 339–343.

375. Su P, Kuan C-C, Kaga K, Sano M, Mima K (2008) Myelination progression in language-correlated regions in the brain of normal children determined by quantitative MRI assessment. Int J Pediatr Otorhinolaryngol 72: 1751–1763.

376. O'Muircheartaigh J, Dean DC 3rd, Dirks H, Waskiewicz N, Lehman K, et al. (2013) Interactions between white matter asymmetry and language during neurodevelopment. J Neurosci 33: 16170–16177.

377. Redcay E, Haist F, Courchesne E (2008) Functional neuroimaging of speech perception during a pivotal period in language acquisition. Dev Sci 11: 237–252.

378. Brauer J, Anwander A, Perani D, Friederici AD (2013) Dorsal and ventral pathways in language development. Brain Lang 127: 289–295.

379. Holowka S, Petitto LA (2002) Left hemisphere cerebral specialization for babies while babbling. Science 297: 1515.

380. Matsuda Y-T, Ueno K, Waggoner A, Erickson D, Shimura Y, et al. (2011) Processing of infant-directed speech by adults. Neuroimage 54: 611–621.

381. Gaab N, Keenan JP, Schlaug G (2003) The effects of gender on the neural substrates of pitch memory. J Cogn Neurosci 15: 810–820.

382. Ruytjens L, Georgiadis JR, Holstege G, Wit HP, Albers FW, Willemsen AT (2007) Functional sex differences in human primary auditory cortex. Eur J Nucl Med Mol Imaging 34: 2073–2081.

383. Hetrick WP, Sandman CA, Bunney WE Jr, Jin Y, Potkin SG, White MH (1996) Gender differences in gating of the auditory evoked potential in normal subjects. Biol Psychiatry 39: 51–58.

384. Loui P, Machorik JP, Li HC, Schlaug G (2013) Effects of voice on emotional arousal. Front Psychol 4: 675.

385. Brun CC, Lepore N, Luders E, Chou Y-Y, Madsen SK, et al. (2009) Sex differences in brain structure in auditory and cingulate regions. Neuroreport 20: 930–935.

386. Kaiser A, Haller S, Schmitz S, Nitsch C (2009) On sex/gender related similarities and differences in fMRI language research. Brain Res Rev 61: 49–59.

387. Burman DD, Bitan T, Booth JR (2008) Sex differences in neural processing of language among children. Neuropsychologia 46: 1349–1362.

388. Lewis J (2013) "A cross-cultural perspective on the significance of music and dance to culture and society," in M. A. Arbib, ed., *Language, Music and the Brain: A Mysterious Relationship* (MIT Press, Cambridge MA), 45–65.

389. Fukui H, Yamashita M (2003) The effects of music and visual stress in testosterone and cortisol in men and women. Neuro Endocrinol Lett 24: 173–180.

390. Fischer-Shofty M, Levkovitz Y, Shamay-Tsoory SG (2012) Oxytocin facilitates accurate perception of competition in men and kinship in women. Soc Cogn Affect Neurosci 8: 313–317.

391. **Lewis JW, Talkington WJ, Walker NA, Spirou GA, Jajosky A**, et al. (2009) Human cortical organization for processing vocalizations indicates representation of harmonic structure as a signal attribute. J Neurosci **29**: 2283–2296.

392. **Peretz I, Vuvan D, Lagrois M-E, Armony JL** (2015) Neural overlap in processing music and speech. Philos Trans R Soc Lond B Biol Sci **370**: 20140090.

393. **Moerel M, De Martino F, Santoro R, Uqurbil K, Goebel R**, et al. (2013) Processing of natural sounds: characterization of multipeak spectral tuning in human auditory cortex. J Neurosci **33**: 11888–11898.

394. **Moerel M, De Martino F, Santoro R, Yacoub E, Formisano E** (2015) Representation of pitch chroma by multi-peak spectral tuning in human auditory cortex. Neuroimage **106**: 161–169.

395. **Zatorre RJ, Gandour JT** (2008) Neural specializations for speech and pitch: moving beyond the dichotomies. Philos Trans R Soc Lond B Biol Sci **363**: 1087–1104.

396. **Cameron DJ, Bentley J, Grahn JA** (2015) Cross-cultural influences on rhythm processing: reproduction, discrimination, and beat tapping. Front Psychol **6**: 366.

397. **Dunbar RIM** (1996) *Grooming, Gossip, and the Evolution of Language.* Faber and Faber, London.

398. **Malouf D** (2008) "The domestic cantata," in *Every Move You Make* (Vintage, London) 213–244.

Chapter Five

1. **Ridley M** (1996) *The Origins of Virtue: Human Instincts and The Evolution of Cooperation.* Penguin, London.

2. **Taborsky M, Frommen JG, Riehl C** (2016) The evolution of cooperation based on direct fitness benefits. Philos Trans R Soc Lond B Biol Sci **371**: 20150472.

3. **Hamilton WD** (1964) The genetical evolution of social behavior. J Theor Biol **7**: 1–52.

4. **Maynard Smith J** (1964) Group selection and kin selection. Nature **201**: 1145–1147.

5. **Kurzban R, Burton-Chellew MN, West SA** (2015) The evolution of altruism in humans. Annu Rev Psychol **66**: 575–599.

6. **Trivers RL** (1971) The evolution of reciprocal altruism. Q Rev Biol **46**: 35–57.

7. **De Waal FMB** (2008) Putting the altruism back into altruism: the evolution of empathy. Annu Rev Psychol **59**: 279–300.

8. **De Waal FB, Suchak M** (2009) Prosocial primates: selfish and unselfish motivations. Philos Trans R Soc Lond B Biol Sci **365**: 2711–2722.

9. **Hrdy SB** (2009) *Mothers and Others: The Evolutionary Origins of Mutual Understanding.* Belknap Press, Cambridge MA.

10. **Silk JB, House BR** (2016) The evolution of altruistic social preferences in human groups. Philos Trans R Soc Lond B Biol Sci **371**: 20150097.

11. **Warneken F, Tomasello M** (2009) Varieties of altruism in children and chimpanzees. Trends Cogn Sci **13**: 397–402.

12. **Hamann K, Warneken F, Greenberg JR, Tomasello M** (2011) Collaboration encourages equal sharing in children but not in chimpanzees. Nature **476**: 328–331.

13. **Grueter CC, Chapais B, Zinner D** (2012) Evolution of multilevel social systems in nonhuman primates and humans. Int J Primatol **33**: 1002–1037.

14. **Muthukrishna M, Henrich J** (2016) Innovation in the collective brain. Philos Trans R Soc Lond B Biol Sci **371**(1690): 20150192.

15. **Fehr E, Fischbacher U** (2003) The nature of human altruism. Nature **425**: 785–791.

16. **Cavalli-Sforza LL, Feldman MW** (1983) Paradox of the evolution of communication and of social interactivity. Proc Natl Acad Sci USA **80**: 2017–2021.

17. **Nowak MA** (2006) Five rules for the evolution of cooperation. Science **314**: 1560–1563.

18. **Boyd R, Richerson PJ** (2009) Culture and the evolution of human cooperation. Philos Trans R Soc Lond B Biol Sci **364**: 3281–3288.

19. **Weingarten CP, Chisholm JS** (2009) Attachment and cooperation in religious groups; an example of a mechanism for cultural group selection. Curr Anthropol **50**: 759–785.

20. **Feldman R** (2016) The neurobiology of mammalian parenting and the biosocial context of human caregiving. Horm Behav **77**: 3–17.

21. **Soley G, Spelke ES** (2016) Shared cultural knowledge: effects of music on young children's social preferences. Cognition **148**: 106–116.

22. **Korn CW, Prehn K, Park SQ, Walter H, Heekeren HR** (2012) Positively based processing of self-relevant social feedback. J Neurosci **32**: 16832–16844.

23. **Rand DG, Greene JD, Nowak MA** (2012) Spontaneous giving and calculated greed. Nature **489**: 427–430.

24. **Boyer P** (2008) Religion: bound to believe? Nature **455**: 1038–1039.

25. **Fehr E, Rockenbach** (2004) Human altruism: economic, neural and evolutionary perspectives. Curr Opin Neurobiol **14**: 784–790.

26. **Hill KR, Walker RS, Bozicević M, Eder J, Headland T**, et al. (2011) Co-residence patterns in hunter-gatherer societies show unique human social structure. Science **331**: 1286–1289.

27. **Henrich J, Boyd R, Bowles S, Camerer C, Fehr E, Gintis H**, et al. (2005) "Economic man" in cross-cultural perspective: behavioral experiments in 15 small-scale societies. Behav Brain Sci **28**: 795–815.

28. **Rilling JK, King-Cass B, Sanfey AG** (2008) The neurobiology of social decision-making. Curr Opin Neurobiol **18**: 159–165.

29. **Izuma K, Saito DN, Sadato N** (2008) Processing of social and monetary rewards in the human striatum. Neuron **58**: 284–294.

30. **Vrticka P** (2012) Interpersonal closeness and social reward processing. J Neurosci **32**: 12649–12650.

31. **Henrich J, Heine SJ, Norenzayan A** (2010) The weirdest people in the world? Behav Brain Sci **33**: 61–83.

32. **Marsh AA, Stoycos SA, Brethel-Haurwitz KM, Robinson P, VanMeter JW, Cardinale EM** (2014) Neural and cognitive characteristics of extraordinary altruists. Proc Natl Acad Sci USA **111**: 15036–15041.

33. **Viding E, McCrory E, Seara-Carduso A** (2014) Psychopathy. Curr Biol **24**: R871–R874.

34. **Grecucci A, Giorgetta C, Bonini N, Sanfey AG** (2013) Reappraising social emotions: the role of inferior frontal gyrus, temporo-parietal junction and insula in interpersonal emotion regulation. Front Hum Neurosci **7**: 523.

35. **Bowles S** (2006) Group competition, reproductive levelling, and the evolution of human altruism. Science **314**: 1569–1572.

36. **Bowles S** (2009) Did warfare among ancestral hunter-gatherers affect the evolution of human social behaviors? Science **324**: 1293–1298.

37. **Johnson B, Cloonan M** (2008) *Dark Side of the Tune: Popular Music and Violence*. Ashgate, Farnham, UK.

38. **Cronin H** (2006) "The battle of the sexes revisited," in **A. Grafen** and **M. Ridley**, eds, *Richard Dawkins: How a Scientist Changed the Way We Think* (Oxford University Press, Oxford), 14–26.

39. **Grueter CC** (2015) Home range overlap as a driver of intelligence in primates. Am J Primatol **77**: 418–424.

40. **Tucker WT, Ferson S** (2008) Evolved altruism, strong reciprocity, and perception of risk. Ann NY Acad Sci **1128**: 111–120.

41. **Shorto R** (2013) *Amsterdam: A History of the World's Most Liberal City.* Abacus, London.

42. **Henrich J, Chudek M, Boyd R** (2015) The Big Man Mechanism: how prestige fosters cooperation and creates prosocial leaders. Philos Trans R Soc Lond B Biol Sci **370**: 1683.

43. **Rilling J, Gutman D, Zeh T, Pagnoni G, Berns G, Kilts C** (2002) A neural basis for social cooperation. Neuron **35**: 395–405.

44. **Cooper JC, Kreps TA, Wiebe T, Pirkl T, Knutson B** (2010) When giving is good: ventromedial prefrontal cortex activation for others' intentions. Neuron **67**: 511–521.

45. **Redcay E, Dodell-Feder D, Pearrow MJ, Mavros PL, Kleiner M, et al.** (2010) Live face-to-face interaction during MRI: a new tool for social cognitive neuroscience. Neuroimage **50**: 1639–1647.

46. **Rice K, Redcay E** (2015) Interaction with others: a perceived social partner alters the neural processing of human speech. Neuroimage **129**: 480–488.

47. **Frith U, Frith CD** (2003) Development and neurophysiology of mentalizing. Philos Trans R Soc Lond B Biol Sci **358**: 459–473.

48. **Coricelli G, Nagel R** (2009) Neural correlates of depth of strategic reasoning in medial prefrontal cortex. Proc Natl Acad Sci USA **106**: 9163–9168.

49. **Yoshida W, Seymour B, Friston KJ, Dolan RJ** (2010) Neural mechanisms of belief inference during cooperative games. J Neurosci **30**: 10744–10751.

50. **Guionnet S, Nadal J, Bertasi E, Sperduti M, Delaveau P, Fossati P** (2011) Reciprocal imitation: toward a neural basis of social interaction. Cereb Cortex **22**: 971–978.

51. **Carter RM, Bowling DL, Reeck C, Huettel SA** (2012) A distinct role of the temporal-parietal junction in predicting socially guided behaviour. Science **337**: 109–111.

52. **Sakaiya S, Shiraito Y, Kato J, Ide H, Okada K, et al.** (2013) Neural correlate of human reciprocity in social interaction. Front Neurosci **7**: 239.

53. **Pardini DA, Raine A, Erickson K, Loeber R** (2014) Lower amygdala volume in men is associated with childhood aggression, early psychopathic traits, and future violence. Biol Psychiatry **75**: 73–80.

54. **Du E, Chang SWC** (2015) Neural components of altruistic punishment. Front Neurosci **9**: 26.

55. **Strobel A, Zimmermann J, Schmitz A, Reuter M, Lis S, et al.** (2011) Beyond revenge: neural and genetic bases of altruistic punishment. Neuroimage **54**: 671–680.

56. **Miric D, Hallet-Mathieu A-M, Amar G** (2005) Etiology of antisocial personality disorder: benefits for society from an evolutionary standpoint. Med Hypotheses **65**: 665–670.

57. **Baumgartner T, Fischbacher U, Feierabend A, Lutz K, Fehr E** (2009) The neural circuitry of a broken promise. Neuron **64**: 756–770.

58. **Stallen M, Smidts A, Sanfey AG** (2013) Peer influence: neural mechanisms underlying in-group conformity. Front Hum Neurosci **7**: 50.

59. **Rushworth MFS, Noonan MP, Boorman ED, Walton ME, Behrens TE** (2011) Frontal cortex and reward-guided learning and decision-making. Neuron **70**: 1054–1069.

60. **Spezio ML, Huang P-Y S, Castelli F, Adolphs R** (2007) Amygdala damage impairs eye contact during conversations with real people. J Neurosci **27**: 3994–3997.

61. **Völlm BA, Taylor AN, Richardson P, Corcoran R, Stirling J, et al.** (2006) Neuronal correlates of theory of mind and empathy: a functional magnetic resonance imaging study in a nonverbal task. Neuroimage **29**: 90–98.

62. **Shamay-Tsoory SG** (2011) The neural basis for empathy. Neuroscientist **17**: 18–24.

63. **Bernardt BC, Singer T** (2012) The neural basis of empathy. Annu Rev Neurosci **35**: 1–23.

64. **Singer T, Seymour B, O-Doherty J, Kaube H, Dolan RJ, Frith CD** (2004) Empathy for pain involves the affective but not the sensory components of pain. Science **303**: 1157–1162.

65. Lamm C, Decety J, Singer T (2011) Meta-analytic evidence for common and distinct neural networks associated with directly experienced and empathy for pain. Neuroimage 54: 2492–2502.

66. Keysers C, Kaas JH, Gazzola V (2010) Somatosensation in social perception. Nature Rev 11: 417–428.

67. Saarela MV, Hlushchuk Y, Williams AC, Schurmann M, Kalso E, Hari R (2007) The compassionate brain: humans detect intensity of pain from another's face. Cereb Cortex 17: 230–237.

68. Ogino Y, Nemoto H, Inui K, Saito S, Kakigi R, Goto F (2007) Inner experience of pain: imagination of pain while viewing images showing painful events forms subjective pain representation in human brain. Cereb Cortex 17: 1139–1146.

69. Lockwood PL, Apps MAJ, Roiser JP, Viding E (2015) Encoding of vicarious reward prediction in anterior cingulate cortex and relationship with trait empathy. J Neurosci 35: 13720–13727.

70. Banissy MJ, Kanai R, Walsh V, Rees G (2012) Inter-individual differences in empathy are reflected in human brain structure. Neuroimage 62: 2034–2039.

71. Mutschler I, Reinbold C, Wankert J, Seifritz E, Ball T (2013) Structural basis of empathy and the domain general region in the anterior insula cortex. Front Hum Neurosci 7: 177.

72. Kanai R, Bahrami B, Duchaine B, Janik A, Banissy MJ, Rees G (2012) Brain structure links loneliness to social perception. Curr Biol 22: 1975–1979.

73. Campbell BG (1985) *Humankind Emerging* (4th edition). Little Brown, Boston, Toronto.

74. Noordzij ML, Newman-Norlund SE, de Ruiter JP, Hagoort P, Levinson SC, Toni I (2009) Brain mechanisms underlying human communication. Front Hum Neurosci 3: 14.

75. Tomasello M, Carpenter M, Call J, Behne T, Moll H (2005) Understanding and sharing intentions: the origins of cultural cognition. Behav Brain Sci 28: 675–691.

76. Nowak MA, Sigmund K (2005) Evolution of indirect reciprocity. Nature 437: 1291–1298.

77. Nowak MA, Karakauer DC (1999) The evolution of language. Proc Natl Acad Sci USA 96: 8028–8033.

78. Lieberman P (1993) *Uniquely Human: The Evolution of Speech, Thought, and Selfless Behavior.* Harvard University Press, Cambridge MA.

79. O'Doherty JP (2004) Reward representations and reward-related learning in the human brain: insights from neuroimaging. Curr Opin Neurobiol 14: 769–776.

80. Gold BP, Frank MJ, Bogert B, Brattico E (2013) Pleasurable music affects reinforcement learning according to the listener. Front Psychol 4: 541.

81. Dumas G, Nadal J, Sousignon R, Martinerie J, Garnero L (2010) Inter-brain synchronization during social interactions. PLoS One 5: e12166.

82. Zahn R, Moll J, Krueger F, Huey ED, Garrido G, Grafman J (2007) Social concepts are represented in the superior anterior temporal cortex. Proc Natl Acad Sci USA 104: 6430–6435.

83. Mitterschiffthaler MT, Fu CHY, Dalton JA, Andrew CM, Williams SCR (2007) A functional MRI study of happy and sad affective states induced by classical music. Hum Brain Mapp 28: 1150–1162.

84. Eres R, Molenberghs P (2013) The influence of group membership on the neural correlates involved in empathy. Front Hum Neurosci 7: 176.

85. Chapin H, Jantzen K, Kelso JAS, Steinberg F, Large E (2010) Dynamic emotional and neural responses to music depend on performance expression and listener experience. PLoS One 12: e13812.

86. Babiloni C, Buffo P, Vecchio F, Marzano N, Del Percio C, et al. (2012) Brains "in concert": frontal oscillatory alpha rythms and empathy in professional musicians. Neuroimage 60: 105–116.

87. Livingstone SR, Thompson WF (2009) The emergence of music from the Theory of Mind. Music Sci (Special Issue 2009–2010): 83–115.

88. Laland K, Wilkins C, Clayton N (2016) The evolution of dance. Curr Biol **26**: R5–R9.

89. Crockett MJ, Apergis-Schoute A, Herrmann B, Lieberman MD, Müller U, et al. (2013) Serotonin modulates striatal responses to fairness and retaliation in humans. J Neurosci **33**: 3505–3513.

90. Bachner-Melman R, Dina C, Zohar AH, Constantini N, Lerer E, et al. (2005) AVPR1a and SLC6A4 gene polymorphisms are associated with creative dance performance. PLoS Genet **1**: e42.

91. Israel S, Lerer E, Shalev I, Uzefovsky F, Reibold M, et al. (2008) Molecular genetic studies of the arginine vasopressin 1a receptor (AVPR1a) and the oxytocin receptor (OXTR) in human behaviour: from autism to altruism with some notes in between. Prog Brain Res **170**: 435–449.

92. Strathearn L, Fonagy P, Amico J, Montague PR (2009) Adult attachment predicts maternal brain and oxytocin response to infant cues. Neuropsychopharmacology **34**: 2655–2666.

93. Rilling JK, Demarco AC, Hackett PD, Thompson R, Ditzen B, et al. (2011) Effects of oxytocin and vasopressin on cooperative behaviour associated with brain activity in men. Psychoneuroendocrinology **37**: 447–461.

94. Neumann ID, Landgraf R (2012) Balance of brain oxytocin and vasopressin: implications for anxiety, depression, and social behaviors. Trends Neurosci **35**: 649–659.

95. Lieberwirth C, Wang Z (2014) Social bonding: regulation by neuropeptides. Front Neurosci **8**: 171.

96. Preckel K, Scheele D, Kendrick KM, Maier W, Hurlemann R (2014) Oxytocin facilitates social approach behaviour in women. Front Behav Neurosci **8**: 191.

97. Hurlemann R, Patin A, Onur OA, Cohen MX, Baumgartner T, et al. (2010) Oxytocin enhances amygdala-dependent, socially reinforced learning and emotional empathy in humans. J Neurosci **30**: 4999–5007.

98. Bethlehem RAI, Baron-Cohen S, Van Honk J, Auyeung B, Bos PA (2014) The oxytocin paradox. Front Behav Neurosci **8**: 48.

99. Marsh N, Scheele D, Gerhardt H, Strang S, Enax L, et al. (2015) The neuropeptide oxytocin induces a social altruism bias. J Neurosci **35**: 15696–15701.

100. Kosfeld M, Heinrichs M, Zak PJ, Fischbacher U, Fehr E (2005) Oxytocin increases trust in humans. Nature **435**: 673–676.

101. Baumgartner T, Heinrichs M, Vonlanthen A, Fischbacher U, Fehr E (2008) Oxytocin shapes the neural circuitry of trust and adaptation in humans. Neuron **58**: 639–650.

102. Israel S, Lerer E, Shalev I, Uzefovsky F, Riebold M, et al. (2009) The oxytocin receptor (OXTR) contributes to prosocial fund allocations in the dictator game and the social value orientations task. PLoS One **4**: e5535.

103. Rodrigues SM, Saslow LR, Garcia N, John OP, Keltner D (2009) Oxytocin receptor genetic variation relates to empathy and stress reactivity in humans. Proc Natl Acad Sci USA **106**: 21437–21441.

104. Dadds MR, Moul C, Cauchi A, Dobson-Stone C, Hawes DJ, et al. (2014) Polymorphisms in the oxytocin receptor gene are associated with the development of psychopathy. Dev Psychopathol **26**: 21–31.

105. Bicknell J (2009) *Why Music Moves Us*. Palgrave Macmillan, London and New York.

106. Nilsson U (2009) Soothing music can increase oxytocin levels during bed rest after open-heart surgery: a randomised control trial. J Clin Nurs **18**: 2153–2161.

107. Keeler JR, Roth EA, Neuser BL, Spitsbergen JM, Waters DJ, Vianney JM (2015) The neurochemistry and social flow of singing: bonding and oxytocin. Front Hum Neurosci **9**: 518.

108. Oubré AY (1997) *Instinct and Revelation: Reflections on the Origins of Numinous Perception* (The World Futures General Evolution Studies—Vol 10). Taylor and Francis, Abingdon (UK) and New York.

109. **Hagen EH, Hammerstein P** (2009) Did Neanderthals and other early humans sing? Seeking the biological roots of music in the territorial advertisements of primates, lions, hyenas and wolves. Music Sci 13: 292.

110. **Jordania J** (2011) *Why Do People Sing? Music in Human Evolution.* Logos, Tbilisi.

111. **Fukui H, Yamashita M** (2003) The effects of music and visual stress in testosterone and cortisol in men and women. Neuro Endocrinol Lett 24: 173–180.

112. **Brothers L** (1997) *Friday's Footprint: How Society Shapes the Human Mind.* Oxford University Press, New York and London.

113. **Pearce E, Launay J, Dunbar RIM** (2015) The ice-breaker effect: singing mediates fast social bonding. R Soc Open Sci 2: 150221.

114. **Fischer R, Callander R, Reddish P, Bulbulia J** (2013) How do rituals affect cooperation? An experimental field study comparing nine ritual types. Hum Nat 24: 115–125.

115. **West-Eberhard MJ** (1979) Sexual selection, social competition and evolution. Proc Am Phil Soc 123: 222–234.

116. **Portin P** (2015) A comparison of biological and cultural evolution. J Genet 94: 155–168.

117. **Mosing MA, Pedersen NL, Madison G, Ullén F** (2014) Genetic pleiotropy explains associations between musical auditory discrimination and intelligence. PloS One 9: e113874.

118. **Plomin R, Deary IJ** (2015) Genetics and intelligence differences: five special findings. Mol Psychiatry 20: 98–108.

119. **Scheinfeld A, Schweitzer MD** (1939) *You and Heredity* (including an original study on the Inheritance of Musical Talent, pp 234–288). Garden City Publishing, New York.

120. **Vinkhuyzen AA, van der Sluis S, Posthuma D, Boomsma DI** (2009) The heritability of aptitude and exceptional talent across different domains in adolescents and young adults. Behav Genet 39: 380–392.

121. **Kraus N, Chandrasekeran B** (2010) Music training for the development of auditory skills. Nat Rev 11: 599–605.

122. **Scott DF, Moffett A** (1977) "The development of early musical talent in famous composers: a biographical review," in M. **Critchley** and R. A. **Henson,** eds, *Music and the Brain: Studies on the Neurology of Music* (Heinemann Medical Books Ltd, London), 174–201.

123. **Ross DA, Marks LE** (2009) "Absolute pitch in children prior to the beginning of musical training," in S. **Dalla Bella** et al., *The Neurosciences and Music III—Disorders and Plasticity,* Ann NY Acad Sci 1169: 199–204 (Wiley-Blackwell, Boston).

124. **Theusch E, Basu A, Gitschier J** (2009) Genome-wide study of families with absolute pitch reveals linkage to 8q24.21 and locus heterogeneity. Am J Hum Genet 85: 112–119.

125. **Seither-Preisler A, Parncutt R, Schneider P** (2014) Size and synchronization of auditory cortex promotes musical, literacy and attentional skills in children. J Neurosci 34: 10937–10949.

126. **Drayna D, Manichaikul A, de Lange M, Sneider H, Spector T** (2001) Genetic correlates of musical pitch recognition in humans. Science 270: 1969–1972.

127. **Oikkonen J, Huang Y, Onkamo P, Ukkola-Vuoti L, Raijas P,** et al. (2014) A genome-wide linkage and association study of musical aptitude identifies loci containing genes related to inner ear development and neurocognitive functions. Mol Psychiatry 20: 275–282.

128. **Granot R, Frankel Y, Gritsenko V, Lerer E, Gritsenko I,** et al. (2007) Provisional evidence that the arginine vasopressin 1a receptor gene is associated with musical memory. Evol Hum Behav 28: 313–318.

129. **Pulli K, Karma K, Norio R, Sistonen P, Göring HH, Järvelä I** (2008) Genome-wide linkage scan for loci of musical aptitude in Finnish families: evidence for a major locus at 4q22. J Med Genet 45: 451–456.

130. **Ukkola LT, Onkamo P, Raijas P, Karma K, Järvelä I** (2009) Musical aptitude is associated with AVPR1A-haplotypes. PLoS One **4**: 5 e5534.

131. **Liu X, Kanduri C, Oikkonen J, Karma K, Raijas P,** et al. (2016) Detecting signatures of positive selection associated with musical aptitude in the human genome. Sci Rep **6**: 21198.

132. **Oikkonen J, Kuusi T, Peltonen P, Raijas P, Ukkola-Vuoti L,** et al. (2016) Creative activities in music—a genome-wide linkage analysis. PLoS One **11**: e0148679.

133. **De Quervain DJ-F, Henke K, Aerni A, Coluccia D, Wollmer MA,** et al. (2003) A functional genetic variation of the 5-HT2a receptor affects human memory. Nat Neurosci **6**: 1141–1142.

134. **Liu B, Song M, Li J, Liu Y, Li K,** et al. (2010) Prefrontal-related functional connectivities within the default network are modulated by COMT val158met in healthy young adults. J Neurosci **30**: 64–69.

135. **Aleman A, Swart M, Van Rijn S** (2008) Brain imaging, genetics and emotion. Biol Psychol **79**: 58–69.

136. **Schmack K, Schlagenhauf F, Sterzer P, Wrase J, Beck A,** et al. (2008) Catechol-O-methyltransferase val158met genotype influences neural processing of reward anticipation. Neuroimage **42**: 1631–1638.

137. **Reuter M, Montag C, Peters K, Kocher A, Kiefer M** (2009) The modulatory influence of the functional COMT Val158Met polymorphism on lexical decisions and semantic priming. Front Hum Neurosci **3**: 20.

138. **Zhang S, Zhang M, Zhang J** (2014) Association of COMT and COMT-DRD2 interaction with creative potential. Front Hum Neurosci **8**: 216.

139. **Blum K, Chen TJ, Chen AL, Madigan M, Downs BW,** et al. (2010) Do dopaminergic gene polymorphisms affect mesolimbic reward activation of music listening response? Therapeutic impact on Reward Deficiency Syndrome (RDS). Med Hypotheses **74**: 513–520.

140. **Pamjav H, Juhász Z, Zalán A, Németh E, Damdin B** (2012) A comparative phylogenetic study of genetics and folk music. Mol Genet Genomics **287**: 337–349.

141. **Brown S, Savage PE, Ko AM, Stoneking M, Ko YC,** et al. (2013) Correlations in the population structure of music, genes and language. Proc Biol Soc **281**(1774): 20132072.

142. **Brown S, Jordania J** (2011) Universals in the world's music. Psychol Music: 1–20.

143. **Le Bomin S, Lecointre G, Heyer E** (2016) The evolution of musical diversity: the key role of vertical transmission. PLoS One **11**: e0151570.

144. **Grauer VA** (2006) Echoes of our forgotten ancestors. World Music **48**: 5–58.

145. **Moffett MW** (2013) Human identity and the evolution of societies. Hum Nat **24**: 219–267.

146. **Storr A** (1992) *Music and the Mind.* Harper Collins Publishers, London.

147. **Brown S** (2000) "The 'musilanguage' model of human evolution," in **N. L. Wallin, B. Merker** and **S. Brown,** eds, *Origins of Music* (MIT Press, Cambridge MA), 271–300.

148. **Cross I** (1999) "Is music the most important thing we ever did? Music, development and evolution," in **S. W. Yi,** ed., *Music, Mind and Science* (Seoul National University Press, Seoul), 10–39.

149. **Cross I** (2003) "Music, cognition, culture and evolution," in **I. Peretz** and **R. L. Zatorre,** eds, *The Cognitive Neuroscience of Music* (Oxford University Press, Oxford), 42–56.

150. **Koelsch S** (2012) *Brain and Music.* Wiley Blackwell, Chichester, UK.

Chapter Six

1. **Storr A** (1992) *Music and the Mind.* Harper Collins Publishers, London.

2. **Merker B, Morley I, Zuidema W** (2015) Five fundamental constraints on theories of the origins of music. Philos Trans R Soc Lond B Biol Sci **370**: 20140095.

3. **Whitehouse H, Lanman JA** (2014) The ties that bind us: ritual, fusion, and identification. Curr Anthropol **55**: 674–695.

4. **Moffett MW** (2013) Human identity and the evolution of societies. Hum Nat **24**: 219–267.

5. **Dawkins CR** (1998) *Unweaving the Rainbow*. Penguin, London.

6. **Medawar PB** (1977) *The Life Science: Current Ideas of Biology*. Wildwood House, London.

7. **Lodge D** (2001) *Thinks*. Secker and Walburg, UK.

8. **Varka A** (2009) Human uniqueness and the denial of death. Nature **460**: 684.

9. **Sharot T, Riccardi AM, Raio CM, Phelps EA** (2007) Neural mechanisms mediating optimism bias. Nature **450**: 102–105.

10. **Sharot T, Korn CW, Dolan RJ** (2011) How unrealistic optimism is maintained in the face of reality. Nat Neurosci **14**: 1475–1479.

11. **Scioli A, Chamberlin CM, Samor CM, Lapointe AB, Campbell TL**, et al. (1997) A prospective study of hope, optimism, and health. Psych Rep **81**: 723–733.

12. **Moll J, Zahn R, de Oliveira-Souza R, Krueger F, Grafman J** (2005) The neural basis of human moral cognition. Nat Rev Neurosci **6**: 799–809.

13. **Tomasello M, Vaish A** (2013) Origins of human cooperation and morality. Annu Rev Psychol **64**: 231–255.

14. **Gargett RH** (1999) Middle Palaeolithic burial is not a dead issue: the view from Qafzeh, Saint-Cézaire, Kebara, Amud, and Dederiyah. J Hum Evol **37**: 27–90.

15. **Pettitt P** (2002) When burial begins. Brit Archaeol 66(August): 8–13.

16. **Freedman L** (2000) *Humankind: Retrospect and Prospect*. Centre for Human Biology, UWA, Perth.

17. **Dunbar R** (2004) *The Human Story: A New History of Mankind's Evolution*. Faber and Faber, London.

18. **Rodriguez-Vidal J, d'Errico F, Giles Pacheco F, Blasco R, Rosell J**, et al. (2014) A rock engraving made by Neanderthals in Gibraltar. Proc Natl Acad Sci USA **111**: 13301–13306.

19. **Lewis-Williams D** (2010) *Conceiving God: The Cognitive Origin and Evolution of Religion*. Thames and Hudson, London.

20. **Mengham R** (1994) *On language: Descent from the tower of Babel*. Little Brown and Company, Boston, New York, Toronto, London.

21. **D'Errico F, Henshilwood C, Lawson G, Vanhaeren M**, Tillier A-M, et al. (2003) Archaeological evidence for the emergence of language, symbolism, and music—an alternative multidisciplinary perspective. J World Prehist **17**: 1–70.

22. **Vanhaeren M, d'Errico F, van Nierkerk KL, Henshilwood CS, Erasmus RM** (2013) Thinking strings: additional evidence for personal ornament use in the Middle Stone Age at Blombos Cave, South Africa. J Hum Evol **64**: 500–517.

23. **Boyer P** (2008) Religion: bound to believe? Nature **455**: 1038–1039.

24. **Tattersall I** (1998) *Becoming Human: Evolution and Human Uniqueness*. Harcourt Brace, Orlando FL.

25. **Bloch M** (2008) Why religion is nothing special but is central. Philos Trans R Soc Lond B Biol Sci **363**: 2055–2061.

26. **Cross I** (2003) "Music, cognition, culture and evolution," in **I. Peretz** and **R. L. Zatorre**, eds, *The Cognitive Neuroscience of Music* (Oxford University Press, Oxford), 42–56.

27. **Mithen S** (2005) *The Singing Neanderthals: The Origins of Music, Language, Mind and Body*. Orion, London.

28. **Oubré AY** (1997) *Instinct and Revelation: Reflections on the Origins of Numinous Perception* (The World Futures General Evolution Studies—Vol 10). Taylor and Francis, Abingdon (UK) and New York.

29. **Jordania J** (2011) *Why Do People Sing? Music in Human Evolution*. Logos, Tbilisi.

30. **Harvey AR** (2008) Music and human evolution. MCA Music Forum **14**: 37–41.

31. **Humphrey N** (2008) The society of selves. Philos Trans R Soc Lond B Biol Sci **362**: 745–754.

32. **Fischer R, Callander R, Reddish P, Bulbulia J** (2013) How do rituals affect cooperation? An experimental field study comparing nine ritual types. Hum Nat **24**: 115–125.

33. **Magowan F** (2007) *Melodies of Mourning: Music and Emotion in Northern Australia*. UWA Press, Crawley WA.

34. **Atkins H, Neumann A** (1978) *Beecham Stories*. Robson Books, London.

35. **Fitch TW** (2000) The evolution of speech: a comparative review. Trends Cogn Sci **4**: 258–267.

36. **Sulaiman AH, Seluakumaran K, Husain R** (2013) Hearing risk associated with the usage of personal listening devices among urban high school students in Malaysia. Public Health **127**: 710–715.

37. **Vickhoff B, Malmgren H, Aström R, Nyberg G, Ekström SR**, et al. (2013) Music structure determines heart rate variability of singers. Front Psychol **4**: 334.

38. **Launay J, Dean RT, Bailes F** (2014) Synchronising movements with the sounds of a virtual partner enhances partner likeability. Cogn Process **15**: 491–501.

Chapter Seven

1. **Green CS, Bavalier D** (2008) Exercising your brain: a review of human brain plasticity and training-induced learning. Psychol Aging **23**: 692–701.

2. **Zatorre RJ** (2005) Music, the food of neuroscience? Nature **434**: 312–315.

3. **Koelsch S** (2011) Towards a neural basis of music perception—a review and updated model. Front Psychol **2**: 1–20.

4. **Morgenstern S** (1956) *Composers on Music* (2nd edition). Pantheon Books, New York.

5. **Peretz I** (2006) The nature of music from a biological perspective. Cognition **100**: 1–32.

6. **Tierney A, Kraus N** (2013) The ability to tap to a beat relates to cognitive, linguistic and perceptual skills. Brain Lang **124**: 225–231.

7. **Tierney A, Kraus N** (2013) The ability to move to a beat is linked to the consistency of neural responses to sound. J Neurosci **33**: 14981–14988.

8. **Hill J, Inder T, Neil J, Dierker D, Harwell J, Van Essen D** (2010) Similar patterns of cortical expansion during human development and evolution. Proc Natl Acad Sci USA **107**: 13135–13140.

9. **Merrett DL, Peretz I, Wilson SJ** (2013) Moderating variables of music training-induced neuroplasticity: a review and discussion. Front Psychol **4**: 606.

10. **Bidelman GM, Krishnan A, Gandour JT** (2011) Enhanced brainstem encoding predicts musicians' perceptual advantages with pitch. Eur J Neurosci **33**: 530–538.

11. **Skoe E, Kraus N** (2012) A little music goes a long way: how the adult brain is shaped by musical training in childhood. J Neurosci **32**: 11507–11510.

12. **Bidelman GM, Alain C** (2015) Musical training orchestrates coordinated neuroplasticity in auditory brainstem and cortex to counteract age-related declines in categorical vowel perception. J Neurosci **35**: 1240–1249.

13. **Abdul-Kareem IA, Stancak A, Parkes LM, V S** (2011) Increased gray matter volume of left pars opercularis in male orchestral musicians correlates positively with years of musical performance. J Magn Reson Imaging **33**: 24–32.

14. **Elmer S, Hänggi J, Meyer M, Jäncke L** (2013) Increased cortical surface area of the left planum temporale in musicians facilitates the categorization of phonetic and temporal speech sounds. Cortex **49**: 2812–2821.

15. **Foster NEV, Zatorre RJ** (2010) Cortical structure predicts success in performing musical transformational judgements. Neuroimage **53**: 26–36.

16. **Groussard M, Viader F, Landau B, Desgranges B, Eustache F, Platel H** (2014) The effects of musical practice on structural plasticity: the dynamics of grey matter changes. Brain Cogn **90**: 174–180.

17. **Klein C, Liem F, Hänggi J, Elmer S, Jäncke L** (2015) The "silent" imprint of musical training. Hum Brain Mapp **37**: 536–546.

18. **Kraus N, Chandrasekaran B** (2010) Music training for the development of auditory skills. Nat Rev **11**: 599–605.

19. **Münte TF, Altenmüller E, Jäncke L** (2002) The musician's brain as a model of neuroplasticity. Nat Rev Neurosci **3**: 473–478.

20. **Pantev C, Lappe C, Herholz SC, Trainor L** (2009) "Auditory-somatosensory integration and cortical plasticity in musical training," in **S. Dalla Bella** et al., *The Neurosciences and Music III—Disorders and Plasticity*, Ann NY Acad Sci **1169**: 143–150 (Wiley-Blackwell, Boston).

21. **Wan CY, Schlaug G** (2010) Music making as a tool for promoting brain plasticity across the lifespan. Neuroscientist **16**: 566–577.

22. **Meyer M, Elmer S, Ringli M, Oechslin MS, Baumann S, Jancke L** (2011) Long-term exposure to music enhances the sensitivity of the auditory system in children. Eur J Neurosci **34**: 755–765.

23. **Lee KM, Skoe E, Kraus N, Ashley R** (2009) Selective subcortical enhancement of musical intervals in musicians. J Neurosci **29**: 5832–5840.

24. **Hyde KL, Lerch J, Norton A, Forgeard M, Winner E,** et al. (2009) Musical training shapes structural brain development. J Neurosci **29**: 3019–3025.

25. **Schlaug G, Marchina S, Norton A** (2009) "Evidence for plasticity in white-matter tracts of patients with chronic Broca's aphasia undergoing intense intonation-based speech therapy," in **S. Dalla Bella** et al., eds, *The Neurosciences and Music III—Disorders and Plasticity*, Ann NY Acad Sci **1169**: 385–394 (Wiley-Blackwell, Boston).

26. **Seither-Preisler A, Parncutt R, Schneider P** (2014) Size and synchronization of auditory cortex promotes musical, literacy and attentional skills in children. J Neurosci **34**: 10937–10949.

27. **Hulshoff Pol HE, Schnack HG, Posthuma D, Mandl RC, Baaré WF,** et al. (2006) Genetic contributions to human brain morphology and intelligence. J Neurosci **26**: 10235–10242.

28. **Robertson D, Irvine DR** (1989) Plasticity of frequency organization in auditory cortex of guinea pigs with partial unilateral deafness. J Comp Neurol **282**: 456–471.

29. **de Villers-Sidani E, Merzenich MM** (2011) Lifelong plasticity in the rat auditory cortex: basic mechanisms and role of sensory experience. Prog Brain Res **191**: 119–131.

30. **Schreiner CE, Polley DB** (2014) Auditory map plasticity: diversity in causes and consequences. Curr Opin Neurobiol **24**: 143–156.

31. **Anomal R, de Villers-Sidani E, Merzenich MM, Panizzutti R** (2013) Manipulation of BDNF signaling modifies the experience-dependent plasticity induced by pure tone exposure during the critical period in the primary auditory cortex. PLoS One **8**: e64208.

32. **Benasich AA, Choudhury NA, Realpe-Bonilla T, Roesler CP** (2014) Plasticity in developing brain: active auditory exposure impacts prelinguistic acoustic mapping. J Neurosci **34**: 13349–13363.

33. **Mithen S** (2008) Singing in the brain. New Sci **197**: 38–39.

34. **Zatorre RJ, Chen JL, Penhune VB** (2007) When the brain plays music: auditory-motor interactions in music perception and production. Nat Rev **8**: 547–558.

35. **Ohnishi T, Matsuda H, Asada T, Aruga M, Hirakata M,** et al. (2001) Functional anatomy of musical perception in musicians. Cereb Cortex **11**: 754–760.

36. **Bangert M, Peschel T, Schlaug G, Rotte M, Drescher D**, et al. (2006) Shared networks for auditory and motor processing in professional pianists: evidence from fMRI conjunction. Neuroimage **30**: 917–926.

37. **Altenmüller E** (2009) "Apollo's gift and curse: brain plasticity in musicians," in *Music and Medicine*, Karger Gazette No. 70: 8–10.

38. **Zimmerman E, Lahav A** (2012) The multisensory brain and its ability to learn music. Ann NY Acad Sci **1252**: 179–184.

39. **Elbert T, Pantev C, Wienbruch C, Rockstroh B, Taub E** (1995) Increased cortical representation of the fingers of the left hand in string players. Science **270**: 305–307.

40. **Gaser C, Schlaug G** (2003) Brain structures differ between musicians and non-musicians. J Neurosci **23**: 9240–9245.

41. **Kim D-E, Shin M-J, Lee K-M, Chu K, Woo SH**, et al. (2004) Musical training-induced functional reorganization of the adult brain: functional magnetic resonance imaging and transcranial magnetic stimulation study on amateur string players. Hum Brain Mapp **23**: 188–199.

42. **Schulz M, Ross B, Pantev C** (2003) Evidence of training-induced crossmodal reorganization of cortical functions in trumpet players. Neuroreport **14**: 157–161.

43. **Schlaug G, Jäncke L, Huang Y, Staiger JF, Steinmetz H** (1995) Increased corpus callosum size in musicians. Neuropsychologia **33**: 1047–1055.

44. **Ridding MC, Brouwer B, Nordstrom MA** (2000) Reduced interhemispheric inhibition in musicians. Exp Brain Res **133**: 249–253.

45. **Steele CJ, Bailey JA, Zatorre RJ, Penhune VB** (2013) Early musical training and white-matter plasticity in the corpus callosum: evidence for a sensitive period. J Neurosci **33**: 1282–1290.

46. **Hutchinson S, Lee LH, Gaab N, Schlaug G** (2003) Cerebellar volume in musicians. Cereb Cortex **13**: 943–949.

47. **Baer LH, Park MT, Bailey JA, Chakravarty MM, Li KZ, Penhune VB** (2015) Regional cerebellar volumes are related to early musical training and finger tapping performance. Neuroimage **109**: 130–139.

48. **Abdul-Kareem IA, Stancak A, Parkes LM, Al-Ameen M, Alghamdi J**, et al. (2011) Plasticity of the superior and middle cerebellar peduncles in musicians revealed by quantitative analysis of volume and number of streamlines based on diffusion tensor tractography. Cerebellum **10**: 611–623.

49. **Tölgyesi B, Evers S** (2014) The impact of cerebellar disorders on musical ability. J Neurol Sci **343**: 76–81.

50. **Herdener M, Esposito F, di Salle F, Boller C, Hilti CC**, et al. (2010) Musical training induces functional plasticity in human hippocampus. J Neurosci **30**: 1377–1384.

51. **Nutley SB, Darki F, Klingberg T** (2014) Music practice is associated with development of working memory during childhood and adolescence. Front Hum Neurosci **7**: 926.

52. **Perani D, Abutalebi J** (2015) Bilingualism, dementia, cognitive and neural reserve. Curr Opin Neurol **28**: 618–625.

53. **Bara-Jimenez W, Catalan MJ, Hallett M, Gerloff C** (1998) Abnormal somatosensory homunculus in dystonia of the hand. Ann Neurol **44**: 828–831.

54. **Altenmüller E, Jabusch HC** (2010) Focal dystonia in musicians: phenomenology, pathophysiology and triggering factors. Eur J Neurol 17(Suppl 1): 31–36.

55. **Konczak J, Abbruzzese G** (2013) Focal dystonia in musicians: linking motor symptoms to somatosensory dysfunction. Front Hum Neurosci **7**: 297.

56. **Rosenkranz K, Butler K, Williamon A, Rothwell JC** (2009) Regaining motor control in musician's dystonia by restoring sensorimotor organization. J Neurosci **29**: 14627–14636.

57. Furuya S, Kalaus M, Nitsche MA, Paulus W, Altenmüller E (2014) Ceiling effects prevent further improvement of transcranial stimulation in skilled musicians. J Neurosci **34**: 13834–13839.

58. Lamb SJ, Gregory AH (1993) The relationship between music and reading in beginning readers. Educ Psychol **13**: 19–26.

59. Chan AS, Ho YC, Cheung MC (1998) Musical training improves verbal memory. Nature **396**: 128.

60. Ho YC, Cheung HC, Chan AS (2003) Music training improves verbal but not visual memory: cross-sectional and longitudinal explorations in children. Neuropsychology **17**: 439–450.

61. Tallal P, Gaab N (2006) Dynamic auditory processing, musical experience and language development. Trends Neurosci **29**: 382–390.

62. Gordon RL, Fehd HM, McCandliss BD (2015) Does music training enhance literacy skills? A meta-analysis. Front Psychol **6**: 1777.

63. White-Schwoch T, Carr KW, Anderson S, Strait DL, Kraus N (2013) Older adults benefit from music training early in life: biological evidence for long-term training-driven plasticity. J Neurosci **33**: 17667–17674.

64. Besson M, Schön D, Moreno S, Santos A, Magne C (2007) Influence of musical expertise and musical training on pitch processing in music and language. Restor Neurol Neurosci **25**: 399–410.

65. Forgeard M, Winner E, Norton A, Schlaug G (2008) Practicing a musical instrument in childhood is associated with enhanced verbal ability and nonverbal reasoning. PLoS One **3**: e3566.

66. Moreno S, Marques C, Santos A, Santos M, Castro SL, Besson M (2009) Musical training influences linguistic abilities in 8-year-old children: more evidence for brain plasticity. Cereb Cortex **19**: 712–723.

67. Lima CF, Castro SL (2011) Speaking to the trained ear: musical expertise enhances the recognition of emotions in speech prosody. Emotion **11**: 1021–1031.

68. Milovanov R, Tervaniemi M (2011) The interplay between musical and linguistic aptitudes: a review. Front Psychol **2**: 321.

69. Zuk J, Benjamin C, Kenyon A, Gaab N (2014) Behavioral and neural correlates of executive functioning in musicians and non-musicians. PLoS One **9**: e99868.

70. Tierney A, Krizman J, Skoe E, Johnston K, Kraus N (2013) High school music classes enhance the neural processing of speech. Front Psychol **4**: 855.

71. Kraus N SJ, Thompson EC, Hornickel J, Strait DL, et al. (2014) Music enrichment programs improve the neural encoding of speech in at-risk children. J Neurosci **34**: 11913–11918.

72. Parbery-Clark A, Skoe E, Kraus N (2009) Musical experience limits the degradative effects of background noise on the neural processing of sound. J Neurosci **29**: 14100–14107.

73. Strait DL, Parbery-Clark A, Hittner E, Kraus N (2012) Musical training during early childhood enhances the neural encoding of speech in noise. Brain Lang **123**: 191–201.

74. Slater J, Skoe E, Strait DL, O'Connell S, Thopson E, Kraus N (2015) Music training improves speech-in-noise perception: longitudinal evidence from a community-based music program. Behav Brain Res **291**: 244–252.

75. Zuk J, Ozernov-Palchik O, Kim H, Lakshminarayanan K, Gabrieli JD, et al. (2013) Enhanced syllable discrimination thresholds in musicians. PLoS One **8**: e80546.

76. Musacchia G, Sams M, Skoe E, Kraus N (2007) Musicians have enhanced subcortical auditory and audiovisual processing of speech and music. Proc Natl Acad Sci USA **104**: 15894–15898.

77. Schellenberg EG (2004) Music lessons enhance IQ. Psych Sci **15**: 511–514.

78. Rauscher FH, Shaw GL, Levine LJ, Wright EL, Dennis WR, Newcomb RL (1996) Music training causes long-term enhancement of preschool children's spatial-temporal reasoning. Neurol Res **19**: 2–8.

79. Rauscher FH, Shaw GL, Ky KN (1993) Music and spatial task performance. Nature **365**: 611.

80. **Sarnthein J, Vonstein A, Rappelsberger P, Petsche H, Rauscher FH, Shaw GL** (1997) Persistent patterns of brain activity—an EEC coherence study of the positive effect of music on spatio-temporal reasoning. Neurol Res **19**: 107–116.

81. **Fudin R, Lembessis E** (2004) The Mozart effect: questions about the seminal findings of Rauscher, Shaw, and colleagues. Percept Mot Skills **98**: 389–405.

82. **Thompson WF, Schellenberg EG, Husain G** (2001) Arousal, mood and the Mozart effect. Psych Sci **12**: 248–251.

83. **Solomon M** (1995) *Mozart: A Life*. Pimlico, London.

84. **Savan A** (1999) The effect of background music on learning. Psych Music **27**: 138–146.

85. **Sluming V, Brooks J, Howard M, Downes JJ, Roberts N** (2007) Broca's area supports enhanced visuospatial cognition in orchestral musicians. J Neurosci **27**: 3799–3806.

86. **Sluming V, Barrick T, Howard M, Cezayirli E, Mayes A, Roberts N** (2002) Voxel-based morphometry reveals increased gray matter density in Broca's area in male symphony orchestra musicians. NeuroImage **17**: 1613–1622.i

87. **Amer T, Kalender B, Hasher L, Trehub SE, Wong Y** (2013) Do older professional musicians have cognitive advantages? PLoS One **8**: e71630.

88. **Douglas KM, Bilkey DK** (2007) Amusia is associated with deficits in spatial processing. Nat Neurosci **10**: 915–921.

89. **Levenson T** (1999) *Measure for Measure: How Music and Science Together Have Explored the Universe*. Oxford University Press, Oxford and New York.

90. **James J** (1993) *The Music of the Spheres: Music, Science and the Natural Order of the Universe*. Grove Press, New York.

91. **Schmithorst VJ, Holland SK** (2004) The effect of musical training on the neural correlates of math processing: a functional magnetic resonance imaging study in humans. Neurosci Lett **354**: 193–196.

92. **Bamberger J** (1991) *The Mind Behind the Musical Ear: How Children Develop Musical Intelligence*. Harvard University Press, Cambridge MA and London.

93. **Kirschner S, Tomasello M** (2009) Joint drumming: social context facilitates synchronization in preschool children. J Exp Child Psychol **102**: 299–314.

94. **Zentner M, Eerola T** (2010) Rhythmic engagement with music in infancy. Proc Natl Acad Sci USA **107**: 5768–5773.

95. **Kirschner S, Tomasello M** (2010) Joint music making promotes prosocial behaviour in 4-year-old children. Evol Hum Behav **31**: 354–364.

96. **Schellenberg EG, Corrigall KA, Dys SP, Malti T** (2015) Group music training and children's prosocial skills. PloS One **10**: e0141449.

97. **Soley G, Spelke ES** (2016) Shared cultural knowledge: effects of music on young children's social preferences. Cognition **148**: 106–116.

98. **Cirelli LK, Einarson KM, Trainor LJ** (2014) Interpersonal synchrony increases prosocial behavior in infants. Dev Sci **17**: 1003–1011.

99. **Karpati FJ, Giacosa C, Foster NE, Penhune VB, Hyde KL** (2016) Sensorimotor integration is enhanced in dancers and musicians. Exp Brain Res **234**: 893–903.

100. **Gerry D, Unrau A, Trainor LJ** (2012) Active music classes in infancy enhance musical, communicative and social development. Dev Sci **15**: 398–407.

101. **Thaut MH** (2009) The musical brain—an artful biological necessity. *Karger Gazette* (Music and Medicine) No. 70: 2–4.

102. **Davies C, Knuiman M, Rosenberg M** (2016) The art of being mentally healthy: a study to quantify the relationship between recreational arts engagement and mental well-being in the general population. BMC Public Heath **16**: 15.

103. Cox A (2001) The mimetic hypothesis and embodied musical meaning. Music Sci **2**: 195–212.

104. Blacking J (1976) *How Musical is Man?* Faber and Faber, London.

105. Fischer R, Callander R, Reddish P, Bulbulia J (2013) How do rituals affect cooperation? An experimental field study comparing nine ritual types. Hum Nat **24**: 115–125.

106. Reddish P, Fischer R, Bulbalia L (2013) Let's dance together: synchrony, shared intentionality and cooperation. PLoS One **8**: e71182.

107. Novembre G, Keller PE (2014) A conceptual review on action-perception coupling in the musician's brain: what is it good for? Front Hum Neurosci **8**: 603.

108. Chen JK, Chuang AY, McMahon C, Hsieh JC, Tung TH, Li LP (2010) Music training improves pitch perception in prelingually deaf children with cochlear implants. Pediatrics **125**: e793–e800.

109. Gfeller K, Driscoll V, Kenworthy M, Van Voorst T (2011) Music therapy for preschool cochlear implant recipients. Music Ther Perspect **29**: 39–49.

110. Rochette F, Moussard A, Bigand E (2014) Music lessons improve auditory perceptual and cognitive performance in deaf children. Front Hum Neurosci **8**: 488.

111. Bonacina S, Cancer A, Lanzi PL, Lorusso ML, Antonietti A (2015) Improving reading skills in students with dyslexia: the efficacy of a sublexical training with rhythmic background. Front Psychol **6**: 1510.

112. Flaugnacco E, Lopez L, Terribili C, Montico M, Zoia S, Schön D (2015) Music training increases phonological awareness and reading skills in developmental dyslexia: a randomized control trial. PLoS One **10**: e0138715.

113. Heaton P, Allen R (2009) " 'With concord of sweet sounds': new perspectives on the diversity of musical experience in autism and other neurodevelopmental conditions," in S. Dalla Bella et al., eds, *The Neurosciences and Music III—Disorders and Plasticity*, Ann NY Acad Sci **1169**: 318–325 (Wiley-Blackwell, Boston).

114. Sacks O (2008) *Musicophilia*. Vintage Books, New York.

115. Eikeseth S, Hayward DW (2009) The discrimination of object names and object sounds in children with autism: a procedure for teaching verbal comprehension. J Appl Behav Anal **42**: 807–812.

116. Eyler LT, Pierce K, Courchesne E (2012) A failure of left temporal cortex to specialize for language is an early emerging and fundamental property of autism. Brain **135**: 949–960.

117. Hinkley LBN, Marco EJ, Brown EG, Bukshpun P, Gold J, et al. (2016) The contribution of the corpus callosum to language lateralization. J Neurosci **36**: 4522–4533.

118. Kliemann D, Dziobek I, Hatri A, Steimke R, Heekeren HR (2010) Atypical reflexive gaze patterns on emotional faces in autism spectrum disorders. J Neurosci **30**: 12281–12287.

119. Bouhuys AL, Bloem GM, Groothuis TGG (1995) Induction of depressed and elated mood by music influences the perception of facial expressions in healthy subjects. J Affect Disord **33**: 215–226.

120. Jeong J-W, Diwadkar VA, Chugani CD, Sinsoongsud P, Muzik O, et al. (2010) Congruence of happy and sad emotion in music and faces modifies cortical audiovisual activation. Neuroimage **54**: 2973–2982.

121. Chanda ML, Levitin DJ (2013) The neurochemistry of music. Trends Cogn Sci **17**: 179–193.

122. Wan CY, Demaine K, Zipse L, Norton A, Schlaug G (2010) From music making to speaking: engaging the mirror neuron system in autism. Brain Res Bull **82**: 161–168.

123. Abrams DA, Lynch CJ, Cheng KM, Phillips J, Supekar K, et al. (2013) Underconnectivity between voice-selective cortex and reward circuitry in children with autism. Proc Natl Acad Sci USA **110**: 12060–12065.

124. **Blank H, Anwander A, von Kriegstein K** (2011) Direct structural connections between voice- and face-recognition areas. J Neurosci **31**: 12906–12915.

125. **Storr A** (1992) *Music and the Mind.* Harper Collins Publishers, London.

126. **Uibel S** (2012) Education through music—the model of the Musikkindergarten Berlin. Ann NY Acad Sci **1252**: 51–55.

127. **Tomalin C** (2002) *Samuel Pepys: The Unequalled Self.* Viking, London.

Chapter Eight

1. **James J** (1993) *The Music of the Spheres: Music, Science, and the Natural Order of the Universe.* Grove Press, New York.

2. **Shapiro N** (1978) *An Encyclopedia of Quotations About Music.* Da Capo Press, New York.

3. **Thaut MH** (2015) Music as therapy in early history. Prog Brain Res **217**: 143–158.

4. **Hindemith P** (1952) *A Composer's World.* Harvard University Press, Cambridge MA.

5. **Salimpoor VN, Benovoy M, Longo G, Cooperstock JR, Zatorre RJ** (2009) The rewarding aspects of music listening are related to degree of emotional arousal. PLoS One **4**: e7487.

6. **Pereira CS, Teixeira J, Figueiredo P, Xavier J, Castro SL, Brattico E** (2011) Music and emotions in the brain: familiarity matters. PLoS One **6**: e27241.

7. **Zatorre RJ, Salimpoor VN** (2013) From perception to pleasure: music and its neural substrates. Proc Natl Acad Sci USA **110**: 10430–10437.

8. **Sachs ME, Damasio A, Habibi A** (2015) The pleasures of sad music: a systematic review. Front Hum Neurosci **9**: 404.

9. **Moore KS** (2013) A systematic review on the neural effects of music on emotion regulation: implications for music therapy practice. J Music Ther **50**: 198–242.

10. **Tarr B, Launay J, Dunbar RIM** (2014) Music and social bonding: "self-other" merging and neurohormonal mechanisms. Front Psychol **5**: 1096.

11. **Fancourt D, Ockelford A, Belai A** (2014) The psychoneuroimmunological effects of music: a systematic review and a new model. Brain Behav Immun **36**: 15–26.

12. **Chanda ML, Levitin DJ** (2013) The neurochemistry of music. Trends Cogn Sci **17**: 179–193.

13. **Okada K, Kurita A, Takase B, Otsuka T, Kodani E**, et al. (2009) Effects of music therapy on autonomic nervous system activity, incidence of heart failure events, and plasma cytokine and catecholamine levels in elderly patients with cerebrovascular disease and dementia. Int Heart J **50**: 95–110.

14. **Fukui H, Toyoshima K** (2008) Music facilitates the neurogenesis, regeneration and repair of neurons. Med Hypotheses **71**: 765–769.

15. **Stefano GB, Zhu W, Cadet P, Salamon E, Mantione KJ** (2004) Music alters consitutively expressed opiate and cytokine processes in listeners. Med Sci Monit **10**: MS18–MS27.

16. **Keeler JR, Roth EA, Neuser BL, Spitsbergen JM, Waters DJ, Vianney JM** (2015) The neurochemistry and social flow of singing: bonding and oxytocin. Front Hum Neurosci **9**: 518.

17. **Ventura T, Gomes MC, Carreira T** (2012) Cortisol and anxiety response to a relaxing intervention on pregnant women awaiting amniocentesis. Psychoneuroendocrinology **37**: 148–156.

18. **Suda M, Morimoto K, Obata A, Koizumi H, Maki A** (2008) Emotional responses to music: towards scientific perspectives on music therapy. Neuroreport **19**: 75–78.

19. **Ueda N, Ishikawa H, Morimoto K, Ishihara R, Narahara H**, et al. (2004) Reduction in salivary cortisol level by music therapy during colonoscopic examination. Hepatogastroenterology **51**: 451–453.

20. **Khalfa S, Bella SD, Roy M, Peretz I, Lupien SJ** (2003) Effects of relaxing music on salivary cortisol level after psychological stress. Ann NY Acad Sci **999**: 374–376.

21. Fukui H, Yamashita M (2003) The effects of music and visual stress in testosterone and cortisol in men and women. Neuro Endocrinol Lett **24**: 173–180.

22. Möckel M, Röcker L, Störk T, Vollert J, Danne O, et al. (1994) Immediate physiological responses of healthy volunteers to different types of music: cardiovascular, hormonal and mental changes. Eur J Appl Physiol **68**: 451–459.

23. Nilsson U (2009) Soothing music can increase oxytocin levels during bed rest after open-heart surgery: a randomised control trial. J Clin Nurs **18**: 2153–2161.

24. McKinney CH, Tims FC, Kumar AM, Kumar M (1997) The effect of selected classical music and spontaneous imagery on plasma beta-endorphin. J Behav Med **20**: 85–99.

25. Salimpoor VN, Benovoy M, Larcher K, Dagher A, Zatorre RJ (2011) Anatomically distinct dopamine release during anticipation and experience of peak emotion in music. Nat Neurosci **14**: 257–264.

26. Gold BP, Frank MJ, Bogert B, Brattico E (2013) Pleasurable music affects reinforcement learning according to the listener. Front Psychol **4**: 541.

27. Kanduri C, Kuusi T, Ahvenainen M, Philips AK, Lähdesmäki H, Järvelä I (2015) The effect of music performance on the transcriptome of professional musicians. Sci Rep **5**: 9506.

28. Gold C, Solli HP, Krüger V, Lie SA (2009) Dose-response relationship in music therapy for people with serious mental disorders: systematic review and meta-analysis. Clin Psych Rev **29**: 193–207.

29. Dingle GA, Gleadhill L, Baker FA (2008) Can music therapy engage patients in group cognitive behaviour therapy for substance abuse treatment? Drug Alcohol Rev **27**: 190–196.

30. Cramer SC, Sur M, Dobkin BH, O'Brien C, Sanger TD, et al. (2011) Harnessing neuroplasticity for clinical applications. Brain **134**: 1591–1609.

31. Bencivelli S (2011) *Why We Like Music: Ear, Emotion, Evolution*. Music World Media, Hudson, New York.

32. Darnley-Smith R, Patey R (2003) *Music Therapy*. Sage Publications, London.

33. Rose J-P, Bartsch HH (2009) Music as therapy. *Karger Gazette* (Music and Medicine) No. 70: 5–7.

34. Baker F, Tamplin J (2006) *Music Therapy Methods in Neurorehabilitation: Clinician's Manual*. Jessica King, London and Philadelphia.

35. Malloch S, Trevarthen C (2008) *Communicative Musicality: Exploring the Basis of Human Companionship*. Oxford University Press, Oxford.

36. Rollnik JD, Altenmüller E (2014) Music in disorders of consciousness. Front Neurosci **8**: 190.

37. Tzovara A, Simonin A, Oddo M, Rossetti AO, De Lucia M (2015) Neural detection of complex sound sequences in the absence of consciousness. Brain **138**: 1160–1166.

38. Castro M, Tillmann B, Luauté J, Corneyllie A, Dailler F, et al. (2015) Boosting cognition with music in patients with disorders of consciousness. Neurorehabil Neural Repair **29**: 734–742.

39. Riganello F, Cortese MD, Arcuri F, Quintieri M, Dolce G (2015) How can music influence the autonomic nervous system response in patients with severe disorder of consciousness? Front Neurosci **9**: 461.

40. Harris KC, Dubno JR, Keren NL, Ahlstrom JB, Eckert MA (2009) Speech recognition in younger and older adults: a dependency on low-level auditory cortex. J Neurosci **29**: 6078–6087.

41. Anderson S, Skoe E, Chandrasekaran B, Kraus N (2010) Neural timing is linked to speech perception in noise. J Neurosci **30**: 4922–4926.

42. Parbery-Clark A, Anderson S, Hittner E, Kraus N (2012) Musical experience strengthens the neural representation of sounds important for communication in middle-aged adults. Front Aging Neurosci **4**: 30.

43. Zendel BR, Alain C (2012) Musicians experience less age-related decline in central auditory processing. Psych Aging **27**: 410–417.

44. **Bidelman GM, Alain C** (2015) Musical training orchestrates coordinated neuroplasticity in auditory brainstem and cortex to counteract age-related declines in categorical vowel perception. J Neurosci **35**: 1240–1249.

45. **Fujii S, Wan CY** (2014) The role of rhythm in speech and language rehabilitation: the SEP hypothesis. Front Hum Neurosci **8**: 777.

46. **Kirschner S, Tomasello M** (2009) Joint drumming: social context facilitates synchronization in preschool children. J Exp Child Psychol **102**: 299–314.

47. **Patel AD** (2011) Why does musical training benefit the neural encoding of speech? A new hypothesis. J Acoust Soc Am **130**: 2398.

48. **Asaridou SS, McQueen JM** (2013) Speech and music shape the listening brain: evidence for shared domain-general mechanisms. Front Psychol **4**: 321.

49. **Jantzen MG, Howe BM, Jantzen KJ** (2014) Neurophysiological evidence that musical training influences the recruitment of right hemispheric homologues for speech perception. Front Psychol **5**: 171.

50. **Verghese J, Lipton RB, Katz MJ, Hall CB, Derby CA**, et al. (2003) Leisure activities and risk of dementia in the elderly. N Engl J Med **348**: 2508–2516.

51. **Bugos JA, Perlstein WM, McCrae CS, Brophy TS, Bedenbaugh PH** (2007) Individualized piano instruction enhances executive functioning and working memory in older adults. Aging Ment Health **11**: 464–471.

52. **Hanna-Pladdy B, Gajewski B** (2012) Recent and past musical activity predicts cognitive aging variability: direct comparison with general lifestyle activities. Front Hum Neurosci **6**: 198.

53. **Hars M, Herrmann FR, Gold G, Rizzoli R, Trombetti A** (2013) Effect of music-based multitask training on cognition and mood in older adults. Age Ageing **43**: 196–200.

54. **Seinfeld S, Figueroa H, Ortiz-Gil J, Sanchez-Vives MV** (2013) Effects of music learning and piano practice on cognitive function, mood and quality of life in older adults. Front Psychol **4**: 810.

55. **Balbag MA, Pedersen NL, Gatz M** (2014) Playing a musical instrument as a protective factor against dementia and cognitive impairment: a population-based twin study. Int J Alzheimers Dis **2014**: 836748.

56. **Zuk J, Benjamin C, Kenyon A, Gaab N** (2014) Behavioral and neural correlates of executive functioning in musicians and non-musicians. PLoS One **9**: e99868.

57. **Metzler MJ, Saucier DM, Metz GA** (2013) Enriched childhood experiences moderate age-related motor and cognitive decline. Front Behav Neurosci **7**: 1.

58. **Clift SM, Hancox G** (2001) The perceived benefits of singing: findings from preliminary surveys of a university college choral society. J R Soc Promot Health **121**: 248–256.

59. **Johnson JK, Louhivuori J, Stewart Al, Tolvanen A, Ross L, Era P** (2013) Quality of life (QOL) of older adult community choral singers in Finland. Int Psychogeriatr **25**: 1055–1064.

60. **Knight WE, Rickard NS** (2001) Relaxing music prevents stress-induced increases in subjective anxiety, systolic blood pressure and heart rate in healthy males and females. J Music Ther **38**: 254–272.

61. **Kunikullaya KU, Goturu J, Muradi V, Hukkari PA, Kunnavil R**, et al. (2015) Combination of music with lifestyle modification versus lifestyle modification alone on blood pressure reduction—a randomized controlled trial. Complement Ther Clin Pract **23**: 102–109.

62. **Jeffries-Stokes C, Stokes A, McDonald L** (2015) Pulkurlkpa: the joy of research in Aboriginal communities. J Paediatr Child Health **51**: 1054–1059.

63. **McCraty R, Atkinson M, Rein G, Watkins A** (1996) Music enhances the effect of positive emotional states on salivary IgA. Stress Med **12**: 167–175.

64. **Kreutz G, Bongard S, Rohrmann S, Hodapp V, Grebe D** (2004) Effects of choir singing or listening on secretory immunoglobulin A, cortisol, and emotional state. J Behav Med **27**: 623–635.

65. **Quiroga Murcia C, Bongard S, Kreutz G** (2009) Emotional and neurohumoral responses to dancing tango argentino. Music Med **1**: 14–21.

66. **Blackburn EH, Epel ES** (2012) Too toxic to ignore. Nature **490**: 169–171.

67. **Cohen EEA, Ejsmond-Frey R, Knight N, Dunbar RIM** (2010) Rowers' high: behavioural synchrony is correlated with elevated pain thresholds. Biol Lett **6**: 106–108.

68. **Tarr B, Launay J, Cohen E, Dunbar R** (2015) Synchrony and exertion during dance independently raise pain threshold and encourage social bonding. Biol Lett **11**: 20150767.

69. **Tarr B, Launay J, Dunbar RI** (2016) Silent disco: dancing in synchrony leads to elevated pain thresholds and social closeness. Evol Hum Behav **37**: 343–349.

70. **Erickson KI, Raji CA, Lopez OL, Becker JT, Rosano C, et al.** (2010) Physical activity predicts gray matter volume in late adulthood: the Cardiovascular Health Study. Neurology **71**: 1415–1422.

71. **Erickson KI, Miller DL, Roecklein KA** (2011) The aging hippocampus: interactions between exercise, depression, and BDNF. Neuroscientist **18**: 82–97.

72. **Yau SY, Li A, Hoo RLC, Ching YP, Christie BR, et al.** (2014) Physical exercise-induced hippocampal neurogenesis and antidepressant effects are mediated by the adipocyte hormone adiponectin. Proc Natl Acad Sci USA **111**: 15810–15815.

73. **Foster PP, Rosenblatt KP, Kuljis RO** (2011) Exercise-induced cognitive plasticity, implications for mild cognitive impairment and Alzheimer's disease. Front Neurol **2**: 28.

74. **Sleiman SF, Henry J, Al-Haddad R, El Hayek L, Abou Haidar E, et al.** (2016) Exercise promotes the expression of brain derived neurotrophic factor (BDNF) through the action of the ketone body β-hydroxybutyrate. ELife **5**: e15092.

75. **Hsiao Y-H, Hung H-C, Chen S-H, Gean P-W** (2014) Social interaction rescues memory deficit in an animal model of Alzheimer's Disease by increasing BDNF-dependent hippocampal neurogenesis. J Neurosci **34**: 16207–16219.

76. **Koelsch S** (2014) Brain correlates of music-evoked emotions. Nat Rev Neurosci **15**: 170–180.

77. **Koelsch S, Skouras S, Jentschke S** (2013) Neural correlates of emotional personality: a structural and functional magnetic resonance imaging study. PLoS One **8**: e77196.

78. **Oechslin MS, Descloux C, Croquelois A, Chanal J, Van De Ville D, et al.** (2014) Hippocampal volume predicts fluid intelligence in musically trained people. Hippocampus **23**: 552–558.

79. **Phillips C, Baktir MA, Srivatsan M, Salehi A** (2014) Neuroprotective effects of physical activity on the brain: a closer look at trophic factor signaling. Front Cell Neurosci **8**: 170.

80. **Fritz J, Poeppel D, Trainor L, Schlaug G, Patel AD, et al.** (2013) "The neurobiology of language, speech, and music," in **M. A. Arbib**, ed., *Language, Music and the Brain: A Mysterious Relationship* (MIT Press, Cambridge MA), 417–459.

81. **Kattenstroth JC, Kalisch T, Holt S, Tegenthoff M, Dinse HR** (2013) Six months of dance intervention enhances postural, sensorimotor, and cognitive performance in elderly without affecting cardio-respiratory functions. Front Aging Neurosci **5**: 5.

82. **Foster PP** (2013) How does dancing promote brain reconditioning in the elderly? Front Aging Neurosci **5**: 4.

83. **Koelsch S** (2010) Towards a neural basis of music-evoked emotions. Trends Cogn Sci **14**: 131–137.

84. **Carter RM, MacInnes JJ, Huettel SA, Adcock RA** (2009) Activation of the VTA and nucleus accumbens increases in anticipation of both gains and losses. Front Behav Neurosci **3**: 21.

85. **Mannella F, Gurney K, Baldassarre G** (2013) The nucleus accumbens as a nexus between values and goals in goal-directed behaviour: a review and a new hypothesis. Front Behav Neurosci **7**: 135.

86. **Koelsch S** (2009) "A neuroscientific perspective on music therapy," in **S. Dalla Bella** et al., eds, *The Neurosciences and Music III—Disorders and Plasticity*, Ann NY Acad Sci **1169**: 374–384. (Wiley-Blackwell, Boston).

87. **Stein MB, Simmons AN, Feinstein JS, Paulus MP** (2007) Increased amygdala and insula activation during emotion processing in anxiety-prone subjects. Am J Psychiatry **164**: 318–327.

88. **Pardini DA, Raine A, Erickson K, Loeber R** (2014) Lower amygdala volume in men is associated with childhood aggression, early psychopathic traits, and future violence. Biol Psychiatry **75**: 73–80.

89. **Erkkilä J, Punkanen M, Fachner J, Ala-Ruona E, Pöntiö I**, et al. (2011) Individual music therapy for depression: randomised controlled trial. Br J Psychiatry **199**: 132–139.

90. **Baker F, Kennelly J, Tamplin J** (2005) Themes within songs written by people with traumatic brain injury: gender differences. J Music Ther **42**: 111–122.

91. **Menon V, Levitin DJ** (2005) The rewards of music listening: response and physiological connectivity of the mesolimbic system. Neuroimage **28**: 175–184.

92. **Osuch EA, Bluhm RL, Williamson PC, Théberge J, Densmore M, Neufeld RW** (2009) Brain activation to favorite music in healthy controls and depressed patients. Neuroreport **20**: 1204–1208.

93. **Zubieta JK, Stohler CS** (2009) "Neurobiological mechanisms of placebo responses," in **M. B. Miller** and **A. Kingstone**, eds, *The Year in Cognitive Neuroscience 2009*, Vol **1156**, 198–210 (Wiley-Blackwell, Boston).

94. **Jeong J-W, Diwadkar VA, Chugani CD, Sinsoongsud P, Muzik O**, et al. (2010) Congruence of happy and sad emotion in music and faces modifies cortical audiovisual activation. Neuroimage **54**: 2973–2982.

95. **Esch T, Guarna M, Bianchi E, Zhu W, Stefano GB** (2004) Commonalities in the central nervous system's involvement with complementary medical therapies: limbic morphinergic processes. Med Sci Monit **10**: MS6–M17.

96. **Eschrich S, Münte TF, Altenmüller EO** (2008) Unforgettable film music: the role of emotion in episodic long-term memory of music. BMC Neurosci **9**: 48.

97. **Jäncke L** (2008) Music, memory and emotion. J Biol **7**: 21.

98. **Herdener M, Esposito F, di Salle F, Boller C, Hilti CC**, et al. (2010) Musical training induces functional plasticity in human hippocampus. J Neurosci **30**: 1377–1384.

99. **Kleber B, Birbaumer N, Veit R, Trevorrow T, Lotze M** (2007) Overt and imagined singing of an Italian aria. Neuroimage **36**: 889–900.

100. **Kraus N SJ, Thompson EC, Hornickel J, Strait DL, Nicol T**, et al. (2014) Music enrichment programs improve the neural encoding of speech in at-risk children. J Neurosci **34**: 11913–11918.

101. **Baddeley A** (2003) Working memory: looking back and looking forward. Nat Rev Neurosci **4**: 29–39.

102. **Schulze K, Koelsch S** (2012) "Working memory for speech and music," in **K. Overy** et al., eds, *The Neurosciences and Music IV—Learning and Memory*, Ann NY Acad Sci **1252**: 229–236 (Wiley-Blackwell, Boston).

103. **Dowling WJ** (1993) "Procedural and declarative knowledge in music cognition and education," in **T. J. Tighe** and **W. J. Dowling**, eds, *Psychology and Music: The Understanding of Melody and Rhythm* (Erlbaum, Hillsdale NJ), 5–18.

104. **Janata P, Tomic ST, Rakowski SK** (2007) Characterization of music-evoked autobiographical memories. Memory **15**: 845–860.

105. **Janata P** (2009) The neural architecture of music-evoked autobiographical memories. Cereb Cortex **19**: 2579–2594.

106. **Omar R, Henley SM, Bartlett JW, Hailstone JC, Gordon E,** et al. (2011) The structural neuoanatomy of music emotion recognition: evidence from frontotemporal lobar dementia. Neuroimage **56:** 1814–1821.

107. **Gosselin N, Peretz I, Hasbourn D, Baulac M, Samson S** (2011) Impaired recognition of musical emotions and facial expressions following anteromedial temporal lobe excision. Cortex **47:** 1116–1125.

108. **Hsieh S, Hornberger M, Piguet O, Hodges JR** (2012) Brain correlates of musical and facial emotion recognition: evidence from the dementias. Neuropsychologia **50:** 1814–1822.

109. **Millard KAO, Smith JM** (1989) The influence of group singing therapy on the behaviour of Alzheimer's Disease patients. J Music Ther **26:** 58–70.

110. **Bannan N, Montgomery-Smith C** (2008) "Singing for the brain": reflections on the human capacity for music arising from a pilot study of group singing with Alzheimer's patients. J R Soc Promot Health **128:** 73–78.

111. **McDermott O, Orrell M, Ridder HM** (2014) The importance of music for people with dementia: the perspectives of people with dementia, family carers, staff and music therapists. Aging Ment Health **18:** 706–716.

112. **Maguire LE, Wanschura PB, Battaglia MM, Howell SN, Flinn JM** (2015) Participation in active singing leads to cognitive improvements in individuals with dementia. J Am Ger Soc **63:** 815–816.

113. **Vanstone AD, Cuddy L, Duffin JM, Alexander E** (2009) "Exceptional preservation of memory for tunes and lyrics: case studies of amusia, profound deafness and Alzheimer's disease," in S. Dalla Bella et al., eds, *The Neurosciences and Music III—Disorders and Plasticity*, Ann NY Acad Sci **1169:** 291–294 (Wiley-Blackwell, Boston).

114. **Finke C, Esfahani NE, Ploner CJ** (2012) Preservation of musical memory in an amnesic professional cellist. Curr Biol **22:** R591–R592.

115. **Groussard M, Viader F, Landau B, Desgranges B, Eustache F, Platel H** (2009) "Neural correlates underlying musical semantic memory," in S. Dalla Bella et al., eds, *The Neurosciences and Music III—Disorders and Plasticity*, Ann NY Acad Sci **1169:** 278–281 (Wiley-Blackwell, Boston).

116. **Jacobsen JH, Stelzer J, Fritz TH, Chételat G, La Joie R, Turner R** (2015) Why musical memory can be preserved in advanced Alzheimer's disease. Brain **138:** 2438–2450.

117. **Foster NA, Valentine ER** (2001) The effect of auditory stimulation on autobiographical recall in dementia. Exp Aging Res **27:** 215–228.

118. **Särkämö T, Laitinen S, Numminen A, Kurki M, Johnson JK, Rantanen P** (2015) Clinical and demographic factors associated with the cognitive and emotional efficacy of regular musical activities in dementia. J Alzheimers Dis **49:** 767–781.

119. **Palisson J, Roussel-Baclet C, Maillet D, Belin C, Ankri J, Narme P** (2015) Music enhances verbal episodic memory in Alzheimer's disease. J Clin Exp Neuropsychol **37:** 503–517.

120. **Thaut MH** (2005) *Rhythm, Music and the Brain.* Taylor and Francis Group, New York and London.

121. **Moussard A, Bigand E, Belleville S, Peretz I** (2014) Learning sung lyrics aids retention in normal ageing and Alzheimer's disease. Neuropsychol Rehabil **24:** 894–917.

122. **Drapeau J, Gosselin N, Gagnon L, Peretz I, Lorrain D** (2009) "Emotional recognition from the face, voice, and music in dementia of the Alzheimer type," in S. Dalla Bella et al., eds, *The Neurosciences and Music III—Disorders and Plasticity*, Ann NY Acad Sci **1169:** 342–345 (Wiley-Blackwell, Boston).

123. **Sampson S, Dellacherie D, Platel H** (2009) "Emotional power of music in patients with memory disorders: clinical implications of cognitive neuroscience," in S. Dalla Bella et al., eds, *The Neurosciences and Music III—Disorders and Plasticity*, Ann NY Acad Sci **1169:** 245–255 (Wiley-Blackwell, Boston).

124. Sacks O (2008) *Musicophilia*. Vintage Books, New York.

125. Zatorre RJ, Chen JL, Penhune VB (2007) When the brain plays music: auditory-motor interactions in music perception and production. Nat Rev **8**: 547–558.

126. Patel AD (2008) *Music, Language and the Brain*. Oxford University Press, New York.

127. Patel AD, Iversen JR (2014) The evolutionary neuroscience of musical beat perception: the Action Simulation for Auditory Prediction (ASAP) hypothesis. Front Syst Neurosci **8**: 57.

128. Thaut MH, Stephan KM, Wunderlich G, Schicks W, Tellman L, et al. (2009) Distinct cortico-cerebellar activations in rhythmic auditory motor synchronization. Cortex **45**: 44–53.

129. Grahn JA, Rowe JB (2013) Finding and feeling the musical beat: striatal dissociations between detection and prediction of regularity. Cereb Cortex **23**: 913–921.

130. Hove MJ, Schwartze M (2014) Deconstructing the ability to move to a beat. J Neurosci **34**: 2403–2405.

131. Nozaradan S, Peretz I, Missal M, Mouraux A (2011) Tagging the neuronal entrainment to beat and meter. J Neurosci **31**: 10234–10240.

132. Brown S, Martinez MJ, Parsons LM (2006) The neural basis of dance. Cereb Cortex **16**: 1157–1167.

133. Merchant H, Grahn J, Trainor L, Rohrmeier M, Fitch WT (2015) Finding the beat: a neural perspective across humans and non-human primates. Philos Trans R Soc Lond B Biol Sci **370**: 20140093.

134. Phillips-Silver J, Trainor LJ (2007) Hearing what the body feels: auditory encoding of rhythmic movement. Cognition **105**: 533–546.

135. Geiser E, Notter M, Gabrieli JDE (2012) A corticospinal neural system enhances auditory perception through temporal cortex context processing. J Neurosci **32**: 6177–6182.

136. Zentner M, Eerola T (2010) Rhythmic engagement with music in infancy. Proc Natl Acad Sci USA **107**: 5768–5773.

137. Corbeil M, Trehub SE, Peretz I (2013) Speech vs. singing: infants choose happier sounds. Front Psychol **4**: 372.

138. Trombetti A, Hars M, Herrmann FR, Kressig RW, Ferrari S, Rizzoli R (2011) Effect of music-based multitask training on gait, balance, and fall risk in elderly people: a randomized controlled trial. Arch Intern Med **171**: 525–533.

139. Schneider S, Askew CD, Abel T, Struder HK (2010) Exercise, music, and the brain: is there a central pattern generator? J Sports Sci **14**: 1–7.

140. Grahn JA, Brett M (2007) Rhythm and beat perception in motor areas of the brain. J Cogn Neurosci **19**: 893–906.

141. Raglio A, Fazio P, Imbriani C, Granieri E (2013) Neuro-scientific basis and effectiveness of music and music therapy in neuromotor rehabilitation. OA Alternative Medicine **1**: 8.

142. Lima CF, Garrett C, Castro SL (2013) Not all sounds sound the same: Parkinson's disease affects differently emotion processing in music and in speech prosody. J Clin Exp Neuropsychol **35**: 373–392.

143. Mattei TA, Rodriquez AH, Bassuner J (2013) Selective impairment of emotion recognition through music in Parkinson's disease: does it suggest the existence of different networks for music and speech prosody processing? Front Neurosci **7**: 161.

144. Thaut MH, McIntosh GC, Rice RR, Miller RA, Rathbun J, Brault JN (1996) Rhythmic auditory stimulation in gait training for Parkinson's disease patients. Mov Disord **11**: 193–200.

145. Satoh M, Kuzuhara S (2008) Training in mental singing while walking improves gait disturbance in Parkinson's Disease patient. Eur Neurol **60**: 237–243.

146. **Bukowska AA, Krezalek P, Mirek E, Bujas P, Marchewka A** (2016) Neurologic music therapy training for mobility and stability rehabilitation with Parkinson's disease—a pilot study. Front Hum Neurosci **9**: 710.

147. **Del Olmo MF, Cudeiro J** (2005) Temporal variability of gait in Parkinson's disease: effects of a rehabilitation programme based on rhythmic sound clues. Parkinsonism Relat Disord **11**: 25–33.

148. **Frazzitta G, Maestri R, Uccellini D, Bertotti G, Abelli P** (2009) Rehabilitation treatment of gait in patients with Parkinson's disease with freezing: a comparison between two physical therapy protocols using visual and auditory cues with or without treadmill training. Mov Disord **24**: 1139–1143.

149. **Bernatzky G, Bernatzky P, Hesse H-P, Staffen W, Ladurner G** (2004) Stimulating music increases motor coordination in patients afflicted with Morbus Parkinson. Neurosci Lett **361**: 4–8.

150. **Sacry L-A R, Clark CAM, Wishaw IQ** (2009) Music attenuates excessive visual guidance of skilled reaching in advanced but not mild Parkinson's disease. PLoS One **4**: e6841.

151. **Coull JT, Hwang HJ, Leyton M, Dagher A** (2012) Dopamine precursor depletion impairs timing in healthy volunteers by attenuating activity in putamen and supplementary motor area. J Neurosci **32**: 16704–16715.

152. **Hackney ME, Kantorovich S, Levin R, Earhart GM** (2007) Effects of tango on functional mobility in Parkinson's disease; a preliminary study. J Neurol Phys Ther **31**: 173–179.

153. **Thaut MH, McIntosh GC, Rice RR** (1997) Rhythmic facilitation of gait training in hemiparetic stroke rehabilitation. J Neurol Sci **151**: 207–212.

154. **Van Wijck F, Knox D, Dodds C, Cassidy G, Alexander G, MacDonald R** (2012) Making music after stroke: using musical activities to enhance arm function. Ann NY Acad Sci **1252**: 305–311.

155. **Schlaug G, Marchina S, Norton A** (2009) "Evidence for plasticity in white-matter tracts of patients with chronic Broca's aphasia undergoing intense intonation-based speech therapy," in S. Dalla Bella et al., eds, *The Neurosciences and Music III—Disorders and Plasticity*, Ann NY Acad Sci **1169**: 385–394 (Wiley-Blackwell, Boston).

156. **Schneider S, Schönle PW, Altenmüller E, Münte TF** (2007) Using musical instruments to improve motor skill recovery following stroke. J Neurol Phys Ther **254**: 1339–1346.

157. **Altenmüller E, Marco-Pallares J, Münte TF, Schneider S** (2009) "Neural reorganization underlies improvement in stroke-induced motor dysfunction by music-supported therapy," in S. Dalla Bella et al., eds, *The Neurosciences and Music III—Disorders and Plasticity*, Ann NY Acad Sci **1169**: 395–405 (Wiley-Blackwell, Boston).

158. **Grau-Sánchez J, Amengual JL, Rojo N, Veciana de Las Heras M, Montero J, et al.** (2013) Plasticity in the sensorimotor cortex induced by music-supported therapy in stroke patients: a TMS study. Front Hum Neurosci **7**: 494.

159. **Ripollés P, Rojo N, Grau-Sánchez J, Amengual JL, Càmara E, et al.** (2015) Music supported therapy promotes motor plasticity in individuals with chronic stroke. Brain Imaging Behav, Dec 26 [epub ahead of print].

160. **Van Vugt FT, Ritter J, Rollnik JD, Altenmüller E** (2014) Music-supported motor training after stroke reveals no superiority of synchronization in group therapy. Front Hum Neurosci **8**: 315.

161. **Tomaino CM** (2012) Effective music therapy techniques in the treatment of nonfluent aphasia. Ann NY Acad Sci **1252**: 312–317.

162. **Özdemir E, Norton A, Schlaug G** (2006) Shared and distinct neural correlates of singing and speaking. Neuroimage **33**: 628–635.

163. **Straube T, Schulz A, Geipel K, Mentzel HJ, Miltner WH** (2008) Dissociation between singing and speaking in expressive aphasia: the role of song familiarity. Neuropsychologia **46**: 1505–1512.

164. Jungblut M, Huber W, Pustelniak M, Schnitker R (2012) The impact of rhythm complexity on brain activation during simple singing: an event-related fMRI study. Restor Neurol Neurosci **30**: 39–53.

165. Stahl B, Henseler I, Turner R, Geyer S, Kotz SA (2013) How to engage the right hemisphere in aphasics without even singing: evidence for two paths of speech recovery. Front Hum Neurosci **7**: 35.

166. Forsblum A, Laitinen S, Särkämö T, Tervaniemi M (2009) "Therapeutic role of music listening in stroke rehabilitation," in S. Dalla Bella et al., eds, *The Neurosciences and Music III—Disorders and Plasticity*, Ann NY Acad Sci **1169**: 426–430 (Wiley-Blackwell, Boston).

167. Bittman B, Croft DT Jr, Brinker J, van Laar R, Vernalis MN, Ellsworth DL (2013) Recreational music-making alters gene expression pathways in patients with coronary heart disease. Med Sci Monit **19**: 139–147.

168. Särkärmö T, Tervaniemi M, Laitinen S, Forsblum A, Soinila S, et al. (2008) Music listening enhances cognitive recovery and mood after middle cerebral artery stroke. Brain **131**: 866–876.

169. Soto D, Funes MJ, Guzmán-Garcia A, Warbrick T, Rotshtein P, Humphreys GW (2009) Pleasant music overcomes the loss of awareness in patients with visual neglect. Proc Natl Acad Sci USA **106**: 6011–6016.

170. Thaut MH, Gardiner JC, Holmberg D, Horwitz J, Kent L, et al. (2009) "Neurologic music therapy improves executive function and emotional adjustment in traumatic brain injury rehabilitation," in S. Dalla Bella et al., eds, *The Neurosciences and Music III—Disorders and Plasticity*, Ann NY Acad Sci **1169**: 406–416 (Wiley-Blackwell, Boston).

171. Bringas ML, Zaldivar M, Rojas PA, Martinez-Montes K, Chongo DM, et al. (2015) Effectiveness of music therapy as an aid to neurorestoration of children with severe neurological disorders. Front Neurosci **9**: 427.

172. Nishimura Y, Onoe H, Onoe K, Morichika Y, Tsukada H, Isa T (2011) Neural substrates for the motivational regulation of motor recovery after spinal cord injury. PLoS One **6**: e24854.

173. Tamplin J, Baker FA, Grocke D, Brazzale DJ, Pretto JJ, et al. (2013) The effect of singing on respiratory function, voice, and mood following quadriplegia: a randomized controlled trial. Arch Phys Med Rehabil **94**: 426–434.

174. Bensmaia SJ, Miller LE (2014) Restoring sensorimotor function through intracortical interfaces: progress and looming challenges. Nat Rev Neurosci **15**: 313–325.

175. Mateo S, Di Rienzo F, Bergeron V, Guillot A, Collet C, Rode G (2015) Motor imagery reinforces brain compensation of reach-to-grasp movement after cervical spinal cord injury. Front Behav Neurosci **9**: 234.

176. Wang CF, Sun YL, Zang HX (2014) Music therapy improves sleep quality in acute and chronic sleep disorders: a meta-analysis of 10 randomized studies. Int J Nurs Stud **51**: 51–62.

177. Picard LM, Bartel LR, Gordon AS, Cepo D, Wu Q, Pink LR (2014) Music as a sleep aid in fibromyalgia. Pain Res Manag **19**: 97–101.

178. Bernatzky G, Presch M, Anderson M, Panksepp J (2011) Emotional foundations of music as a non-pharmacological pain management tool in modern medicine. Neurosci Behav Rev **35**: 1989–1999.

179. Henson RA (1977) "Neurological aspects of musical experience," in M. Critchley and R. A. Henson, eds, *Music and the Brain: Studies on the Neurology of Music* (Heinemann Medical Books Ltd, London), 3–21.

180. Roy M, Pertez I, Rainville P (2008) Emotional valence contributes to music-induced analgesia. Pain **134**: 140–147.

181. Zhao H, Chen AC (2009) Both happy and sad melodies modulate tonic human heat pain. J Pain **10**: 953–960.

182. **Younger J, Aron A, Parke S, Chatterjee N, Mackey S** (2010) Viewing pictures of a romantic partner reduces experimental pain: involvement of neural reward systems. PLoS One **5**: e13309.

183. **Gardner WJ, Licklider JC, Weisz AZ** (1960) Suppression of pain by sound. Science **132**: 32–33.

184. **Voss JA, Good M, Yates B, Baun NM, Thompson A, Herzog M** (2004) Sedative music reduces anxiety and pain during chair rest after open-heart surgery. Pain **112**: 197–203.

185. **Good M, Anderson GC, Ahn S, Cong X, Stanton-Hicks M** (2005) Relaxation and music reduce pain following intestinal surgery. Res Nurs Health **28**: 240–251.

186. **Nilsson U** (2008) The anxiety- and pain-reducing effects of music interventions: a systematic review. AORN J **87**: 780–807.

187. **Nilsson U, Unosson M, Rawal N** (2005) Stress reduction and analgesia in patients exposed to calming music postoperatively: a randomized controlled trial. Eur J Anaesthesiol **22**: 92–102.

188. **Nilsson S, Kokinsky E, Nilsson U, Sidenvall B, Enskär K** (2009) School-aged children's experiences of postoperative music medicine on pain, distress, and anxiety. Paediatr Anaesth **19**: 1184–1190.

189. **Schneider N, Schedlowski M, Schürmeyer TH, Becker H** (2001) Stress reduction through music in patients undergoing cerebral angiography. Neuroradiology **43**: 472–476.

190. **Nilsson U** (2012) Effectiveness of music interventions for women with high anxiety during coronary angiographic procedures: a randomized controlled trial. Eur J Cardiovasc Nurs **11**: 150–153.

191. **O'Callaghan CC** (1996) Pain, music creativity and music therapy in palliative care. Am J Hosp Pall Care **13**: 43–49.

192. **Klassen JA, Liang Y, Tjosvold L, Klassen TP, Hartling L** (2008) Music for pain and anxiety in children undergoing controlled medical procedures: a systematic review of randomized control trials. Ambul Pediatr **8**: 117–128.

193. **Hoare DJ, Searchfield GD, El Refaie A, Henry JA** (2014) Sound therapy for tinnitus management: practicable options. J Am Acad Audiol **25**: 62–75.

194. **Argstatter H, Grapp M, Plinkert PK, Bolay HV** (2012) "Heidelberg Neuro-Music Therapy" for chronic-tonal tinnitus—treatment outline and psychometric evaluation. Int Tinn J **17**: 34–44.

195. **Grapp M, Hutter E, Argstatter H, Plinkert PK, Bolay HV** (2013) Music therapy as an early intervention to prevent chronification of tinnitus. Int J Clin Exp Med **6**: 589–593.

196. **Krick CM, Grapp M, Daneshvar-Talebi J, Reith W, Plinkert PK, Bolay HV** (2015) Cortical reorganization in recent-onset tinnitus patients by the Heidelberg Model of Music Therapy. Front Neurosci **9**: 49.

197. **Penhune VB, Cismaru R, Dorsaint-Pierre R, Petitto L-A, Zatorre RJ** (2003) The morphometry of auditory cortex in the congenitally deaf measured using MRI. Neuroimage **20**: 1215–1225.

198. **Ullal-Gupta S, Vanden Bosch der Nederlanden CM, Tichko P, Lahav A, Hannon EE** (2013) Linking prenatal experience to the emerging musical mind. Front Syst Neurosci **7**: 48.

199. **McMahon E, Wintermark P, Lahav A** (2012) Auditory brain development in premature infants: the importance of early experience. Ann NY Acad Sci **1252**: 17–24.

200. **Lorch CA, LorcH V, Diefendorf AO, Earl PW** (1993) Effect of stimulative and sedative music on systolic blood pressure, heart rate and respiratory rate in premature infants. J Music Ther **31**: 105–118.

201. **Standley JM, Moore RS** (1995) Therapeutic effects of music and mother's voice on premature infants. Pediatr Nurs **21**: 509–512.

202. **Kaminski J, Hall W** (1996) The effect of soothing music on neonatal behavioral states in the hospital newborn nursery. Neonatal Netw **15**: 45–54.

203. **Arnon S, Shapsa A, Forman L, Regev R, Bauer S, et al.** (2006) Live music is beneficial to preterm infants in the neonatal intensive care environment. Birth **33**: 131–136.

204. **Standley J** (2012) Music therapy research in the NCIU: an updated meta-analysis. Neonatal Netw **31**: 311–316.

205. **Keith DR, Weaver BS, Vogel RL** (2012) The effect of music-based listening interventions on the volume, fat content, and caloric content of breast milk-produced by mothers of premature and critically ill infants. Adv Neonatal Care **12**: 112–119.

206. **Kamioka H, Tsutani K, Yamada M, Park H, Okuizumi H,** et al. (2014) Effectiveness of music therapy: a summary of systematic reviews based on randomized controlled trials of music interventions. Patient Prefer Adherence **8**: 727–754.

207. **Linnemann A, Strahler J, Nater UM** (2016) The stress-reducing effect of music listening varies depending on social context. Psychoneuroendocrinology **72**: 97–105.

208. **Magee WL, Stewart L** (2015) The challenges and benefits of a genuine partnership between Music Therapy and Neuroscience: a dialog between scientist and therapist. Front Hum Neurosci **9**: 223.

209. **Osborne N** (2012) Neuroscience and "real world" practice: music as a therapeutic resource for children in zones of conflict. Ann NY Acad Sci **1252**: 69–76.

Chapter Nine

1. **Parry R** (2014) *"Episteme and Techne," The Stanford Encyclopedia of Philosophy* (Fall 2014 edn), E. N. Zalta, ed., http://plato.stanford.edu/archives/fall2014/entries/episteme-techne/

2. **Gribben J** (2005) *The Fellowship: The Story of a Revolution*. Allen Lane, London.

3. **Snow CP** (1961) *The Two Cultures and the Scientific Revolution*. Cambridge University Press, New York.

4. **Cross I** (2001) Music, mind and evolution. Psychol Music **29**: 95–102.

5. **Davies C, Knuiman M, Rosenberg M** (2016) The art of being mentally healthy: a study to quantify the relationship between recreational arts engagement and mental well-being in the general population. BMC Public Health **16**: 15.

6. **Storr A** (1992) *Music and the Mind*. Harper Collins Publishers, London.

7. **Humphrey N** (2008) The society of selves. Philos Trans R Soc Lond B Biol Sci **362**: 745–754.

8. **Pearce E, Launay J, Dunbar RIM** (2015) The ice-breaker effect: singing mediates fast social bonding. R Soc Open Sci **2**: 150221.

9. **Freeman W** (2000) "A neurological role of music in social bonding," in **N. L. Wallin, B. Merker** and **S. Brown**, eds, *The Origins of Music* (MIT Press, Cambridge MA), i411–424.

10. **Shaw R** (2004) *The Robert Shaw Reader*, **R. Blocker**, ed, Yale University Press, Yale, p 38.

11. **Cross I** (1999) "Is music the most important thing we ever did? Music, development and evolution," in **S. W. Yi**, ed., *Music, Mind and Science* (Seoul National University Press, Seoul), 10–39.

12. **Morley I** (2014) A multi-disciplinary approach to the origins of music: perspectives from anthropology, archaeology, cognition and behavior. J Anthrop Sci **92**: 147–177.

13. **Pahlen K** (1949) *Music of the World: A history*. Translated by **JA Galston**. Spring Books, London.

Index

Notes: Page numbers suffixed by *f* denotes material in figures.